Gynecological Emergencies

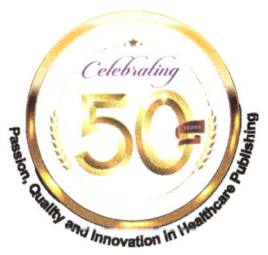

Gynecological Emergencies

SECOND EDITION

Editor
Kamini A Rao
DGO DORCP DCh FRCOG (UK) MCh (UK) FRCOG PGDMLE (Law) FNAMS
Medical Director
Milann—The Fertility Center
Bengaluru, Karnataka, India

Co-Editor
Arveen Vohra
MBBS MS (Obs & Gyn) Fellowship in Reproductive Medicine (FRM)
Fertility Specialist
Senior Consultant in Reproductive Medicine
Clinical Director, Milann—The Fertility Center, Indiranagar
Bengaluru, Karnataka, India

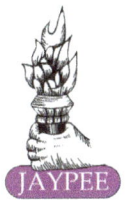

JAYPEE BROTHERS MEDICAL PUBLISHERS
The Health Sciences Publisher
New Delhi | London

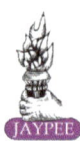 **Jaypee Brothers Medical Publishers (P) Ltd**

Headquarters
Jaypee Brothers Medical Publishers (P) Ltd
4838/24, Ansari Road, Daryaganj
New Delhi 110 002, India
Phone: +91-11-43574357
Fax: +91-11-43574314
E-mail: jaypee@jaypeebrothers.com

Overseas Office
JP Medical Ltd
83 Victoria Street, London
SW1H 0HW (UK)
Phone: +44 20 3170 8910
Fax: +44 (0)20 3008 6180
E-mail: info@jpmedpub.com

Website: www.jaypeebrothers.com
Website: www.jaypeedigital.com

© 2020, Jaypee Brothers Medical Publishers

The views and opinions expressed in this book are solely those of the original contributor(s)/author(s) and do not necessarily represent those of editor(s) of the book.

All rights reserved. No part of this publication may be reproduced, stored or transmitted in any form or by any means, electronic, mechanical, photocopying, recording or otherwise, without the prior permission in writing of the publishers.

All brand names and product names used in this book are trade names, service marks, trademarks or registered trademarks of their respective owners. The publisher is not associated with any product or vendor mentioned in this book.

Medical knowledge and practice change constantly. This book is designed to provide accurate, authoritative information about the subject matter in question. However, readers are advised to check the most current information available on procedures included and check information from the manufacturer of each product to be administered, to verify the recommended dose, formula, method and duration of administration, adverse effects and contraindications. It is the responsibility of the practitioner to take all appropriate safety precautions. Neither the publisher nor the author(s)/editor(s) assume any liability for any injury and/or damage to persons or property arising from or related to use of material in this book.

This book is sold on the understanding that the publisher is not engaged in providing professional medical services. If such advice or services are required, the services of a competent medical professional should be sought.

Every effort has been made where necessary to contact holders of copyright to obtain permission to reproduce copyright material. If any have been inadvertently overlooked, the publisher will be pleased to make the necessary arrangements at the first opportunity. The **CD/DVD-ROM** (if any) provided in the sealed envelope with this book is complimentary and free of cost. **Not meant for sale.**

Inquiries for bulk sales may be solicited at: jaypee@jaypeebrothers.com

Gynecological Emergencies

First Edition: 2015

Second Edition: **2020**

ISBN 978-93-89587-18-0

Contributors

Anu Joseph
MBBS DNB (OBG) Fellowship in Fetal and Maternal Medicine
Medical Director and Consultant Obstetrics and Gynecology and Fetal Medicine
Department of Obstetrics and Gynecology
Trinity Healthcare Clinic, Electronic City
Bengaluru, Karnataka, India

Aradhana Kalra Dawar
MBBS MS DNB PGD USG Fellowship Reproductive Medicine
Consultant Obstetrician and Gynecologist
Department of Reproductive Medicine
Milann—The Fertility Center, New Delhi
Eva Care, Faridabad, Haryana, New Delhi, India

Arunima Halder
MBBS MS DNB FNB (Reproductive Medicine)
Consultant, Department of Reproductive Medicine
Milann—The Fertility Center
Bengaluru, Karnataka, India

Arveen Vohra
MBBS MS (Obs & Gyn) Fellowship in Reproductive Medicine (FRM)
Fertility Specialist
Senior Consultant in Reproductive Medicine
Clinical Director, Milann—The Fertility Center
Indiranagar
Bengaluru, Karnataka, India

Arya Rajendran MBBS MD DNB FNB
Consultant Reproductive Medicine
Department of Reproductive Medicine
NIMS Fertility Centre, NIMS Welcare Hospital
Palakkad, Kerala, India

B Ramesh MBBS MS DGO DFP ICOG
Chief Laparoscopic Surgeon and Director
Altius Hospital
Bengaluru, Karnataka, India

Harpreet Kaur
MD DNB (Obs & Gyne) Fellowship in Reproductive Medicine (FNB) MRCOG (UK)
Senior Consultant
Department of Gynecology and Reproductive Medicine
Milann—The Fertility Center, Chandigarh

Ipsita Batra MBBS MS (OBG) FRM
Fellow
Department of Reproductive Medicine
International Institute for Training and Research in Reproductive Health and Milann—The Fertility Center
Bengaluru, Karnataka, India

Jahnavi Esanakula MBBS MS (OBG) FRM
Consultant Reproductive Medicine
Department of Reproductive Medicine
Subhashini Fertility Centre
Puttur, Andhra Pradesh, India

Karthigayeni R
MBBS MS (Obs & Gyne) Fellowship in Reproductive Medicine DNB (Obs & Gyne)
Consultant
Department of Reproductive Medicine
Milann—The Fertility Center
Bengaluru, Karnataka, India

Kavita Manchanda
MBBS MS DNB (Obs & Gyne)
FNB Fellow
Department of Reproductive Medicine
Milann—The Fertility Center
Bengaluru, Karnataka, India

Meghana V Nyapathi MS (OBG) FRM
Consultant
Department of Reproductive Medicine
Milann—The Fertility Center
Bengaluru, Karnataka, India

Mekhala B Dwarakanath MBBS DGO MS FRM
Consultant, Department of Reproductive Medicine
Milann—The Fertility Center
Bengaluru, Karnataka, India

Nivedita Shetty
MD FRCOG (UK) Fellowship in Reproductive Medicine
(National Board, New Delhi)
Director, Assisted Reproduction Medicine
Columbia Asia Hospital
Mysuru, Karnataka, India

Priyanka Yadav MBBS DGO DNB
Attending Consultant, Fortis Escorts Jaipur
Department of Reproductive Medicine
Jaipur, Rajasthan, India

Ravishankar P
MBBS MS (OBG) FRM DMAS (Germany)
Consultant Gynecologist and Fertility Specialist
Department of Reproductive Medicine
The Nest Woman Wellness and Fertility Clinic
Thiruvananthapuram, Kerala, India

Shashikala KT
MBBS DGO Fellowship in Reproductive Medicine
Fellowship in Minimal Access Surgery
Infertility Specialist, Obstetrician and
Gynecologist
Department of Reproductive Medicine
Milann—The Fertility Center
Bengaluru, Karnataka, India

Sonal Agarwal
MBBS MS DNB FNB (RM) FMAS MNAMS
Infertility Specialist and Consultant
Department of Reproductive Medicine
Shanti Mukand Hospital, New Delhi, India

Sowmya Davuluri
MBBS MS (OBG) FRM DMAS
Consultant Reproductive Medicine
Department of Reproductive Medicine
Milann Fertility Centre
MS Ramaiah Memorial Hospital
Bengaluru, Karnataka, India

Taswin Kaur Reddy
MBBS DGO FRM FMAS
Consultant
Department of Obstetrics, Gynecology,
and Reproductive Medicine
Chandra Superspecialty Hospital
Andhra Pradesh, India

Tejaswi K MBBS DGO
Fellow
Department of Reproductive Medicine
Milann—The Fertility Center
Bengaluru, Karnataka, India

Varsha Rengaraj
MS (OBG) FMAS FRM PGDHHM
Consultant Gynecologist
Laparoscopic Surgeon and
Infertility Specialist
Department of Obstetrics and Gynecology
Treetop Hospital, Hulhumale, Maldives

Vyshnavi A Rao
MBBS MS (Obs & Gyne) Fellowship in Reproductive
Medicine
Infertility Specialist, Gynecologist and
Obstetrician
Department of Reproductive Medicine
Milann—The Fertility Center
Bengaluru, Karnataka, India

Preface to the Second Edition

Gynecological Emergencies is an invaluable reference guide for busy practitioners and students who want to optimize their practice of gynecological emergency management. This book holds promise for all gynecologists as it covers in depth, yet succinctly, the entire armamentarium of gynecological emergencies for adolescent, reproductive age and post-menopausal age group.

Clinical gynecology is very important to improve the health of women in our country. Ethical practice guided by evidence-based investigations and management is still a challenge posed to the gynecological health of women. In this book clinical emergencies associated with puberty, menstruation and menopause with the appropriate investigations and management strategies have been very well elucidated by the authors in a very streamlined fashion.

In the rapidly advancing age of technology and changing trends in diagnosis, management, and procedures, it is of paramount importance to update books periodically. We have added many new chapters like post coital bleeding, management of ovarian mass in pre-menopausal and postmenopausal women. Special emphasis is given to the ethical and medicolegal issues related to gynecological emergencies like assault and rape. We have modernized and reworked a few chapters completely to incorporate the new evidence-based practice guidelines.

The first edition of the book was very well received as a reference book by practicing gynecologists for clinical practice as well as post graduate students for examination purposes. Now, four years later we have carefully updated the book in a second edition using the same concise yet updated algorithms that were the hallmark of success for the first edition. Relevance of the content and the clinical approach is the intention of this book.

We hope that this book will provide an effective learning experience and serve as an outstanding reference manual for all current and future gynecologists and practitioners, leading to improved patient care.

Kamini A Rao
Arveen Vohra

Preface to the First Edition

In our day-to-day practice, we come across gynecological emergencies, which can be in different age groups. As students and as practitioners, we have experienced difficulties in going through lots of textbooks, and to concise the gynecological emergencies separately, this book is very important both from the examination point of view and, more importantly, from clinical practice viewpoint.

This textbook is meant to be a concise and also a ready-reckoner for gynecological emergencies, be it for preparation of examination or for clinical practice.

We have tried our best to make this book very precise, simple, with lots of tables and flowcharts, so that it can be used for quick reference.

We hope our students and colleagues will appreciate our efforts, and this book will be of great help to them.

The last couple of decades have not only witnessed significant changes and advancement in the practice of gynecology but also seen the publication of several books on this subject. Despite, there is lack of books that are solely dedicated to the management of emergencies in gynecology.

This textbook provides a lucid description of evidence-based management of gynecological emergencies. Each chapter has been painstakingly researched to provide concise and comprehensive information on current practices.

The inclusion of user-friendly flowcharts and tabulated data has turned this book into a very useful teaching tool and invaluable reference guide for the busy practitioners.

Kamini A Rao
Divyashree PS

Acknowledgments

This book is a culmination of the sincere efforts of all the authors who very enthusiastically came forward to write the chapters. We would like to express our sincerest thanks to all of them for their time, effort and commitment to sharing their knowledge and expertise. As always, the publication team of Jaypee Brothers has gone out on a limb to bring out the book and ensure its timely release. We thank them for their constant support in making this happen. Special thanks to Mrs Kala Diwakar for coordinating the entire effort, interacting with both the contributors and the publishers at every stage, and generally following up with all stakeholders until the book was finally a reality. Lastly of course to both our families, especially our Mothers—Mrs Parimala Desai and Mrs Harvinder Vohra—thank you for standing by us and supporting us in all our endeavors.

Contents

SECTION 1: ADOLESCENTS

1. **Common Gynecologic and Urinary Problems in Pediatric and Adolescent Females** 3
   Meghana V Nyapathi
2. **Sexual Abuse and Assault in Pediatric Patient** 17
   Priyanka Yadav

SECTION 2: REPRODUCTIVE AGE GROUP

3. **Early Pregnancy: Miscarriage** 23
   Vyshnavi A Rao
4. **Gestational Trophoblastic Diseases** 34
   Arunima Halder
5. **Ectopic Pregnancy** 47
   Harpreet Kaur
6. **Leiomyoma Uterus Presenting as Emergency** 53
   Arya Rajendran
7. **Dysmenorrhea** 59
   Arveen Vohra
8. **Abnormal Uterine Bleeding** 69
   Mekhala B Dwarakanath, Jahnavi Esanakula
9. **Postcoital Bleeding** 76
   Sowmya Davuluri
10. **Infections** 81
    Karthigayeni R
11. **Pelvic Mass** 109
    Ravishankar P, Tejaswi K
12. **Ovarian Hyperstimulation Syndrome** 119
    Nivedita Shetty
13. **Ovarian Torsion** 126
    B Ramesh

14. **Management of Ovarian Mass in Premenopausal Women**   133
    Kavita Manchanda, Jahnavi Esanakula

15. **Emergencies and Complications Related to Contraception**   144
    Shashikala KT

SECTION 3: POSTMENOPAUSAL AGE GROUP

16. **Pyometra**   155
    Arveen Vohra

17. **Postmenopausal Bleeding**   159
    Arveen Vohra

18. **Management of Ovarian Mass in Postmenopausal Women**   167
    Sonal Agarwal

19. **Gynecological Emergencies in Postmenopausal Women with Mass per Vaginum**   180
    Anu Joseph

SECTION 4: EMERGENCIES IN GYNECOLOGICAL SURGERIES

20. **Complications in Open Gynecological Surgery**   187
    Jahnavi Esanakula, Varsha Rengaraj

21. **Complications in Laparoscopy**   196
    Kavita Manchanda, Varsha Rengaraj

22. **Gynecological Oncology Emergencies**   206
    Ipsita Batra

23. **Imaging in Gynecological Emergencies**   214
    Aradhana Kalra Dawar, Jahnavi Esanakula

SECTION 5: MISCELLANEOUS GYNECOLOGICAL EMERGENCIES

24. **Acute Retention of Urine**   227
    Arveen Vohra

25. **Sexual Assault**   232
    Priyanka Yadav

26. **Miscellaneous Gynecological Emergencies**   236
    Sowmya Davuluri

27. **Medicolegal and Ethical Issues in Gynecological Emergencies**   242
    Taswin Kaur Reddy

Index   *251*

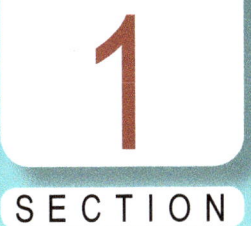

SECTION

Adolescents

- Common Gynecologic and Urinary Problems in Pediatric and Adolescent Females
  Meghana V Nyapathi
- Sexual Abuse and Assault in Pediatric Patient
  Priyanka Yadav

CHAPTER 1

Common Gynecologic and Urinary Problems in Pediatric and Adolescent Females

Meghana V Nyapathi

INTRODUCTION

About 13.1% of Indian population is in the 0-6 years age group.[1] About 236.5 billion people in India are adolescents in the age group of 10-19 years.[2] Children **(Box 1)** and adolescents **(Flowchart 1)** are a unique subset of patients in our outpatient clinic with varied complaints requiring tact and a different line of management in comparison to the adult population.

EXAMINATION OF A PEDIATRIC PATIENT (TABLE 1)

- Good communication skills to make the child comfortable.
- Drugs like meperidine 50 mg, chlorpromazine hydrochloride (Thiozine) 12.5 mg, or promethazine hydrochloride 12.5 mg can be given to sedate the patient. Examination under anesthesia is an option in noncooperative children.
- *Breast examination*: Evaluated for Tanner staging. Slight bilateral asymmetry is a common finding.
- *Abdominal examination:* To look for tenderness and any palpable mass.
- *Examination of the external genitalia:* Tanner staging, skin lesions and to look

BOX 1: Common gynecological complaints in pediatric population.
- Labial agglutination
- Vulvovaginitis
  - Infectious origin
  - Noninfectious origin
- Dermatological conditions
  - Lichen sclerosus
  - Lichen simplex lichenification
  - Lichen planus
  - Psoriasis
  - Seborrheic dermatitis
  - Atopic dermatitis
- Obstructive vaginal disorders
  - Septate vagina
  - Transverse septum
- Ambiguous genitalia
- Bleeding per vaginum

TABLE 1: Problems in pediatric population.[4-12]

Condition	Age	Cause	Symptoms	Physical examination	Anatomical area	Treatment	Long-term outcome
Labial agglutination Incidence: 0.6–3%[4]	13–23 months	Hypoestrogenic state, inflammation	Irritation, urinary tract infections, dribbling of urine	Thin vertical lucent line seen in central area of labia	Commonly posterior aspect of the labia minora	Estrogen cream BDX 2–4 weeks, zinc oxide ointment, perineal hygiene, sitz baths, bland creams, manual separation under sedation (acute cases and those not responsive to medical management)[6]	Spontaneous resolution within 18 months. Recurrence in 40%.[5] Iatrogenic precocious puberty due to estrogen use
Vulvo-vaginitis (noninfective/nonspecific) MC (74–80%)[7]	Prepubertal	External irritants and poor hygiene Trauma to the sensitive mucosa by chemical, environmental causes Neutral vaginal pH	Itching, foul smelling discharge, pain, dysuria, bleeding	Tanner staging, presence of erythema, edema, discharge noted. Sometimes foreign body may be seen. Wet mount examination and culture of discharge if any.	Labia majora and minora, clitoris, introitus and vagina	Pesonal hygiene, proper fitting undergarments, sitz bath, mild steroid cream in acute cases for about 2 weeks	Recurrence common
Vulvovaginitis (infectious)	Prepubertal	Poor hygiene, sexual abuse	Discharge, ulcerative lesions	Wet mount examination and culture of discharge	Labia majora and minora, clitoris, introitus and vagina	Antibiotic based on culture report, personal hygiene	Recurrence common with low personal hygiene

Contd...

Chapter 1: Common Gynecologic and Urinary Problems in Pediatric and Adolescent Females

Contd...

Condition	Age	Cause	Symptoms	Physical examination	Anatomical area	Treatment	Long-term outcome
Dermatological conditions	Beyond 24 months usually	Autoimmune	Vulvar irritation, pruritus	Tiny pink-white papules (lichen sclerosus), pale lesions with increased skin margin markings (lichen simplex lichenification), well-demarcated erythematous papules with scales (psoriasis)	Labia majora and minora. Also in nongenital areas	Personal hygiene, emollients, mild steroid cream like clobetasol ointment for 2–4 weeks and then tapered[8] Vulvar biopsy in cases resistant to treatment	Prolonged steroid use in some cases
Congenital disorders	From birth	Chromosomal disorders, maternal drug intake, congenital adrenal hyperplasia, pseudohermaphroditism	Detected at birth, may be associated with other symptoms	Look for abnormalities of clitoris/phallus, palpate for gonads in the inguinal/labioscrotal folds (undescended gonads), lower abdominal mass, blood tests as required	Inguinal region, labioscrotal folds	Surgical correction in amenable cases Symptomatic management	Proper counseling
Precocious puberty	Onset before 8 years	GnRH dependent, GnRH independent	vaginal bleeding, breast development, pubic hair	Tanner staging, hormonal evaluation	Breast, external genitalia	Treatment of the cause (tumors, CAH), hormonal therapy (GnRH agonist)	

Contd...

Contd...

Condition	Age	Cause	Symptoms	Physical examination	Anatomical area	Treatment	Long-term outcome
Genital trauma (0.2–0.8% of trauma and accidents in children[10]	Mean age: 7.1 years[9] Peak age: 6 years[8]	MC-straddle injury (70–81%) leading to lacerations[8]	Bleeding from genital tract, pain	Examination under anesthesia in all cases to avoid missing periurethral and perianal injuries[10]	Abrasions over labia minora and fourchette Bruising of mons pubis and labia majora[10]	Conservative—analgesics, cold packs, catheterization in cases of urinary retention Surgical—required in 9–20% of cases[11] Associated anal sphincter, bladder and urethral injuries, deep penetrating injuries with persistent bleeding requiring suturing	Long-term follow-up
Urethral prolapse	5–8 years	Hypoestrogenism. Usually resolves around puberty with estrogenization	Painless vaginal bleeding. Vaginal irritation and discharge are usually absent	Mass per vaginum, surrounding genital anatomy is normal	Urethra protruding through vagina	Observation till puberty Topical estrogen over the area BDX2—4 weeks Resection of the necrotic area may be rarely required[12]	Recurrence can be seen till puberty

Contd...

Contd...

Condition	Age	Cause	Symptoms	Physical examination	Anatomical area	Treatment	Long-term outcome
Ulcers	Rare in premenarchal age	Solitary ulcer—syphilis, Crohn's disease, chancroid, cancer Multiple ulcers—secondary syphilis, scabies, Varicella zoster virus, Behçet syndrome, infectious mononucleosis[13]	Painful and recurrent in cases due to herpes and Behçet syndrome. Painless in syphilis. Can be associated with malaise, fever (Epstein-Barr virus, cancer) or GI symptoms (Crohn's)	Examine vulva and perineum for erosion of both dermis and epidermis. Presence of fluid filed vesicles causing erosion of skin. Also look for oral ulcers. Swabs taken and biopsy from the edge of the lesion including normal skin done for diagnosis[6,14]	Vulva, perineum	Depending upon the culture and biopsy report	Relapse can occur in cases of Behçet's syndrome, herpes shingles, Crohn's disease, etc.

(CAH: congenital adrenal hyperplasia; GnRH: gonadotropin-releasing hormone; MC: most common)

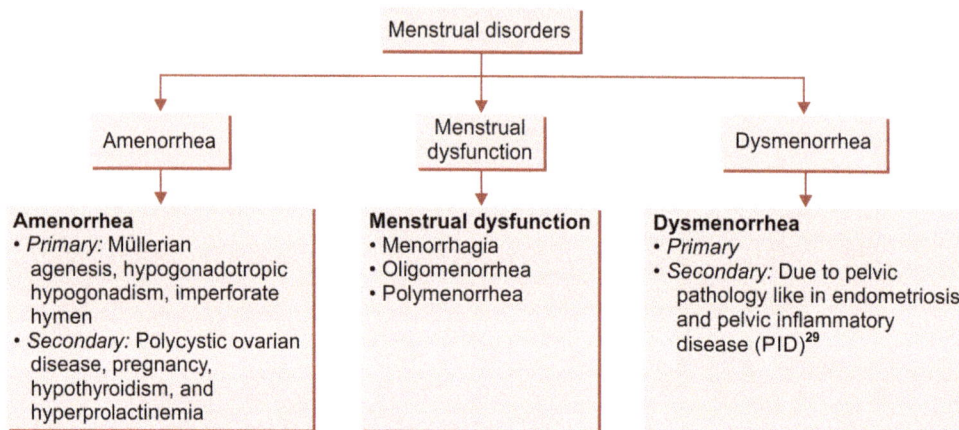

Flowchart 1: Gynecological complaints in adolescents.

- for any disfigurements. Also look for the presence of hypertrophied clitoris and urethral abnormalities.
- *Pelvic examination*: Performed with the child in frog-leg or knee-chest position to visualize the vulvovaginal area. Look for discharge, edema, erythema, foreign body, and congenital anomalies.
- Examination of the hymen.
- Wet preparation of the discharge for management in cases of infective vulvovaginitis
- *Rectal examination:* When abdominopelvic mass is suspected (can be substituted by ultrasound evaluation).[3]

Vulvovaginitis is the most common gynecological complaint in the pediatric population.[6,15] Causes and management enumerated in **Tables 2 to 4**. Most of the cases are nonspecific and usually present with vaginal discharge and soreness in the region as the most common complaint. Other symptoms include itching in the vulva and vagina, dysuria. Bleeding and pain are less frequent symptoms.

ETIOLOGY

- Thin vaginal mucosa due to nonestrogenized state
- Thin vulval skin
- Vaginal pH which is alkaline
- Short distance from the vagina to the anus
- Poor hygiene
- Placement of foreign bodies in the vagina
- Chronic constipation.[4,6]

GYNECOLOGICAL PROBLEMS IN ADOLESCENT POPULATION

By World Health Organization (WHO) definition, adolescents are individuals in the age group of 10–19 years. In the Southeast Asian region, adolescents comprise approximately 22% of the population.[17] India has the distinction of having the largest population of adolescent girls (20%).[18,19] Early adolescent period extends from 10 years to 13 years, middle adolescents are girls between 14 years and 16 years and late adolescence comprises the ages from 17 years to 19 years.[20,21] The physical and psychological problems

Chapter 1: Common Gynecologic and Urinary Problems in Pediatric and Adolescent Females

TABLE 2: Organisms causing vulvovaginitis.[4,15]

Commensals	Nonsexually transmitted	Sexually transmitted
Staphylococcus epidermidis Diphtheroids Lactobacilli Anaerobic bacteria like *Bacteroides*	Bacteria—*Streptococcus pyogenes* (59%), *Escherichia coli* *Shigella* (enteric transmission) *Haemophilus influenzae* (respiratory contact) Viral—adenovirus, varicella-zoster Helminths—*Enterobius vermicularis* Fungal—*Candida albicans* (rare)	*Neisseria gonorrheae* (5–20%) *Chlamydia trachomatis* (2–13%) *Trichomonas vaginalis* *Mycoplasma hominis* *Ureaplasma urealyticum* Herpesvirus 1 and 2 Human papillomavirus Molluscum contagiosum

TABLE 3: Vulvovaginitis and its management in pediatric population.[3,16]

Condition	Causative agent	Symptoms	Physical examination	Investigation	Treatment
Noninfective	Chemical irritants, poor hygiene, foreign body in the vagina, pin worm infestations, dermatological conditions	Pain, itching, dysuria, discharge (usually thin and copious)	Obese girls, vulvar erythema, inflammation, excoriation, foreign body	Vaginal swab for culture	• Vaginal irrigation for removal of foreign body, • Lukewarm sitz bath BD • Application of emollients and zinc ointment • Personal hygiene, proper cleaning of the area after bowel movement (wiping from front to back), • Antibiotics in cases with secondary infection • Topical steroids in severe cases • Antihistamines to relieve pruritus
Infective (nonsexual)	*Streptococcus pyogenes* (MC), *Staphylococcus aureus*, *Proteus mirabilis*, etc.	Itching, persistent vaginal discharge		Vaginal swab for c/s	Specific antibiotic, personal hygiene

Contd...

Contd...

Condition	Causative agent	Symptoms	Physical examination	Investigation	Treatment
Infective (sexually transmitted)	Neisseria gonorrheae, Chlamydia trachomatis, Trichomonas vaginalis	Itching, persistent vaginal discharge with history of sexual abuse	Purulent (*N. gonorrheae*)/ serous (*C. trachomatis*) vaginal discharge. Look for other signs of sexual abuse	Vaginal swab for c/s	Specific antibiotic, personal hygiene, psychological counseling

(MC: most common)

TABLE 4: Management of pediatric patients with gynaecological problems.[6,7,9,14]

History:
- Proper history from the child and attendant
- History of trauma, foreign body insertion, sexual abuse, chronic infections and illness, immunocompromised state
- Duration of symptoms
- Any previous medications
- Questions pertaining to Personal hygiene

- General physical examination
- Tanner staging
- Local examination in frog-leg position of external genitalia for hygiene, erythema, excoriation, ulcers, signs of trauma
- Vaginal examination when required with or without sedation to look for discharge, foreign body, swab for culture
- Rectoabdominal examination in suspected mass

Nonspecific vulvovaginitis:
- Personal hygiene
- Proper cleaning of the anal region after bowel movement (cleaning from front to back)
- Sitz bath
- Emollients/barrier creams
- Proper fitting cotton undergarments.

Infective vulvovaginitis:
- Specific antibiotic
- Sitz bath
- Personal hygiene

Foreign body in the vagina:
- Vaginal irrigation using saline with moderate pressure
- Removal under sedation/anesthesia

Dermatologic complaints:
- Treatment of specific cause

of adolescents are different from the adult population and needs to be dealt accordingly **(Box 2)**.

The most commonly encountered gynecological problem in this age group is menstrual disorders which may vary from amenorrhea to menstrual dysfunction **(Box 3)**.[22,23]

As recommended by the American College of Obstetricians and Gynecologists (ACOG), the initial visit to the gynecologist should occur between the ages of 13 and 15 years **(Box 4)**.[24,25]

Menstrual disorders are the most commonly encountered problem in the adolescent girls. It comprises about 45–58% of complaints in adolescent girls seeking treatment.[30,31] Amongst the various causes for menstrual disturbances, anovulatory dysfunctional uterine bleeding (DUB) accounts for the majority.[23] This is mostly due to the immaturity

Chapter 1: Common Gynecologic and Urinary Problems in Pediatric and Adolescent Females

BOX 2: Problems in adolescent population.[22,23,28]
- Menstrual disorders
- Dysmenorrhea
- White discharge per vaginum
- Mass in the abdomen
- Urogenital malformations
- Teenage pregnancies
- Sexual assault
- Sexually transmitted diseases

BOX 3: Common causes of menstrual dysfunction in adolescents.[24-26,34]
- Anovulatory DUB due to immaturity of HPO axis
- Coagulation disorders—factor viii deficiency, Von Willebrand disease
- Endocrine abnormalities like hypothyroidism and hyperprolactinemia
- Androgen disorders like Cushing's syndrome, late onset CAH, and adrenal tumors
- Primary amenorrhea due to gonadal dysgenesis, Müllerian agenesis, and imperforate hymen
- Secondary amenorrhea due to polycystic ovarian disease, pregnancy, and premature ovarian failure
- Teenage pregnancy and associated problems
- Stress

(CAH: congenital adrenal hyperplasia; DUB: dysfunctional uterine bleeding; HPO: hypothalamic–pituitary–ovarian)

BOX 4: History taking in an adolescent.

History taking for an adolescent girl in gynecologist outpatient department (OPD) should include:
- The clinician eliciting history should be gentle and empathetic. The patient should be assured about the maintenance of confidentiality[26]
- The consent of the parent or guardian should be obtained. The parent/guardian could be made a part of history taking when required
- The age of the adolescent should be ascertained
- Questions should be directed toward eliciting symptoms like pain abdomen, mass per abdomen, menstrual cycle abnormalities, bowel, and bladder symptoms
- History of previous illness and surgeries, and medications in the past and present should be elucidated
- All adolescents should be gently questioned about substance abuse and sexual activity[27]

of the hypothalamic–pituitary–ovarian (HPO) axis and it may be 5 years before normal and regular ovulatory cycles are established.[32]

Vaginal discharge is the second most common complaint in the adolescent age group and is mostly due to physiological leukorrhea.[33,34] Leukorrhea accounts for approximately 25% of gynecological complaints of adolescent girls.[35]

Dysmenorrhea is a common complaint in girls attending outpatient with the onset usually 6–12 months following menarche. Postpubertal girls usually present with lower abdominal or pelvic pain with or without pain radiating to the back or legs occurring with the onset of menstrual bleeding.[36] In this age-group, dysmenorrhea is usually of the primary type with no obvious pelvic pathology. Dysmenorrhea persisting in spite of medications usually of secondary type indicating underlying pelvic organ disease which needs investigation.[37,38] A pelvic pathology like endometriosis or uterine pathology is noted in about 10% of adolescents suffering with dysmenorrhea.[38]

Mass per abdomen is a relatively uncommon complaint in adolescent girls. Ovarian masses are estimated to have an incidence of 0.0026% **(Box 5)**. Majority of ovarian tumors are benign with mature cystic teratoma being the most common neoplastic

BOX 5: Causes of mass per abdomen in adolescent girls.[40]
- Ovarian masses—benign/malignant
- Pregnancy
- Tubal and paratubal lesions
- Pelvic inflammatory disease and tubo-ovarian masses
- Müllerian anomalies like vaginal agenesis, segmental vaginal atresia, and imperforate hymen
- Nongynecological conditions like peritoneal inclusion cysts, appendicitis, and appendicular abscess

tumor seen in adolescents. In women less than 20 years, mature cystic teratoma accounts for more than half of the ovarian neoplasms.[39]

Adolescent pregnancy is an important social issue in recent times. It is defined as pregnancy in an underaged or teenage girl between 13 years and 19 years.[41] In India, teenage pregnancies vary between 5% and 33% as shown by various studies.[42] A teenage pregnancy poses great risk to the pregnant mother and the fetus in terms of increased rates of unsafe abortions, anemia, preeclampsia and eclampsia, preterm delivery, cephalopelvic disproportion leading to cesarean section, low birth weight, and complications due to prematurity.

Reproductive tract abnormalities can be seen in 7% of females which might be diagnosed before or after puberty.[43] Urogenital malformations in adolescents requiring visit to the gynecology OPD includes imperforate hymen, vaginal atresia with or without the presence of urogenital sinus, and transverse vaginal septum leading to hematocolpos.[44] The girls usually present with pain, mass per abdomen, and primary amenorrhea. There can be an increased incidence of renal and spinal abnormalities in these girls and should be looked for.[43]

Many adolescents are victims of sexual abuse. Studies reveal that 1 in 4 girls are victims of sexual assault.[45] The incidence of sexual abuse in children worldwide is about 18–20%.[46] Though sexual assault is an underrated complaint amongst the girls attending the hospital, clinicians should be sensitized to this condition, which requires skill and tactful approach.

In sexually active adolescents, sexually transmitted diseases (STDs) can be a problem in about 30% having had at least one sexual partner **(Table 5)**.

TABLE 5: Organisms causing sexually transmitted diseases.[47]

Organism	%
Chlamydia trachomatis	>10%
Neisseria gonorrhoeae	0–12%
Trichomoniasis	5–34%
Herpes simplex virus-2	5.6%
Human immunodeficiency virus (HIV) infection	Increased

High-risk factors for STDs:[48,49]
- Level of education (more in school dropouts)
- Alcohol and drug abusers
- Lack of knowledge about STDs
- Peer pressure
- Low usage of barrier contraceptives
- Western influence.

Other conditions requiring hospital visit may include appendicitis and appendicular abscess, urinary tract infections, and anorectal malformations leading to chronic constipation and cachexia. Though anorectal malformations are usually identified at birth, approximately 20% might not be detected till about pubertal age.[50]

Investigations should include:
- Routine blood work up, which includes complete blood count to rule out anemia, blood group and typing, and fasting blood sugar.
- Platelet count, bleeding and clooting time, and coagulation factors in girls with menorrhagia and suspected coagulation disorders.
- Transabdominal ultrasound of the pelvic organs in cases of menstrual abnormalities, dysmenorrhea, and mass and pain abdomen. A transvaginal ultrasound examination can be done in sexually active girls after due consent.

Chapter 1: Common Gynecologic and Urinary Problems in Pediatric and Adolescent Females

- Magnetic resonance imaging (MRI)—abdomen and pelvis in cases presenting with pain and mass in the abdomen to diagnose conditions like benign/malignant ovarian tumors, appendicular abscess, tubo-ovarian abscess, hematocolpos/hematometra, endometriosis, etc.
- Chromosomal analysis as and when required (cases of primary and some cases of secondary amenorrhea)
- A high vaginal swab is indicated in sexually active adolescents with symptoms of pelvic inflammatory disease. Vaginal swab can also be taken in sexually active girls without symptoms to rule out infections.
- Hysteroscopy can be performed in cases of intractable and nonresponsive menorrhagia.[51]
- Laparoscopy might be required in the diagnosis and treatment of mass per abdomen, intractable dysmenorrhea, and management of large endometrioma.[52]

Treatment of the gynecological conditions in the adolescents will be according to the condition they present with as enumerated in **Table 6**.

TABLE 6: Treatment for various gynecological conditions in pediatric and adolescent girls.

Condition	Treatment
Menstrual abnormalities	- Reassurance (in view of immaturity of HPO axis) - Management of specific cause (coagulopathies, anemia) - Tranexamic acid can reduce menstrual blood loss by 50% due to its antifibrinolytic property. C/I—personal/family history of thromboembolic diseases - Mefenamic acid can help to reduce menstrual blood loss by about 20% along with being an effective drug for management of dysmenorrhea. Most effective when started before the onset of menstruation. C/I—asthma and renal diseases - Low dose oral contraceptive pills to reduce menstrual blood loss in both ovulatory and nonovulatory DUB). Useful in girls with PCOS - Oral progestogens (nonovulatory DUB) - Medroxyprogesterone acetate—given once every 12 weeks as an intramuscular injection. Can cause decrease in bone mineral density on prolonged usage. Should be used with caution in girls below 18 years.[53] Intrauterine levonorgestrel implant inserted under sedation in refractory DUB[51]
Dysmenorrhea	- NSAIDs for pain relief - If no relief with NSAIDs in three cycles—low dose OCP can be used[38] - Nonpharmacological therapies like topical heat application, acupuncture, yoga, nutritional interventions, etc. (without sufficient evidence)[36] - Management of specific condition like endometriosis, imperforate hymen, etc.
Leukorrhea	- Personal hygiene - Avoid use of chemicals and harsh detergents - Specific treatment in cases of pathological white discharge
Mass per abdomen	Treatment of the specific condition, mostly surgical intervention
Pregnancy	Management depends upon the stage of pregnancy

Contd...

Contd...

Condition	Treatment
Urogenital malformations	• Cruciate incision, trimming of the hymen and marsupialization in cases of imperforate hymen[54,55] • Creation of neovagina in cases of vaginal atresia • Resection of the transverse vaginal septum
Sexually transmitted diseases	• Treatment of the specific cause • Advice on contraceptive usage and safe sexual practices • Counseling against promiscuous sexual behavior
Other nongynecological conditions	Treatment directed at the cause

(C/I: contra indications; DUB: dysfunctional uterine bleeding; HPO: hypothalamus–pituitary–ovary; NSAIDs: Nonsteroidal anti-inflammatory drugs; OCP: oral contraceptive pills; PCOS: polycystic ovary syndrome)

CONCLUSION

With about 13.5% of the indian population in the 0–6 years age group and 236.5 billion adolescents, we will often come across pediatric gynecological problems in our outpatient clinics. With a sound knowledge of the problems affecting girls of this age group and good communication skills, gynecologists can successfully treat many of the conditions affecting these young girls and adolescents.

REFERENCES

1. Ministry of Statistics and Programme Implementation. (2018). Children in India: A Statistical Appraisal. [online] Available from http://www.mospi.gov.in/sites/default/files/publication_reports/Children%20in%20India%202018%20%E2%80%93%20A%20Statistical%20Appraisal_26oct18.pdf [Last accessed September, 2019].
2. United Nations, Department of Economic and Social Affairs, Population Division. (2013). World Population Prospects: The 2012 Revision. [online] Available from https://www.un.org/en/development/desa/publications/world-population-prospects-the-2012-revision.html [Last accessed September, 2019].
3. Davis VJ. What the paediatrician should know about paediatric and adolescent gynecology: The perspective of a gynecologist. J Sex Reprod Med. 2003;3(3):103-7.
4. Sanfilippo JS, Syed TS, Murray PJ. Pediatric Gynecology. New York: CRC Press; 2004.
5. Bacon JL. Prepubertal labial adhesions: Evaluation of a referral population. Am J Obstet Gynecol. 2002;187:327-31.
6. Eyk NV, Allen L, Giesbrecht E, et al. Pediatric vulvovaginal disorders: a diagnostic approach and review of the literature. J Obstet Gynecol Can. 2009;31(9):850-62.
7. Stricker T, Navratil F, Sennhauser FH. Vulvovaginitis in prepubertal girls. Arch Dis Child. 2003;88:324-26.
8. Dowlut-Mcelroy T, Higgins J, Williams KB, et al. Patterns of treatment of accidental genital trauma in girls. J Pediatric Adolesc Gynecol. 2018;31:19-22.
9. Bercaw-Pratt JL, Boardman LA, Simms-Cendan JS. Clinical recommendation: pediatric lichen sclerosus. J Pediatr Adolesc Gynecol. 2014;27:111-6.
10. Casey JT, Bjurlin MA, Cheng EY. Pediatric genital injury: an analysis of the national electronic injury surveillance system. Urology. 2013;82(5):1125-30.
11. Saxena AK, Steiner M, Hollwarth ME. Straddle injuries in female children and adolescents: 10-year accident and management analysis. Indian J Pediatr. 2014;81(8):766-9.
12. Iqbal CW, Jrebi NY, Zielinski MD, et al. Patterns of accidental genital trauma in young girls and indications for operative management. J Pediatr Surg. 2010;45:930-3.
13. Vunda A, Vandertiun L, Gervaix A. Urethral prolapse: an overlooked diagnosis of

urogenital bleeding in pre-menarcheal girls. J Pediatr. 2011;158:682-3.
14. Trager JDK. Recurrent oral and vulvar ulcers in a fifteen-year-old girl. J Pediatr Adolesc Gynecol. 2004;17:397-401.
15. Black M, McKay M. Obstetric and Gynecologic Dermatology, 2nd edition. London: Mosby; 2002.
16. Hertweck P, Yoost J. Common problems in pediatric and adolescent gynecology. Expert Rev Obstet Gynecol. 2010;5(3):311-28.
17. Randhawa AJ, Abdul MA, Umar HS. Pattern of childhood gynaecological presentations in a Nigerian tertiary health facility. Afr J Paediatr Surg. 2008;5:73-5.
18. World Health Organization. (2018). Child and adolescent health and development. [online] Available from http://www.searo.who.int/entity/child_adolescent/en/ [Last accessed September, 2019].
19. Omidvar S, Amiri FN, Bakhtiari A, et al. A study on menstruation of Indian adolescent girls in an urban area of South India. J Family Med Prim Care. 2018;7:698-702.
20. Registrar General of India. Provisional Population Totals: census of India 2001. New Delhi: Ministry of Home Affairs, Government of India; 2001.
21. Kumar AS, Amrita NS, Sreedhar M. Nutritional status of adolescent girls of urban slums of Hyderabad. Indian J Basic Applied Med Res. 2014;4(1):457-61.
22. Nair A, Doibale MK, Kuril BM, et al. Study of nutritional status of adolescent girls in a rural area of a district of Maharashtra. Int J Community Med Public Health. 2017;4(12):4617-22.
23. Goswami S, Dutta R, Sengupta S. A profile of adolescent girls with gynecological problems. J Obstet Gynecol India. 2005;55(4):353-5.
24. Rathod AD, Chavan RP, Pajai SP, et al. Gynecological problems of adolescent girls attending outpatient department at tertiary care center with evaluation of cases of puberty menorrhagia requiring hospitalization. J Obstet Gynaecol India. 2016;66(Suppl 1):400-6.
25. Murat OZ, Yakut HI, Ozgu BS, et al. Adolescent gynaecology: satisfying the needs for special patients. OA Women's Health. 2014;2(1):1.
26. ACOG Committee Opinion no. 598: Committee on Adolescent Health Care: The initial reproductive health visit. Obstet Gynecol. 2014;123:1143-7.
27. Sacks D, Westwood M. An approach to interviewing adolescents. Paediatr Child Health. 2003;8(9):554-6.
28. Vo D. Taking a history with newcomer children and adolescents. Paediatr Child Health. 2014;19(2):87-8.
29. Sheela WG, Chellatamizh M, Mohanamba M, et al. Adolescent gynaecology problems in rural South India: a review of hospital admission in a tertiary care teaching hospital in Ammapettai, Tamil Nadu, India. Int J Reprod Contracept Obstet Gynecol. 2017;6(5):1920-3.
30. Ramaraju HE, Shivakumar HC, Khazi AA. Adolescent gynaecological problems in a tertiary care centre. Indian J Basic Appl Med Res. 2015;4(4):649-53.
31. Jacks TH, Obed JY, Agida ET, et al. Dysmenorrhoea and menstrual abnormalities among post menarcheal secondary school girls in Maideguri Nigeria. Afr J Med Sci. 2005;34:87-9.
32. Prasad D, Singh K, Pankaj S. Clinical spectrum of adolescent girls in tertiary care centre. Int J Sci Study. 2014;2(4):46-9.
33. Rimsza ME. Dysfunctional uterine bleeding. Pediatr Rev. 2002;23(7):227-33.
34. Berry PL, Schubiner H, Giblin PT. Issues in adolescent gynaecological care. Obstet Gynaecol Clin N Am. 1990;17(4):837-49.
35. Kumari A. Adolescent gynaecological problems: a clinical study. J Evol Med Dent Sci. 2013;2(9):1111-5.
36. Kapoor J. A descriptive study to assess the knowledge regarding leucorrhoea among adolescent girls in govt. Int J Curr Res Life Sci. 2018;7(2):942-5.
37. Osayande AS, Mehulic S. Diagnosis and initial management of dysmenorrhea. Am Fam Physician. 2014;89(5):341-6.
38. De Sanctis V, Soliman A, Bernasconi S, et al. primary dysmenorrhea in adolescents: prevalence, impact and recent knowledge. Pediatr Endocrinol Rev. 2015;13(2):512-20.
39. Harel Z. Dysmenorrhea in adolescents. Ann N Y Acad Sci. 2008:1135:185-95.

40. Tanksale S, Bendre K, Niyogi G. Adolescent ovarian tumours: a gynecologist's dilemma. Int J Reprod Contracept Obstet Gynecol. 2015;4(3):833-6.
41. Eskander RN, Bristow RE. Adnexal masses in pediatric and adolescent females: a review of the literature. Curr Obstet Gynecol Rep. 2012;1:25-32.
42. Emmanuel JJ. (2011). Adolescent Pregnancy in India: An issue of life and death. [online] Available from https://www.researchgate.net/publication/233741747_Adolescent_Pregnancy_in_India_An_issue_of_life_and_death' [Last accessed September, 2019].
43. Dutta I, Dutta DK, Joshi P. Outcome of teenage pregnancy in rural India with particular reference to obstetrical risk factors and perinatal outcome. Journal of SAFOG. 2013;5(3):102-6.
44. Dietrich JE, Millar DM, Quint EH. Obstructive reproductive tract anomalies. J Pediatr Adolesc Gynecol. 2014;27(6):396-402.
45. Boruah DB, Yadav RR, Mahanta K, et al. MR imaging evaluation of obstructing vaginal malformations with hematocolpos or hematometra in adolescent girls: a cross sectional study. The Egyptian Journal of Radiology and Nuclear Medicine. 2017;48(4):1187-96.
46. Moles RL, Levanthal JM. Sexual abuse and assault in children and teens: time to prioritize prevention. J Adolesc Health. 2014;55(3):312-3.
47. Haffejee S, Theron L. Resilience processes in sexually abused adolescent girls: A scoping review of the literature. S Afr J Sci. 2017;113(9-10):1-9.
48. Bunnell RE, Dahlberg L, Rolfs R, et al. High prevalence and incidence of sexually transmitted diseases in urban adolescent females despite moderate risk behaviors. J Infect Dis. 1999;180(5):1624-31.
49. Darj E, Mirembe FM, Rassjo EB. STI-prevalence and differences in social background and sexual behavior among urban and rural young women in Uganda. Sex Reprod Healthc. 2010;1(3):111-5.
50. Avuvika E, Masese LN, Wanje G, et al. Barriers and Facilitators of Screening for Sexually Transmitted Infections in Adolescent Girls and Young Women in Mombasa, Kenya: A Qualitative Study. PLoS One. 2017;12(1):e0169388.
51. Rawat J, Singh S, Pant N. Anorectal Malformations in Adolescent Females: A Retrospective Study. J Indian Assoc Pediatr Surg. 2018;23(2):57-6.
52. Hickey M, Balen A. Menstrual disorders in adolescence: investigation and management. Hum Reprod Update. 2003;9(5).493-504.
53. Yogini KD, Balasubramaniam D, Palanivelu C, et al. Laparoscopic approach to adnexal mass in adolescents: a retrospective analysis. J Datta Meghe Inst Med Sci Univ. 2017;12(1):55-60.
54. Williams CE, Creighton SM. Menstrual Disorders in Adolescents: Review of Current Practice. Horm Res Paediatr. 2012;78(3):135-43.
55. Ramareddy RS, Kumar A, Alladi A. Imperforate Hymen: Varied Presentation, New Associations, and Management. J Indian Assoc Pediatr Surg. 2017;22(4):207-10.

CHAPTER 2

Sexual Abuse and Assault in Pediatric Patient

Priyanka Yadav

■ DEFINITION AND INTRODUCTION

World Health Organization (WHO) defines "Child sexual assault as the involvement of child in sexual activity that he or she does not fully comprehend, is unable to give consent to, or for which the child is not developmentally prepared and cannot give consent, or that violates the laws or social taboos of society".[1]

There are different terminologies used for sexual contact:[2]

Sexual assault: It is a comprehensive term which includes physical force with or without penetration in which victim is unable to give consent. This includes touching the victim's intimate parts or touching clothes covering intimate parts. Stranger is usually involved in this type.

Sexual abuse: The abuser is usually the known person they can be relative, sibling, step parents, or own parents. This is more dangerous type as the victim finds it difficult to talk about it.

Date/acquaintance rape: The abuser is usually victim's current or past partner, classmate, or friend.

The age for giving consent varies from country to country, but any case where victim is younger than 18 years must be reported.

■ INCIDENCE

Sexual abuse against pediatric age group is a major problem in both developed and developing countries.

Stoltenborgh et al.[3] reported one out of every eight young people around the world has been abused in their lifetime and in India one-third of the rape case reported are usually of child abuse.

Children with mental disabilities or any other physical deformities, female child are at increased risk of sexual assault with incidence of 1.5–2 times than general population.[4]

Those who have milder cognitive disabilities are at the higher risk.[5,6]

CLINICAL MANIFESTATION

Sexual or physical abuse is suspected when the injury is unexplained, implausible or misdiagnosed.

Physical symptoms with which victim usually presents with are penile, vaginal and rectal pain, abnormal discharge, skin bruises, pelvic pain, and dysuria.

The adolescent may present with anxiety, nightmares, aggressive behavior, disturbed sleep, depression, post-traumatic stress syndrome, less self-esteem, eating disorders, and drug abuse.

INVESTIGATION

- Complete blood count (CBC)
- Throat culture
- Vaginal culture
- Cervical culture
- Urethral culture
- Anorectal swab culture
- Human immunodeficiency virus (HIV)
- Hepatitis B surface antigen (HBsAg)
- Venereal disease research laboratory (VDRL).

EXAMINATION

- Detailed history related to incident happened.
- The victim should be allowed to give history and narrate the incidence.
- Forensic examination will include history, documentation, and collection of evidence.
- The victim should undergo forensic medical examination to find out local wounds and signs of infection.
- The oral cavity should be examined properly for abrasions or signs of trauma, if present bite marks can be measured and wax impression is made for identifying the perpetrator.
- The abdominal examination should be done to find out if victim is already pregnant, thorough genital/rectal examination is done to examine signs of trauma.
- Female child can be examined in supine frog position or knee chest position under good lighting. Genital examination should be examined thoroughly which includes inspection of labia, fourchette, introitus, vestibule, edge of hymen, also anus and urethra.
- The examination is useful within 4 days postassault with use of deoxyribonucleic acid (DNA) amplification technique.[7]
- After 4 days forensic experts can be approached to find out if it is still useful to collect evidence.
- After 1 week forensic collection is not required victim should undergo counseling and treatment.

MANAGEMENT

Immediate Care

- The physician should treat the nongenital injuries, which may require immediate attention depending on severity of injury.
- Prevention of pregnancy should also be priority.
- A baseline urine pregnancy test should be done for female adolescent victim.
- Emergency contraception to be given to adolescent female victim.
- Progestin only pills and contraception pills are most preferred in postpubertal females.[8]

RECOMMENDATIONS

Prophylactic treatment for chlamydia and gonorrhea should be recommended to adolescent sexual assault victims who have been vaginally or anally penetrated (with or without ejaculation) or orally penetrated (with ejaculation) **(Box 1)**.

According to Centers for Disease Control and Prevention (CDC)[10]

Human papilloma virus (HPV) vaccination is recommended for female victims of age between 9 years and 26 years and male victims aged between 9 years and 21 years.

> **BOX 1:** Current recommendations according to Centers for Disease Control and Prevention.[9]
> - 125 mg of ceftriaxone intramuscularly
> - 2 g of metronidazole once orally
> - Either 1 g of azithromycin once orally or 100 mg doxycycline twice daily for 1 week
> - Hepatitis B immunization should be offered
>
> (If available, cefixime 400 mg once orally can be used instead of ceftriaxone).

Human immunodeficiency virus (HIV) prophylaxis is not universally recommended, but should be considered when there is mucosal membrane exposure (oral, vaginal, and anal) or through broken skin.

On the Basis of Current Guideline[11,12]

- Zidovudine (AZT) 200 mg thrice daily or 250 mg twice daily plus
- Lamivudine 150 mg twice daily plus
- Indinavir 800 mg thrice daily taken for 4 weeks.

Postexposure prophylaxis is most effective within 2 hours after exposure, but is recommended up to 72 hours after the assault **(Flowchart 1)**.

FOLLOW-UP

- Visit within 1 week to assess healing of injury.
- Sexually transmitted infections should be reassessed depending on treatment given initially and the history of sexual activity.

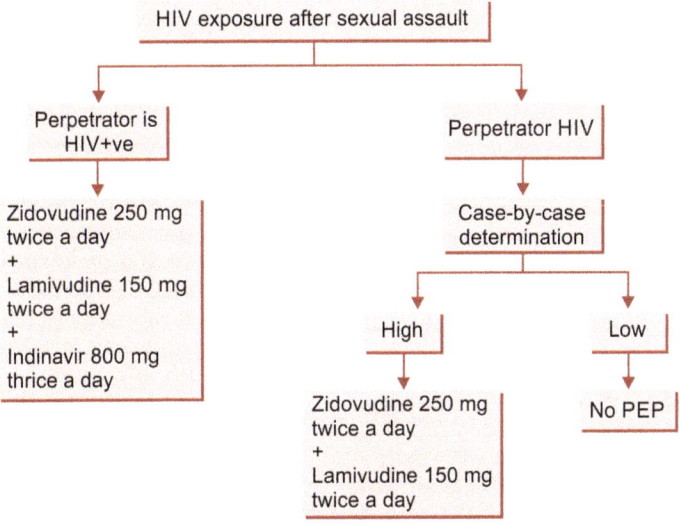

Flowchart 1: Treatment of HIV exposure after sexual assault with evidence of penetration.[13]

(HIV: human immunodeficiency virus; PEP: postexposure prophylaxis)

Recommendations from Centers for Disease Control and Prevention[14]

- Human immunodeficiency virus test to be repeated at 6 weeks and thereafter 3 and 6 months.
- Syphilis test should be repeated after 4–6 weeks and 3–6 months.

SUMMARY

- Thorough history, examination, screening, treatment, and follow-up are required for the child.
- Parents should see their child needs and requirement.
- Trauma focused "cognitive behavioral therapy" is useful in these cases.[15]

CONCLUSION

- Sexual abuse in pediatric patient is a major problem and it has to be diagnose on high suspection.
- It requires detail investigation and examination.
- Management includes immediate care and other prophylactic treatment and follow-up with greater emphasis on psychosocial therapy.

REFERENCES

1. WHO. (1999) Report of the consultation on child abuse prevention. [online] Available from https://apps.who.int/iris/handle/10665/65900 [Last accessed September, 2019].
2. American Academy of Pediatrics: Committee on Adolescence. Care of the adolescent sexual assault victim. Pediatrics. 2001;107(6):1476-9.
3. Stoltenborgh M, Van Ijzendoorn MH, Euser EM, et al. A global perspective on child sexual abuse: Meta-analysis of prevalence around the world. Child Maltreat. 2011;16(2):79-101.
4. Nosek MA. Sexual abuse of women with physical disabilities. In: Krotoski D, Nosek M, Turk M (Eds). Women with Physical Disabilities: Achieving and Maintaining Health and Well-being. Baltimore: Paul Brookes Publishing Co; 1996. pp. 153-73.
5. Sobsey D, Doe T. Patterns of sexual abuse and assault. Sex Disabil. 1991;9(3):243-60.
6. Ticoll M, Panitch M. Opening the doors: Addressing the sexual abuse of women with an intellectual disability. Can Womens Stud. 1993;13(4):84-7.
7. Hall A, Ballantyne J. Novel Y-STR typing strategies reveal the genetic profile of the semen donor in extended interval postcoital cervicovaginal samples. Forensic Sci Int. 2003;136(1-3):58-72.
8. Randomized controlled trial of levonorgestrel versus the Yuzpe regimen of combined oral contraceptives for emergency contraception. Task Force on Postovulatory Methods of Fertility Regulation. Lancet. 1998;352(9126):428-33.
9. Centers for Disease Control and Prevention. (2006). Sexually transmitted diseases: Treatment guidelines, 2006. [online] available from www.cdc.gov/std/treatment/2006/sexual-assault.htm [Last accessed September, 2007].
10. Workowski KA, Bolan GA, Centers for disease control and prevention. Sexually transmitted diseases treatment guidelines, 2015. MMWR Recomm Rep. 2015;64(RR-03):1-137.
11. Bamberger JD, Waldo CR, Gerberding JL, et al. Postexposure prophylaxis for human immunodeficiency virus (HIV) infection following sexual assault. Am J Med. 1999;106(3):323-6.
12. Centers for Disease Control. Updated US Public Health Service guidelines for the management of occupational exposures to HBV, HCV, and HIV and recommendations for postexposure prophylaxis. MMWR Recomm Rep. 2001;50(RR-11):1-42.
13. Smith DK, Grohskopf LA, Black RJ, et al. Antiretroviral postexposure prophylaxis after sexual, injection drug use, or other non occupational exposure to HIV in United States: recommendations from the U.S. Department of Health and Human Services. MMWR Recomm Rep. 2005;54(RR-02):1-20.
14. Evidence papers for the CDC sexually transmitted diseases treatment guidelines. Clin Infect Dis. 2015;61(Suppl 8):S759-62.
15. Saywitz KJ, Mannarino AP, Berliner L, et al. Treatment for sexually abused children and adolescents. Am Psychol. 2000;55(9):1040-9.

SECTION 2

Reproductive Age Group

- Early Pregnancy: Miscarriage
  Vyshnavi A Rao
- Gestational Trophoblastic Diseases
  Arunima Halder
- Ectopic Pregnancy
  Harpreet Kaur
- Leiomyoma Uterus Presenting as Emergency
  Arya Rajendran
- Dysmenorrhea
  Arveen Vohra
- Abnormal Uterine Bleeding
  Mekhala B Dwarakanath, Jahnavi Esanakula
- Postcoital Bleeding
  Sowmya Davuluri
- Infections
  Karthigayeni R
- Pelvic Mass
  Ravishankar P, Tejaswi K
- Ovarian Hyperstimulation Syndrome
  Nivedita Shetty
- Ovarian Torsion
  B Ramesh
- Management of Ovarian Mass in Premenopausal Women
  Kavita Manchanda, Jahnavi Esanakula
- Emergencies and Complications Related to Contraception
  Shashikala KT

CHAPTER 3

Early Pregnancy: Miscarriage

Vyshnavi A Rao

INTRODUCTION

Miscarriage (abortions) is defined as the spontaneous or induced termination of pregnancy before the period of fetal viability (or) expulsion of an embryo or fetus weighing 500 g or less[1] before the period of viability before 20 weeks (28 weeks in India).

The terms abortion or miscarriage are often used synonymously. On the other hand, induced abortion implies surgical or medical termination. Serum human chorionic gonadotropin (hCG) measurements can identify very early pregnancies. With the advent of transvaginal sonography:
- The earlier detection of pregnancy in which no products are seen in ultrasonography (USG)
- Pregnancy that display a gestational sac but no embryo
- Those in which a dead fetus can be detected.

ETIOLOGY

Cause of spontaneous abortion is multifactorial:
- Chromosomal anomalies[2]
- Metabolic and endocrine abnormalities
- *Anatomical factors*: Cervical incompetence, congenital anomalies of the uterus, uterine adhesions, and uterine fibroids
- *Others*: Infections (5–10%), immunological causes (5–10%), ABO blood group incompatibility, advanced maternal age, stress-related factors, extremes of age can lead to abortions.[3-5]

There are a few terminologies which need to be defined:
- *Biochemical pregnancy*: Denotes a positive serum beta hCG with pregnancy not being located on scan
- *Fetal loss*: Previous crown rump length (CRL) measurement with loss of fetal cardiac activity

- *Early pregnancy loss*: Confirmation of an empty sac or fetus on USG but no fetal cardiac activity <12 weeks of gestation
- *Delayed miscarriage/late pregnancy loss*: Loss of fetal cardiac activity >12 weeks of gestation
- *Pregnancy of unknown location (PUL)*: Serum beta hCG being positive with no identifiable pregnancy on scan.

TYPES OF MISCARRIAGE

Different types of miscarriages are given in **Table 1**.

Implantation Bleeding

Cyclical bleeding that may happen up to 12 weeks of pregnancy until the decidual space is obliterated by the fusion of decidua capsularis with decidua vera.

Bleeding is minimal lasts for lesser duration than her usual and usually corresponds to the date of the expected period.

Prerequisites on Approaching a Case of Miscarriage

- Detailed history with respect to last menstrual period to ascertain the period of gestation, whether the pregnancy occurred due to a contraceptive failure (use of emergency contraception) or whether it was a planned one
- Previous obstetric and gynecological procedures

TABLE 1: Types of miscarriage.

Type	Definition	Clinical presentation
Spontaneous miscarriage	Miscarriage occurring without medical (or) mechanical intervention to empty the uterus	Bleeding per vagina Cramping pain abdomen
Threatened miscarriage	Miscarriage which causes minimal spotting/bleeding but has not progressed to a stage where recovery is impossible	Light bleeding Cervical os closed Uterus corresponds to dates *Scan:* Fetal cardiac activity present
Inevitable miscarriage	Miscarriage where the changes have progressed to a state from where continuation of pregnancy is impossible	Cramping lower abdominal pain, uterus being tender on examination Heavy bleeding, uterus corresponds to dates, dilated cervix
Incomplete miscarriage	Miscarriage where products of conception are partially expelled	Heavy bleeding, dilated cervix, uterus smaller than dates
Complete miscarriage	Miscarriage where the products of conception are completely expelled	Light bleeding, closed cervical os, uterus smaller than dates, softer than normal
Missed miscarriage	When the fetus is dead in utero and retained inside for a variable length of time	Cervical os closed, no bleeding, fetal cardiac activity which was previously present but presently no cardiac activity seen on ultrasonography (USG)
Septic miscarriage	Miscarriage associated with clinically detectable infection of uterus and its contents	Tachycardia and fever General malaise, sweating, headache, features suggestive of endotoxic shock, reduced urine output, dryness of tongue

- Contraceptive history and to educate the woman regarding repeated abortions/ dilatation and evacuation can result in infertility in the later years to be emphasized upon
- Drugs taken (over the counter) and anticoagulant medication if taken
- Complete medical/surgical history
- Any concomitant comorbidities for which the patient is already on medications has to be enquired into.

Clinical Examination

- *General physical examination*: To look for pallor, icterus, cyanosis, clubbing, lymphadenopathy, and edema.
- Examination of breast, thyroid, and spine along with vitals like pulse rate, blood pressure, respiratory rate, and temperature is to must to be performed.
- *Pelvic examination*: To determine the size of the pregnant uterus, uterus anteverted/ retroverted, and presence of any other pelvic pathology (leiomyoma/ectopic pregnancy or adnexal mass) have to be ruled out.
- With the advent of ultrasound, the diagnosis and management of abortions have become much more precise.

Laboratory Investigations

Blood grouping and Rh typing:
- Complete blood picture determining the hemoglobin (Hb), total leukocyte count, differential count erythrocyte sedimentation rate (ESR), packed cell volume, red blood cell RBC indices, and thyroid-stimulating hormone (TSH).
- To look for infection and the general health of the patient has to be considered.

- Urine routine and microanalysis along with urine albumin and sugar.
- *Serology:* Human immunodeficiency virus (HIV), hepatitis B surface antigen (HBsAg), hepatitis C virus (HCV), and venereal disease research laboratory (VDRL).
- Vaginal swabs if there is suspicion of reproductive tract infection.
- Pelvic ultrasound is a must, in order to confirm the pregnancy is intrauterine in origin, and pelvic USG is mandatory before performing a medical termination of pregnancy (MTP).

Complete Abortion

Clinical presentation includes:
- Pregnancy test is positive
- Cervical os is closed as the products of conception are expelled completely
- Pain may be present or absent
- Vaginal bleeding is present/absent
- Signs and symptoms of pregnancy coincide with the weeks of gestation.

Management

- A pelvic USG is required in order to check if the uterine cavity is empty
- If patient complains of pain, analgesics may be prescribed
- Contraception advice.

Threatened Abortion

Clinical presentation includes:
- Ultrasound shows a live fetus
- Pregnancy test is positive
- Cervical os is closed
- Pain is absent or slight
- Vaginal bleeding is minimal, bright red color, bleeding followed by pain
- Signs and symptoms coincide with the weeks of gestation.

Management

- Bed rest is advocated until bleeding subsides.
- Intercourse should be avoided.
- Progestogens, e.g. hydroxyprogesterone caproate 250 mg intramuscular (IM) 1 dose if excessive bleeding is detected.
- The meta-analysis of all women, suggests that there is probably a reduction in the number of miscarriages for women given progestogen supplementation compared to placebo/controls [average risk ratio (RR) 0.69, 95% confidence interval (CI) 0.51–0.92, 11 trials, 2,359 women, moderate-quality evidence].[6,7]
- Micronized progesterone 400 mg vaginal BID up to 16 weeks if conception as occurred as a result of assisted reproductive techniques (ART).
- *Roles of hemostatics*: First trimester decidual hemorrhage leads to adverse outcomes including pregnancy loss, pre-eclampsia, abruption, intrauterine growth restriction (IUGR), and preterm births (PTBs). Decidual hemorrhage generates excess thrombin that binds to decidual cell-expressed protease-activated receptors (PARs) to induce chemokines promoting shallow placentation; such bleeding later in pregnancy generates thrombin to downregulate decidual cell progesterone receptors and upregulate cytokines and matrix metalloproteinases (MMPs) linked to PTB. Endometria of progestin-only, long-acting, reversible contraception (pLARC) users display ischemia-induced excess vasculogenesis and progestin inhibition of spiral artery vascular smooth muscle cell proliferation and migration leading to dilated fragile vessels prone to bleeding.
- Perivascular decidualized human endometrial stromal cells (HESCs) promote endometrial hemostasis during placentation yet facilitate menstruation through progestational regulation of hemostatic, proteolytic, and vasoactive proteins. Pathological endometrial hemorrhage elicits excess local thrombin generation, which contributes to pLARC-associated abnormal uterine bleeding (AUB), endometriosis, and adverse pregnancy outcomes through several biochemical mechanisms.[8]

Inevitable Abortion

Clinical presentation includes:
- Symptoms and signs of pregnancy coincide its duration
- Vaginal bleeding is excessive and may be associated with clots
- Colicky pain is present in the suprapubic region, which radiates to the back
- Dilated internal os with products of conception may be felt through the os
- Rupture of membranes between 12 weeks and 28 weeks, which represents a sign of inevitability
- Ultrasonography may or may not show a live fetus.

Management

- Any attempt to continue pregnancy may be not useful
- On per speculum examination, products at os are present—remove using sponge holding forceps/ovum forceps, check curettage may be required
- Ultrasonography pelvis to confirm if there are retained products of conception (RPOC)
- Prophylactic antibiotics are to be administered

- Postmiscarriage counseling—grief counseling and correction of anemia if present
- Contraception advice.

Incomplete Abortion

When there is presence of RPOC in the uterine cavity, it is called incomplete abortion.

Clinical Presentation

- Patient gives history of passage of a part of products of conception
- Bleeding per vaginal (PV) is continuous
- Ultrasonography shows products of conception retained inside uterine cavity
- On examination, uterus is less than the period of amenorrhea.

Treatment

- On speculum examination, if products of conception are seen, it is removed using sponge holding/ovum forceps
- Misoprostol 400 µg vaginal/sublingual dose (or) 600 µg orally/rectally
- Products of conception needs to be expelled completely
- Analgesics, antipyretics should be given if needed
- Postmiscarriage counseling
- Repeat scan in order to confirm that the uterine cavity is empty
- Contraceptive advice.

Missed Abortion

Clinical Presentation

- Regression of pregnancy-associated symptoms like nausea, vomiting, and breast tenderness
- Fetal movements are not perceived or ceases if present before
- Uterus does not corresponds to the period of gestation
- Cervical os is closed
- Dark brownish vaginal discharge is present.

Management

- Ultrasonography will reveal a collapsed gestational sac and absent fetal heart/movement
- *Diagnosis:* Based on two transvaginal/transabdominal (TV/TA) USG at least 7 days apart shows an embryo >7 weeks of gestation (CRL >6 mm diameter and gestational sac >20 mm in diameter) with absent fetal cardiac activity
- Complete blood picture to rule out sepsis and disseminated intravascular coagulation (DIC).

Evacuation of uterus becomes essential when:
- There is presence of excessive bleeding PV
- Spontaneous expulsion does not occur within 5 weeks
- Infection or DIC sets in.

Dilatation and evacuation is the treatment of choice in first trimester missed abortions.

Medical management:
- Misoprostol 600 µg vaginal/sublingually 3 hourly maximum of two doses
- 800 µg vaginally 3 hourly maximum of two doses
- Prophylactic antibiotics to be administered for 5 days
- Analgesics and antipyretics may be needed
- Postmiscarriage counseling
- Contraceptive advice.

Septic Abortion

Septic abortion is characterized by infection of uterus and its contents, which usually follows unsafe abortion or incomplete abortion. The infection may spread to and involve myometrium, parametrium, tubes, ovaries, and peritoneum.

Retained products of conception form a good culture media for organisms like *Escherichia coli*, streptococci, and anaerobes responsible for causing septic abortion.

It may occur due to criminal interference.

Types of Septic Abortion

Grade 1: The infection is confined to decidua—80%

Grade 2: The infection extended to myometrium—15%

Grade 3: The infection extends to pelvis, generalized peritonitis, and endotoxic shock present.
- Detailed history of the patient needs to be obtained—where, how, by whom, was the case previously handled, and use of abortifacients
- Pyrexia, tachycardia, general malaise, sweating, headache, and joint aches
- Bleeding—duration, amount, and presence of clots
- Cramping—duration severity, any history of fainting episodes (suggestive of ectopic pregnancy)
- Previous obstetric/gynecological history.

Clinical Examination
- Suprapubic pain and tenderness
- Absent bowel sound as in paralytic ileus
- Abdominal rigidity and distension indicates peritonitis due to bowel perforation.

Local Examination
- Vaginal bleeding
- Offensive vaginal discharge
- Uterus is tender
- Fullness and tenderness of pouch of Douglas (POD) points out towards pelvic abscess associated with diarrhea.

Investigations and Management of a Case of Septic Abortion (Flowchart 1)
- Close monitoring of pulse rate, blood pressure, temperature, and bleeding PV is mandatory
- Intravenous (IV) therapy is continued until patient is afebrile for 48 hours and has to be followed by oral medication, tablet doxycycline 100 mg twice a day for 2 weeks
- Tetanus immunoprophylaxis is recommended
- Follow-up and contraception advice
- Anti-D immunoglobulin is given to Rh-negative women, 300 µg[9]
- Ampicillin 1g IV every 6 hours
- Gentamicin 80 mg IV every 12 hours
- Metronidazole 500 mg IV every 8 hours
- Retained products of conceptions were evacuated under antibiotic cover and sent for histopathology
- A booster dose of tetanus toxoid 0.5 mL to be given
- Septic abortion with septic shock, generalized peritonitis, and suspected renal failure.

Management of Shock[10,11]
- *Universal measures:*
  - Airway—should be open
  - Keep the patient nil per oral
  - Keep the patient warm
  - Maintain circulation by leg elevation so that the vital organs remain perfused
- *Oxygen:* By mask at 6–8 L/minute
- *Fluid therapy:* To be maintained for hydration. Normal saline or ringer lactate started at the rate of 1 liter in 20–30 minutes, gradually titrated as per requirement
- *Blood transfusion:* To maintain Hb between 7 g% and 9 g%[10]

Flowchart 1: Investigations and management of septic abortion.

Investigations:
- Complete blood count, blood grouping and Rh typing
- Cervical swabs for culture and sensitivity
- Coagulation profile, serum electrolytes blood culture if pyrexia >38.5°C

↓

Treatment:
- Isolate patient, bed rest in semiprone position
- Establish an intravenous (IV) line, in case of shock, central venous pressure (CVP) line to help in administering
- Fluid/blood products if needed

↓

Monitoring vital signs:
- Pulse rate, blood pressure, and temperature
- Intake output chart

↓

- *Antibiotics:* Effective against gram-negative, gram-positive, anaerobic organism and chlamydia
- *Uterine evacuation:*
  - Vacuum aspiration is avoided if there is prior interference
  - Oxytocin (20 units in 500 mL of IV fluid) and methylergometrine (0.2 mg IM)
  - For uterine atony
- Products of conception are sent for histopathology

- *Vasopressors:* Used to maintain mean arterial pressure of at least 65 mm Hg
  - Dopamine is started at the rate of 5–10 µg/kg/min IV and the infusion is adjusted according to blood pressure
  - Epinephrine is used when blood pressure is poorly responsive to norepinephrine or dopamine
- *Inotropes:* Recommended when cardiac output remains low despite fluid resuscitation and vasopressors[10]
- *Steroids:* Used when blood pressure is poorly responsive to fluid and vasopressor therapy hydrocortisone 200 mg/day in four divided doses for 7 days or more[12]
- *Monitoring:* Pulse rate, blood pressure, respiratory rate, and intake/output charting. CVP is monitored and maintained at 8–10 cm of water
  - Injection ceftriaxone 2 g IV every 12 hours and injection metronidazole 500 mg IV every 8 hours were started
  - A booster dose of tetanus toxoid was given
  - In view of suspected gut/uterine perfusion patient was taken up for urgent laparotomy

Prognosis

- Prognosis depends upon the degree of infection present, intervention, and presence of complications.
- In India, 13–25% of the cases admitted to hospital succumb to complications due to septic shock, DIC, and hepatorenal failure.[3,4]
- Late complications include tubal block and infertility, pelvic inflammatory disease, and chronic pelvic pain.

Induced Abortion

Indications

- Pregnancy as a result of rape
- When continuation of pregnancy endangers the life of a pregnant woman in conditions like:
  - Persistent heart disease after cardiac decompensation
  - Invasive carcinoma of cervix
- When continuation of pregnancy may cause severe physical deformities or mental retardation of the child.

Medical Methods

Antiprogesterone (RU486):
- *Contraindications*:
  - Intrauterine contraceptive device (IUCD) in situ
  - Hypertension, glaucoma, asthmatic, and anemia
  - Lactating women
  - Previous uterine scar
- *Complications*:
  - Nausea, vomiting, and gastrointestinal cramping
  - *Failure to abort:* 1%
  - *Mobius syndrome:* In fetus (congenital facial palsy, limb defects, and hydrocephalus)
  - Termination of pregnancy is mandatory if medical methods fail
  - In case the woman bleeds profusely, emergency evacuation is mandatory
  - Subsequent menstruation may be delayed.

Prostaglandins:
- The prostaglandins (PGs) are a group of physiologically active lipid compounds having diverse hormone-like effects
- Prostaglandins have been found in almost every tissue in humans and other animals
- They are derived enzymatically from fatty acids

MEDICAL TERMINATION OF PREGNANCY

Protocol

- Obtaining an informed consent is mandatory
- Performing an USG prior to administration of MTP drugs is vital in order to confirm the presence of intrauterine pregnancy, its duration and to rule out ectopic pregnancy.

For Pregnancies up to 9 weeks Gestation (63 days)

- Medical termination with mifepristone 200 mg orally followed by vaginal misoprostol 24–48 hours later.
- For vaginal route, the recommended dose is 800 µg. It can also be administered through the sublingual/buccal routes.
- Up to 7 weeks of gestation, misoprostol can be administered by vaginal, buccal, and sublingual routes. After week 7, oral misoprostol should not be used.
- Up to 9 weeks of gestation, misoprostol is given by vaginal and buccal/sublingual routes.

For Pregnancies between 9 weeks and 12 weeks (63–84 Days)

- 200 mg mifepristone orally followed by 36–48 hours later by 800 µg of misoprostol vaginally.
- Misoprostol should be given 400 µg vaginally or sublingually every 3 hours up to four doses until products of conception are expelled.

For Pregnancies above 12 weeks of Gestation

- 200 mg mifepristone orally followed by 36–48 hours later administration of misoprostol
- Gestations between 12 weeks and 24 weeks, the initial misoprostol dose followed by oral mifepristone should be either 800 µg vaginally or 400 µg orally
- Subsequent doses of misoprostol 400 µg given by the vaginal/sublingual routes every 3 hours up to four doses
- For pregnancies beyond 24 weeks, because of greater sensitivity of the uterus to PGs, misoprostol usage must be decreased.

Recommended Methods for Medical Abortion in Situations where Mifepristone is not Available

- For pregnancies of gestational age up to 12 weeks (84 days)
- *For medical abortions*: The recommended dose of misoprostol is 800 µg given either vaginally or sublingually, up to three doses of 800 µg can be administered at a given gap of 3–4 hours, but not longer than 12 hours
- *For pregnancies of gestational age over 12 weeks*: 400 µg of misoprostol given vaginally or sublingually repeated every 3 hourly up to five doses is acceptable
- *For pregnancies beyond 24 weeks*: Misoprostol dose should be decreased considerably due to the higher sensitivity of the uterus to PGs, but lack of clinical studies precludes specific dosing recommendations
- *Between 12 weeks and 24 weeks*: Dilatation and evacuation and medical methods (mifepristone and misoprostol; misoprostol alone) are both recommended for miscarriages for gestation over 12–14 weeks.

THE MEDICAL TERMINATION OF PREGNANCY ACT, 1971

An Act to provide for the termination of certain pregnancies by registered medical practitioners and for matters connected therewith or incidental thereto. Be it enacted by Parliament in the Twenty-second Year of the Republic of India.

This Act aims to improve the maternal health scenario by preventing large number of unsafe abortions and consequent high incidence of maternal mortality and morbidity. This Act legalizes abortion services and promotes access to safe abortion services to women.

Medical Grounds

When the continuation of pregnancy is likely to endanger the life of the pregnant women (or) cause grievous injury to her physical and/or mental health, as in cases of severe hypertension, cardiac disease, diabetes, psychiatric illnesses, and genital and breast cancer.

Eugenic Grounds

When there is an increased risk of the child being born with serious physical (or) mental abnormalities.

Humanitarian Grounds

When the pregnancy is caused by rape or incest.

Social Grounds

When in the actual or reasonably foreseeable future, her environment (social/economic) might lead to risk of injury to her health (or) pregnancy has resulted due to a failure of a contraceptive device/method.

Authorized Place for Conducting Medical Termination of Pregnancy

- A hospital established or maintained by Government
- A place for the time being approved for the purpose of this Act by Government.

■ DEPARTMENT OF HEALTH AND WELFARE DRAFT MEDICAL TERMINATION OF PREGNANCY (AMENDMENT) BILL, 2014

The Government took cognizance of the challenges faced by women in accessing safe abortion services and in 2006 constituted an expert group to review the existing provisions of the MTP Act to propose draft amendments. A series of expert group meetings were held from 2006–2010 to identify strategies for strengthening access to safe abortion services. In 2013, a national consultation was held which was attended by a range of stakeholders further emphasized the need for amendments to the MTP Act. The proposed amendments to the MTP Act were primarily based on increasing the availability of safe and legal abortion services for women in the country.

- Expanding the provider base
- Increasing the upper gestation limit for legal MTPs
- Increasing access to legal abortion services for women
- Increasing clarity of the MTP law.

■ CONTRACEPTION ADVICE: POSTABORTION

- The informed choice of the available methods of contraception needs to be offered to the patient after detailed counseling regarding the side effects and failure rates of each method. This is called cafeteria approach.
- With the advent of an active sexual life, particularly in adolescent age group, advice regarding contraception is the need of the hour.
- Pregnancy, abortion, and gynecologic pathology including sexually transmitted infections (STIs) and acquired immunodeficiency syndrome (AIDS) must be discussed in detail as each can have a significant impact on long-term physical, mental, and social well-being of women.

■ CONCLUSION

- Abortion is a process where the fetus is expelled either spontaneously or induced as discussed above causing tremendous physical, mental, and emotional turmoil in women. As clinicians we need to address all aspects involved in a very sympathetic yet scientific and rational manner.
- Safe abortion saves lives.

■ REFERENCES

1. Cunningham FG, Kenneth JL, Bloom SL, et al. Abortion. Williams Obstetrics, 22nd edition. India: Mcgraw Hill; 2005. pp. 232-51.
2. Kajii T, Ferrier A, Niikawa N, et al. Anatomic and chromosomal anomalies in 639 spontaneous abortuses. Hum Genet. 1980;55:87-98.
3. Arck PC, Rucke M, Rose M, et al. Early risk factors for miscarriage: A prospective cohort study in pregnant women. Reprod Biomed Online. 2008;17:101-13.
4. Maconochie N, Doyle P, Prior S, et al. Risk factors for first trimester miscarriage results from a UK population-based case-control study. BJOG. 2007;114:170-86.
5. Gracia CR, Sammel MD, Chittams J, et al. Risk factors for spontaneous abortion in early

symptomatic first trimester pregnancies. Obstet Gynecol. 2005;106:993-9.
6. Haas DM, Hathaway TJ, Ramsey PS. Progestogen for preventing miscarriage in women with recurrent miscarriage of unclear etiology. Cochrane Database Syst Rev. 2018;10:CD003511.
7. Ku CW, Allen JC Jr, Lek SM, et al. Serum progesterone distribution in normal pregnancies compared to pregnancies complicated by threatened miscarriage from 5 to 13 weeks gestation: a prospective cohort study. BMC Pregnancy Childbirth. 2018;18(1):360.
8. Schatz F, Guzeloglu-Kayisli O, Arlier S, et al. The role of decidual cells in uterine hemostasis, menstruation, inflammation, adverse pregnancy outcomes and abnormal uterine bleeding. Hum Reprod Update. 2016;22(4):497-515.
9. FOGSI. (2009). Guidelines for the use of Anti-D immunoglobulin for Rh Prophylaxis. [online] Available from www.fogsi.org/anti_d_immunoglobulin.pdf
10. Dellinger RP, Levy MM, Carlet JM, et al. Surviving Sepsis Campaign: International guidelines for management of severe sepsis and septic shock: 2008. Crit Care Med. 2008;36:296-327.
11. WHO. Clinical management of abortion complications: A practical guide. Geneva: World Health Organization; 1994.
12. Marik PE, Pastores SM, Annane D, et al. Recommendations for the diagnosis and management of corticosteroid insufficiency in critically ill adult patients: consensus statements from an international task force by the American College of Critical Care Medicine. Crit Care Med. 2008;36:1937-49.

CHAPTER 4

Gestational Trophoblastic Diseases

Arunima Halder

■ INTRODUCTION

Gestational trophoblastic tumor is an all-inclusive term including a spectrum of benign and malignant disorders **(Flowchart 1)**. The incidence of gestational trophoblastic diseases is about 1 in 40,000 pregnancies with preponderance in the Asian population as compared to the European or the American counterparts.[1] Gestational trophoblastic neoplasia (GTN) is one of the most curable gynecological cancers. With proper chemotherapy, not only can patients be completely cured but can undergo pregnancy subsequently without any potential harm to the developing fetus.

■ PATHOGENESIS OF GESTATIONAL TROPHOBLASTIC DISEASES

Risk factors for developing gestational trophoblastic diseases are given in **Table 1**.

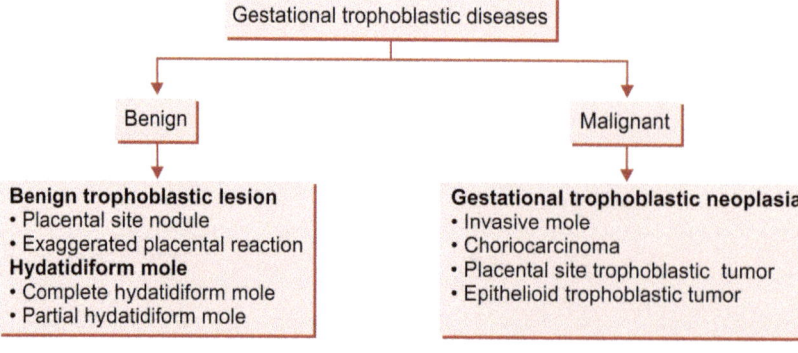

Flowchart 1: Classification of gestational trophoblastic diseases.[2]

Chapter 4: Gestational Trophoblastic Diseases

TABLE 1: Risk factors associated with gestational trophoblastic diseases.

S. No.	Factors	Description	Remarks
1.	Age	• Hydatidiform mole appears to be more common in extremes of gestational age and the distribution has been shown to follow a J-shaped curve[3] • Possible pathogenesis behind this could be abnormal gametogenesis and abnormal fertilization in both advanced maternal and paternal age	The risk between maternal age and the development of hydatidiform mole is better established for complete moles than partial moles
2.	Reproductive history	• Previous history of hydatidiform mole increases chance of developing molar pregnancy subsequently. Most of the time it is the same type of mole which had appeared previously • Previous spontaneous abortion may double the risk of molar pregnancy[5]	There is 1% increased chance of molar pregnancy in previous 1 hydatidiform mole and 25% chance in previous 2 moles[4]
3.	Diet	Several studies have suggested an increased incidence of complete mole with decreasing consumption of animal fat and beta-carotene. This may explain geographical variations[6]	Studies show conflicting results
4.	Others	• *Oral contraceptive pills:* Development of molar pregnancy has been attributed to prior usage of oral contraceptive pills (OCPs), its duration, and conception in the similar cycle[7] • High education, irregular menses, only male infants previously, smoking[8]	Weak association Linkage mainly to partial mole[8]

GENETICS OF GESTATIONAL TROPHOBLASTIC DISEASE

Complete Hydatidiform Mole

Complete moles are paternal in origin and are diploid. Eighty percent of them develop from the duplication of haploid sperm in an egg which has lost its maternal nuclear material before or after fertilization. Twenty percent of these may arise from the fertilization of two sperms. Though the nuclear deoxyribonucleic acid (DNA) is of paternal origin, the mitochondrial DNA remains maternal **(Figs. 1A to D)**.[9]

CLINICAL FEATURES

Previously, complete hydatidiform mole used to present with an array of symptoms like vaginal bleeding, hyperemesis gravidarum, preeclampsia, and more for gestational age uterine size. However, in the present era, such presentation is rare as detection of the molar pregnancy is quite early due to increased awareness regarding early pregnancy scans and beta-human chorionic gonadotropin (β-hCG) levels. Partial moles on the other hand, usually present with missed miscarriage or vaginal bleeding. Partial mole is usually diagnosed in histology.

PATHOLOGY

The gestational trophoblastic tumors are derived from different parts of a normal placenta itself.

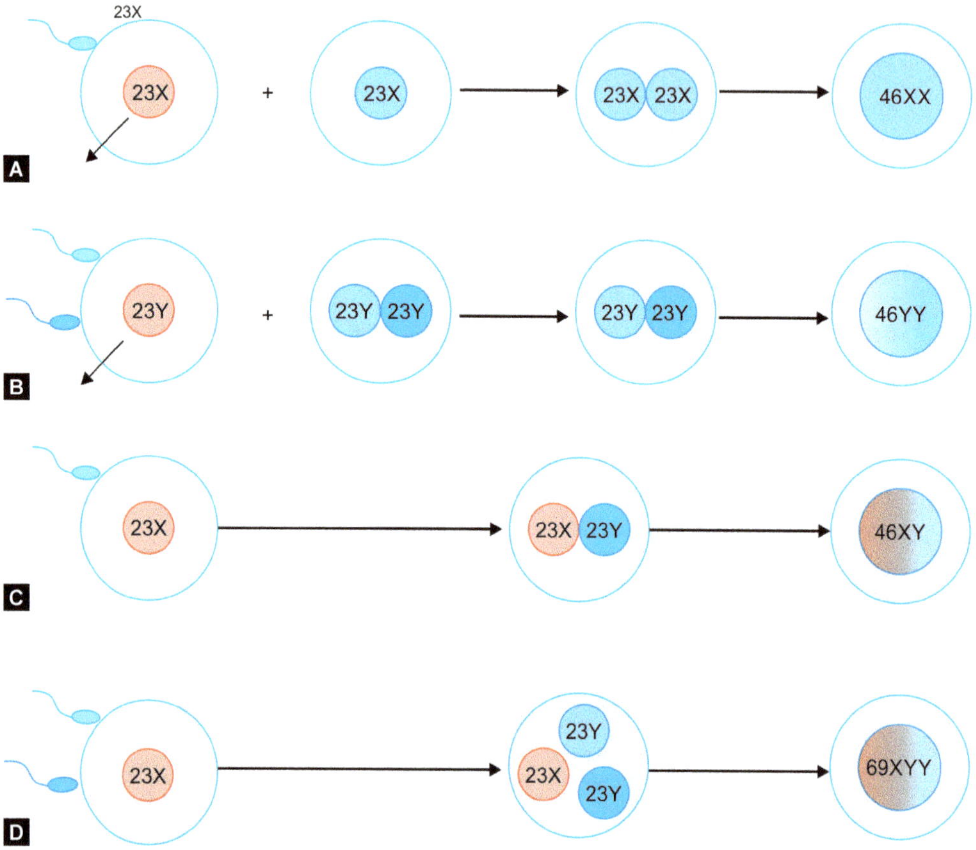

Figs. 1A to D: Genetic origins of the hydatidiform mole. (A) Loss of maternal chromosome with duplication of 23X from sperm; (B) Loss of maternal chromosome with duplication of 23Y from sperm; (C) Biparental complete hydatidiform mole (CHM) in females who are homozygous or compound heterozygous for mutations NLRP7 and KHDC3L; (D) Partial mole.

TABLE 2: Origins of various gestational tumors.

Derived from villous trophoblast	Derived from extravillous (interstitial) trophoblast
• Complete hydatidiform mole • Partial hydatidiform mole • Choriocarcinoma	• Placental site trophoblastic tumor • Epithelioid trophoblastic tumor

The origins of various gestational tumors are as per **Table 2**.

Complete hydatidiform moles exhibit a villous structure with the following features **(Fig. 2)**:[10]

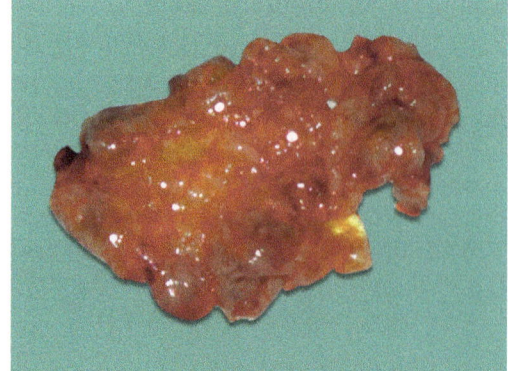

Fig. 2: Early complete hydatidiform mole.
Courtesy: Dr Soundarya Raghuram, Ganesamoni Hospital, Nagercoil

- Abnormal trophoblastic hyperplasia
- Stromal hypercellularity
- Stromal karyotypic debris
- Collapsed blood vessels.

Partial hydatidiform mole shows:[10]
- Patchy villous hydropic changes
- Scattered abnormally-shaped villi
- Trophoblastic pseudoinclusions
- Localized trophoblastic hyperplasia.

IMMUNOHISTOCHEMISTRY IN HYDATIDIFORM MOLE

When a pregnancy is aborted in the early first trimester, it is difficult to distinguish between complete mole, partial mole, and hydropic chromosomally normal abortuses that mimic molar pregnancy. This distinction can be done by p57KIP2 immunostaining. The *p57KIP2* gene is paternally imprinted and maternally expressed. As a result, it is strongly expressed in a normal placenta. It also gets expressed in partial moles and hydropic fetuses. However, in complete moles, it remains unexpressed as the entire genome is of paternal origin. Fluorescent in situ hybridization, flow cytometry, and molecular genotyping can be used to do the immunostaining. In a summary, though histology is the primary diagnostic modality to differentiate between the types of moles, immunostaining remains an adjuvant especially for borderline histological diagnoses.

DETERMINATION OF PLOIDY

Ploidy helps in the determination of the number of complete set of chromosomes that might be present. It can be measured using flow cytometry or automated image cytometry. Automated image cytometry is however, more sensitive in the former.

TRANSVAGINAL ULTRASONOGRAPHY

Transvaginal ultrasonography is the primary mode of clinical diagnosis. Usually it presents as an enlarged heterogeneous mass of complex echogenicity. The lesion is typically called as "snowstorm appearance" or granular owing to the heteroechoic nature **(Fig. 3)**.[11] Transvaginal sonography (TVS) can also detect the extent of myometrial invasion if any. In the first trimester, the fluid-filled areas (which are actually the hydropic villi) are approximately 1 mm up to 30 mm in size. These spaces increase in size with the gestational age making a molar pregnancy more easily detectable in the second trimester. Another important thing is the measurement of uterine volume, which helps in determining the tumor burden and hence risks stratification.[12]

Partial moles, on the other hand, are associated with a growth-retarded fetus along with an enlarged placenta with heteroechoic areas or cystic areas. Partial moles can be differentiated from a dizygotic diploid twin pregnancy with concurrent complete mole by

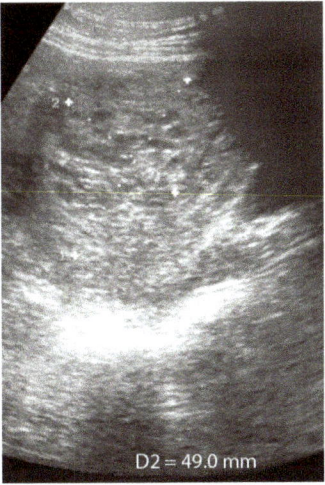

Fig. 3: Snowstorm appearance on USG.
Courtesy: Dr Vydehi. Dwarakamayi Hospital. Srikakulam.

identification of a normal placental structure in the latter.[12,13] In the presence of cystic spaces in the placenta, a ratio of transverse to anteroposterior diameter of the gestation sac of greater than 1.5 contributes to the reliable diagnosis of partial moles.[14]

Bilateral theca lutein cysts is a common finding occur as a result of high circulating hCG levels in the body.

Although ultrasonography may be the primary diagnostic modality, histopathology along with immunochemistry clinches the diagnosis of molar pregnancy.[15]

TREATMENT OF MOLAR PREGNANCY

Most of the time, the diagnosis of a molar pregnancy is made preoperatively. However, if it is diagnosed prior to evacuation a proper treatment plan can be chalked out. Necessary investigations prior to evacuation have been enumerated in **Table 3**.

TABLE 3: List of pre-evacuation investigations.[16]

S. No.	Investigations	Rationale
1.	Chest X-ray	Postevacuation trophoblastic infiltration into lungs may occur. Pre-evacuation X-ray will prevent any confusion postoperatively
2.	CBC	Preoperative hemoglobin status
3.	BG and Rh typing	Anti-D in case of Rh-negative
4.	β-hCG	Postevacuation surveillance
5.	LFT	

(BG: blood group; β-hCG: beta-human chorionic gonadotropin; CBC: complete blood count; LFT: liver function test; Rh: rhesus)

Suction and Evacuation

Suction evacuation is the most preferred method of termination of a molar pregnancy. It is usually done under general anesthesia.

The steps while performing suction evacuation are as follows:[17]
- Oxytocin infusion to be started prior to induction of anesthesia.
- Serial cervical dilatation to be done. Misoprostol ripening of cervix to be avoided to prevent the embolization of the trophoblastic tissue.
- Suction evacuation to be carried out followed by gentle sharp curettage.
- In case of excessive intraoperative bleeding, the process of suction evacuation should be expedited.
- In case, the need for suction evacuation is precluded by the size of fetus especially in cases of partial mole, medical termination can be done. However in these cases, the chance of persistent trophoblastic disease is higher.[14,17]
- Anti-D prophylaxis to be given to those who have Rh-negative type of blood group.

Hysterectomy

In women who do not desire to preserve their fertility, hysterectomy could be an option.

Chemotherapy

Providing prophylactic chemotherapy at the time of evacuation remains controversial. In a Cochrane meta-analysis, three randomized controlled trials (RCTs) involving 613 women were analyzed. This study suggested that prophylactic chemotherapy decreases the number of women developing cancer after a molar pregnancy. However, this was more relevant in case of complete moles. The study further suggested that prophylactic chemotherapy actually delays the diagnosis of cancer and leads to increased requirements of anticancer agents to treat the disease.[18]

Chemotherapy may be given in the following situations:
- Stagnant or rising beta-hCG levels
- Histopathologically proven choriocarcinoma
- Distant metastases in the brain, liver, gastrointestinal (GI) tract or lungs (chest X-ray showing metastases >2 cm in diameter)
- Transvaginal or intraperitoneal or GI hemorrhage
- Vaginal metastases or lung metastases
- Serum β-hCG levels are >20,000 IU/L even after 4 weeks of evacuation (repeat evacuation has increased chance of uterine perforation).

COMPLICATIONS OF HYDATIDIFORM MOLE[19]

- *Metastases*: The metastases of molar pregnancy may happen in lungs, brain, vagina, and liver. If present in the lungs, patient may present with hemoptysis, shortness of breath, and chest pain. If in brain, they may present with dizziness, fainting, seizure, and headache. Vaginal metastases can present with vaginal bleeding or pus discharge. Liver metastases may present with signs and symptoms of jaundice and abdominal pain.
- *Anemia*: Excessive vaginal bleeding may result in lowered hemoglobin to up to less than 10 in patients with molar pregnancy.
- *Hyperthyroidism*: Associated hyperthyroidism could be seen in approximately 7% of patients with molar pregnancy. Beta sympathetic blockers are to be given in these patients before induction of anesthesia to prevent thyroid storm during a surgical procedure.
- Preeclampsia
- Pulmonary distress is seen in 2% of the cases.

POSTMOLAR SURVEILLANCE

- Postmolar surveillance is strictly individualized.
- Following evacuation, titers of β-hCG should be monitored every week or 2 weeks.
- If hCG has come back to normal within a period of 56 days following the pregnancy, follow-up has to be done for a period of 6 months from the date of evacuation. If hCG has not returned to normal within 56 days of pregnancy then follow-up for 6 months from normalization of the hCG levels.
- To prevent confusion regarding the β-hCG levels women are advised to use contraception till its levels fall below 5 mIU/L, though pregnancies during the surveillance remain more or less uneventful.

Gestational Trophoblastic Neoplasia

This is a group of disorders which is characterized by the proliferation and invasion of trophoblastic cells in the endometrium and myometrium **(Table 4)**. Although these diseases are characterized histologically, very little tissue is usually available. Most of the times, the diagnosis is made by β-hCG levels. Most of the times, an antecedent pregnancy cannot be confirmed with certainty. Most of the cases occur after molar pregnancy.

Diagnosis of GTN can be made in the following situations:[20,21]

TABLE 4: Comparison of various gestational trophoblastic tumors.

Characteristics	Invasive mole	Gestational choriocarcinoma	PSTT	ETT
Antecedent event	Complete or partial molar pregnancy	Molar pregnancy (majority), nonmolar pregnancy	Any type of pregnancy (term gestation most commonly)	Remote pregnancy event or in most cases prior gestation cannot be confirmed
Histopathology	Syncytiotrophoblastic or cytotrophoblastic hyperplasia with presence of chorionic villi	Sheets of anaplastic trophoblastic tissue with syncytiotrophoblastic and cytotrophoblastic cells without any chorionic villi	Nests and sheets of intermediate trophoblastic cells invading between myometrial cells and fibers	Intermediate trophoblasts in sheets and nests forming tumor nodules in myometrium
Immunohistochemistry	Positive for β-hCG	Positive for β-hCG	50–100% positive for hPL. <10% positive for β-hCG	Positive for multiple markers like cytokeratin and inhibin A
Invasive nature/metastases (Figs. 4A to D)	Local invasion into the vagina	Hematogenous spread to lungs, liver, and brain	Hematogenous spread to lungs, liver, and brain	Hematogenous spread to lungs, liver, and brain
Clinical features	Irregular vaginal bleeding, uterine subinvolution, theca lutein cysts, persistent vaginal bleeding, uterine perforation, and intraperitoneal hemorrhage	Vaginal bleeding, most commonly diagnosed during surveillance	Hemoptysis, headache, vaginal bleeding (signs and symptoms of metastatic event)	Hemoptysis, headache, vaginal bleeding (signs and symptoms of metastatic event)
Ultrasonography	Sonographically indistinguishable from one another. May be echogenic, hypoechoic, complex or multicystic mass within the myometrium. On Doppler they appear hypovascular or at times hypervascular			
Treatment	Single dose of chemotherapy	Chemotherapy	Hysterectomy	Hysterectomy

(β-hCG: beta-human chorionic gonadotropin; ETT: epithelioid trophoblastic tumor; hPL: human placental lactogen; PSTT: placental site trophoblastic tumor)

- Four β-hCG values that have plateaued over a period of 3 weeks (on days 1, 7, 14, and 21)
- A rising β-hCG value of greater than 10% noted over a period of 2 weeks (day 1, 7, and 14)
- β-hCG levels still persisting after a period of 6 months postevacuation of the hydatidiform mole.
- Diagnosis of choriocarcinoma on histopathology.

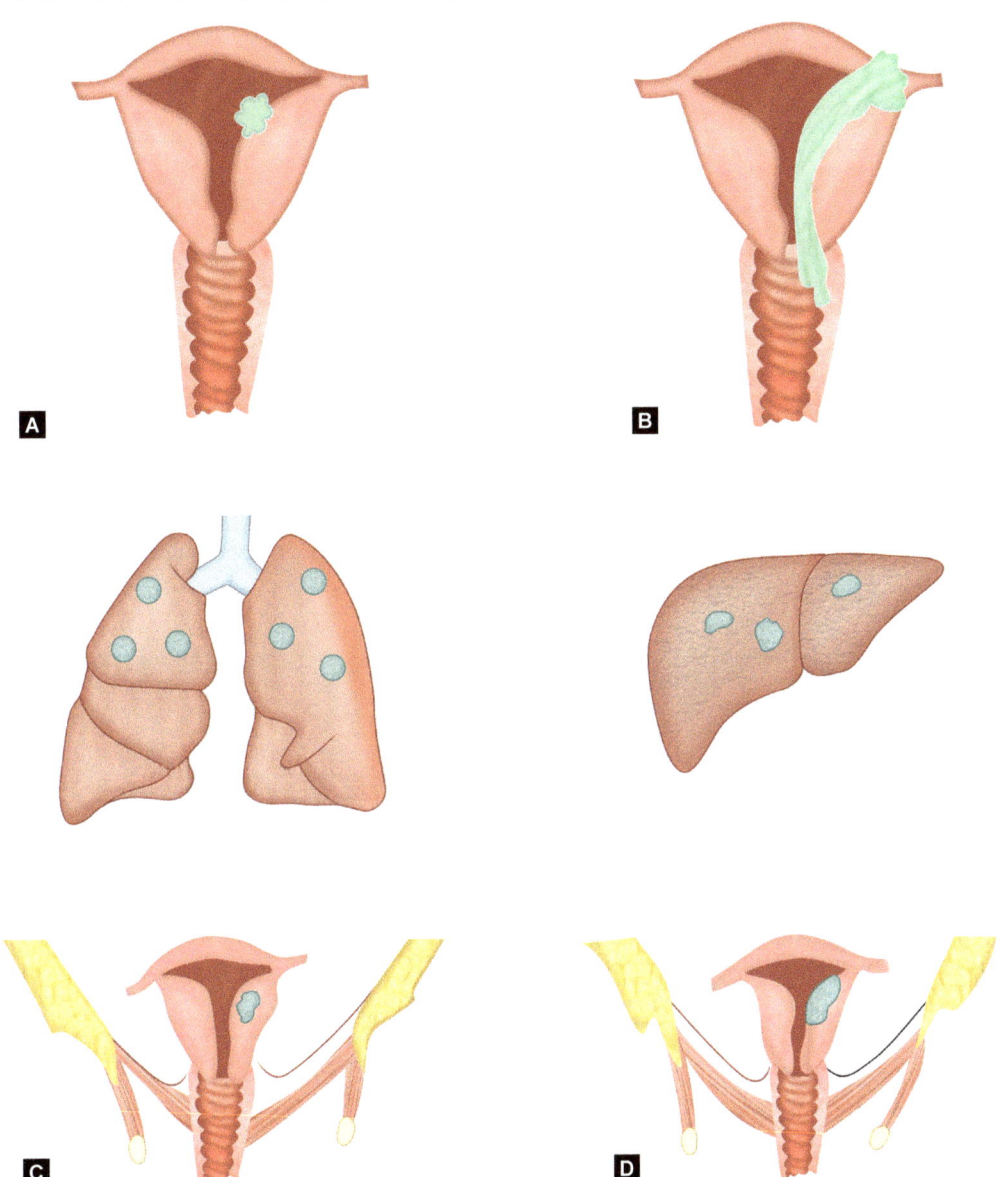

Figs. 4A to D: Various stages of gestational trophoblastic neoplasia (GTN). (A) *Stage I:* Disease confined to uterus; (B) *Stage II:* GTN extended beyond the uterus but limited to genital structures; (C) *Stage III:* GTN extends to the lungs with or without extension to other genital organs; (D) *Stage IV:* All other metastatic sites.

- Clinical or radiological evidence of metastasis.

Investigations to determine treatment strategies for a patient with GTN are as per **Table 5**.[4]

TREATMENT OF GESTATIONAL TROPHOBLASTIC NEOPLASIA

The treatment of GTN depends upon the prognostic scoring **(Table 6)** and stratifies the

TABLE 5: Investigations to determine treatment strategies for a patient with gestational trophoblastic neoplasia (GTN).

S. No.	Evaluation	Rationale
1.	Clinical history	
2.	Examination	
3.	Measurement of serum beta-human chorionic gonadotropin (β-hCG)	
4.	Doppler ultrasound	• To the absence of pregnancy • To look for the size of the uterus, volume, and spread of the disease and its vascularity • Vascularity which is measured by Doppler pulsatility index is an independent risk factor for resistance to single dose methotrexate therapy[22]
5.	Chest X-ray (CXR)	Pulmonary metastases are most common
6.	Magnetic resonance imaging (MRI)	MRI brain is done to look or metastases if the CXR is positive

TABLE 6: The International Federation of Gynecology and Obstetrics (FIGO) scoring system.[23]

Score	0	1	2	4
Age in years	<40 years	≥40 years	–	–
Antecedent pregnancy	Male	Abortion	Term	–
Time interval in months between the end of the antecedent pregnancy and start of treatment	<4	4 to less than 7	7 to less than 13	≥13
Human chorionic gonadotropin (hCG) levels prior to the treatment	<10^3	10^3 to less than 10^4	10^4 to less than 10^5	≥10^5
Largest tumor size (including uterus)	<3	3 to less than 5	≥5	–
Metastatic sites	Lung	Kidney and spleen	Gastrointestinal	Liver, brain
Number of metastases	–	1–4	5–8	>8
Previous failed chemotherapy	–	–	Single drug	2 or more drug

Note: A score of 6 or lower is considered as low risk and a score of 7 or higher is considered as high risk.

patient into a low risk category and a high risk category. The management of GTN primarily depends upon the clinical presentation rather than the histology.

About 95% of the patients diagnosed with GTN after hydatidiform mole have low risk neoplasia.[4] The role of D&C in the treatment of GTN is only valuable when the hCG levels is below 5,000 IU/L with disease confined to the endometrium and no invasion to the myometrium. However, the role of second D&C in decreasing the need for chemotherapy

Chapter 4: Gestational Trophoblastic Diseases

> **BOX 1:** Chemotherapy for low-risk gestational trophoblastic neoplasia (GTN).
>
> *Chemotherapy regimen for low-risk diseases:*
> - *Methotrexate (MTX)*:* 50 mg by intramuscular infection repeated every 48 hours for a total of four doses
> - *Folinic acid*:* 15 mg orally 30 hours after each injection of MTX
>
> *Alternative regimens with methotrexate:*
> - *Methotrexate:* 30–50 mg/m² intramuscular (IM) weekly
> - *Methotrexate:* 0.3–0.5 mg/kg intravenous (IV) or IM daily for 5 days every 2 weeks (maximum 25 mg per dose)
>
> *Methotrexate*
> - MTX 100 mg/m² IV over 30 minutes followed by MTX 200 mg/m² IV infusion over 12 hours
>
> *Folinic acid*
> - 15 mg every 12 hours in six doses IM or orally beginning 24 hours after starting MTX
>
> *Alternative regimens with actinomycin-D:*
> - Actinomycin-D 10–12 mg/kg IV push daily for 5 days
> - Actinomycin-D 1.25 mg/m² IV push every 2 weeks
>
> **Courses every 2 weeks*

remains controversial. Meanwhile there are some people who have completed their families and request hysterectomy.

Single agent chemotherapy regimen with methotrexate (MTX) or actinomycin-D (ActD) is traditionally considered as the primary chemotherapy for low risk GTN **(Box 1)**. The MTX/folinic acid regimen developed at Charring Cross Hospital is effective, well tolerated and well accepted. However, it was common to have treatment resistance or side effects. In 2016, an updated Cochrane review[24] was conducted wherein the authors concluded that ActD was more likely to cure disease in the first instance as compared to MTX and was less likely to fail. Also the side effects for both the treatment regimens were similar which were commonly nausea fatigue and anemia. In another Cochrane study published in the same year[25] it was deduced that for cases resistant to MTX or recurrent low risk GTN, a 5-day dactinomycin followed by methotrexate, actinomycin-D, and cyclophosphamide (MAC) or etoposide, methotrexate, actinomycin-D, cyclophosphamide, vincristine (EMA/CO) if required may be given. It was also suggested that dactinomycin for 5 days had more side effects than pulsed dactinomycin. However, RCTs regarding this were still lacking.

Step-by-Step Outline for the Management of Low-risk Gestational Trophoblastic Neoplasia[26,27]

Flowchart 2 presents outline for the management of low-risk GTN.

Management of High-risk Gestational Trophoblastic Neoplasia

High-risk cases of GTN are usually uncommon. A score equal to or above 7 is considered high risk for GTN.[4] These patients are typically at a high risk of developing drug resistance and typically single agent chemotherapy does not work for them. Hence, several different therapies have been developed for them **(Table 7)**.[28]

The EMA/CO regimen was first developed at the Charring Cross Hospital and has been widely accepted.[4] It has a predictable and short-term toxicity profile which is relatively easier to deal with. In a Cochrane study published in 2013, the authors concluded that CHAMOCA regimen was extremely toxic and not better as compared to the MAC regimen. The study could not establish that EMA/CO was the best and the least toxic regimen as compared to others though it suggested that it remains the most widely used regimen in the world for high-risk GTN **(Box 2)**.[29]

Section 2: Reproductive Age Group

Flowchart 2: Outline for the management of low risk GTN.

Initiate single agent chemotherapy with either methotrexate or actinomycin-D. Consider hysterectomy if fertility is not required

↓

Monitor hematologic, renal and hepatic parameters before each cycle of chemotherapy. Also monitor β-hCG during the treatment. In case severe toxicity or resistance develops, consider switching to alternative regimen

↓

If resistance also develops for alternative regimen:
- Repeat metastatic evaluation
- Consider hysterectomy is disease is confined to uterus
- Multiagent therapy like EMA/CO

(β-hCG: beta-human chorionic gonadotropin; EMA/CO: etoposide, methotrexate, actinomycin-D, cyclophosphamide, vincristine; GTN: gestational trophoblastic neoplasia)

TABLE 7: Various regimens for treatment of high-risk gestational trophoblastic neoplasia (GTN).

S. No.	Therapy	Short form
1.	Methotrexate (MTX), folinic acid, and actinomycin-D	MFA
2.	MTX, actinomycin-D, cyclophosphamide, doxorubicin, melphalan, hydroxyurea, and vincristine	CHAMOCA
3.	MTX, actinomycin-D, cyclophosphamide	MAC
4.	Etoposide, MTX, actinomycin-D, cyclophosphamide, vincristine	EMA/CO

BOX 2: The EMA/CO regimens.

Regimen 1
Day 1:
- Etoposide 100 mg/m² intravenous infusion over 30 minutes
- Actinomycin-D 0.5 mg intravenous bolus
- Methotrexate 100 mg/m² intravenous bolus 200 mg/m² intravenous infusion over 12 hours

Day 2:
- Etoposide 100 mg/m² intravenous infusion over 30 minutes
- Actinomycin-D 0.5 mg intravenous bolus
- Folinic acid rescue 15 mg intramuscularly or orally every 12 hours for four doses (starting 24 hours after beginning the methotrexate infusion)

Regimen 2
Day 8:
- Vincristine 1 mg/m² intravenous bolus (maximum 2 mg)
- Cyclophosphamide 600 mg/m² intravenous infusion over 30 minutes
- The two regimens are given alternate weekly.

(EMA/CO: etoposide, methotrexate, actinomycin-D, cyclophosphamide, vincristine)

With the EMA/CO regimen the complete reversal rate was near to 85%. The 5 years survival rates in these cases were 75–80%. However, in those who had distant metastases like in the brain or the liver, prognosis appeared to be somewhat poorer.[29-31]

SUMMARY

- Pre-evacuation diagnosis of molar pregnancy may be made by trends of β-hCG and sonography. However, a definitive diagnosis may be reached only after histological examination.
- Suction curettage is the method of choice of evacuation for complete as well as partial molar pregnancies except when the size of the fetal parts deters the use

of suction curettage and then medical evacuation can be used.
- Follow-up after gestational trophoblastic disease (GTD) is of prime importance.
- If hCG has reverted to normal within 56 days of the pregnancy event then follow up will be for 6 months from the date of uterine evacuation.
- If hCG has not reverted to normal within 56 days of the pregnancy event then follow-up will be for 6 months from normalization of the hCG level.
- In those patients with gestational trophoblastic neoplasia, the risk stratification according to FIGO scoring should be done and treatment regimen should be chosen accordingly.

CONCLUSION

Gestational trophoblastic diseases are a rare group of diseases wherein majority of them are completely treatable. The key to the treatment here is strict follow-up with beta hCG and early diagnosis of neoplasia. If diagnosed to have neoplasia, risk stratification should be done corresponding treatment should be given.

REFERENCES

1. Bruce S, Sorosky J. Gestational trophoblastic disease. [Updated 2019 Jul 30]. In: StatPearls [Internet]. Treasure Island (FL): StatPearls Publishing; 2019 Jan-. Available from: https://www.ncbi.nlm.nih.gov/books/NBK470267/
2. Bouchard-Fortier G, Covens A. Gestational trophoblastic disease hydatidiform mole, nonmetastatic and metastatic gestational trophoblastic tumor: Diagnosis and management. Comprehensive Gynecology, 7th edition. Amsterdam, Netherlands: Elsevier; 2016. pp. 787-99.
3. Sebire NJ, Foskett M, Fisher RA, et al. Risk of partial and complete hydatidiform molar pregnancy in relation to maternal age. BJOG. 2002;109:99-102.
4. Seckl MJ, Sebire NJ, Fisher RA, et al. Gestational trophoblastic disease: ESMO Clinical Practice Guidelines for diagnosis, treatment and follow-up. Ann Oncol. 2013;24(Suppl 6):vi39-50.
5. Parrazini F, Mangili G, La Vecchia C, et al. Risk factors for gestational trophoblastic disease: a separate analysis of complete and partial hydatidiform moles. Obstet Gynecol. 1991;78:1039-45.
6. Berkowitz RS, Cramer DW, Bernstein MR, et al. Risk factors for complete molar pregnancy from a case-control study. Am J Obstet Gynecol. 1985;152(8):1016-20.
7. Parazzini F, Cipriani S, Mangili G, et al. Oral Contraceptive Pills and risk of gestational trophoblastic disease. Contraception. 2002;65:425-7.
8. Hoffman BL, Schorge JO, Schaffer JL, et al. William's Gynecology, Second edition. The McGraw Hill Companies Inc; 2012.
9. Seckl MJ, Sebire NJ, Berkowitz RS. Gestational trophoblastic disease. Lancet. 2010;376:717-29.
10. Sebire NJ, Seckl MJ. Immunohistochemical staining for diagnosis and prognostic assessment of hydatidiform moles: current evidence and future directions. J Reprod Med. 2010;55:236-46.
11. Wagner BJ, Woodward PJ, Dickey GE. From the archives of the AFIP. Gestational trophoblastic disease: radiologic-pathologic correlation. Radiographics. 1996;16(1):131-48.
12. Allen SD, Lim AK, Seckl MJ, et al. Radiology of gestational trophoblastic neoplasia. Clin Radiol. 2006;61(4):301-13.
13. Dhanda S, Ramani S, Thakur M. Gestational trophoblastic disease: A multimodality imaging approach with impact on diagnosis and management. Radiol Res Pract. 2014;2014:842751.
14. RCOG. (2010). Gestational Trophoblastic Disease (Green-top guideline No. 38). [online] Available from https://www.rcog.org.uk/en/guidelines-research-services/guidelines/gtg38/ [Last accessed September, 2019].
15. Fowler DJ, Lindsay I, Seckl MJ, et al. Routine pre-evacuation ultrasound diagnosis of hydatidiform mole: experience of more than

16. Berek JS. Berek and Novak's Gynecology. Fifteenth edition. Philadelphia. Wolters Kluwer India Private Limited; 2012.
17. Gerulath AH, Ehlen TG, Bessette P, et al. Gestational Trophoblastic Disease. J Obstet Gynaecol Can. 2002;24:434-9.
18. Wang Q, Fu J, Hu L, et al. Prophylactic chemotherapy for hydatidiform mole to prevent gestational trophoblastic neoplasia. Cochrane Database Syst Rev. 2017;9:CD007289.
19. Jelly P, Rakesh S. Gestational trophoblastic disease (GTD). Int J Med Paediatr Oncol. 2016;2(2):70-3.
20. Ngan HY, Seckl MJ, Berkowitz RS, et al. Update on the diagnosis and management of gestational trophoblastic disease. Int J Gynecol Obstet. 2015;131 (Suppl 2):S123-6.
21. Kani KK, Lee JH, Dighe M, et al. Gestational trophoblastic disease: multimodality imaging assessment with special emphasis on spectrum of abnormalities and value of imaging in staging and management of disease. Curr Probl Diagn Radiol. 2012;41(1):1-10.
22. Agarwal R, Harding V, Short D, et al. Uterine artery pulsatility index: a predictor of methotrexate resistance in gestational trophoblastic neoplasia. Br J Cancer. 2012;106:1089-94.
23. FIGO Oncology Committee. FIGO staging for gestational trophoblastic neoplasia 2000. Int J Gynecol Obstet. 2002;77:285-7.
24. Lawrie TA, Alazzam M, Tidy J, et al. First-line chemotherapy in low-risk gestational trophoblastic neoplasia. Cochrane Database Syst Rev. 2016;(6):CD007102.
25. Alazzam M, Tidy J, Osborne R, et al. Chemotherapy for resistant or recurrent gestational trophoblastic neoplasia. Cochrane Database Syst Rev. 2016;(1):CD008891.
26. Soper JT, Spillman M, Sampson JH, et al. High-risk gestational trophoblastic neoplasia with brain metastases: individualized multidisciplinary therapy in the management of four patients. Gynecol Oncol. 2007;104(3):691-4.
27. Deng L, Yan X, Zhang J, et al. Combination chemotherapy for high-risk gestational trophoblastic tumour. Cochrane Database Syst Rev. 2009;(2):CD005196.
28. Deng L, Zhang J, Wu T, et al. Combination chemotherapy for primary treatment of high-risk gestational trophoblastic tumour. Cochrane Database Syst Rev. 2013;(1):CD005196.
29. Ahamed E, Short D, North B, et al. Survival of women with gestational trophoblastic neoplasia and liver metastases: is it improving? J Reprod Med. 2012;57(5-6):262-9.
30. Neubauer NL, Latif N, Kalakota K, et al. Brain metastasis in gestational trophoblastic neoplasia: an update. J Reprod Med. 2012;57(7-8):288-92.
31. Newlands ES, Holden L, Seckl MJ, et al. Management of brain metastases in patients with high-risk gestational trophoblastic tumors. J Reprod Med. 2002;47(6):465-71.

CHAPTER 5

Ectopic Pregnancy

Harpreet Kaur

INTRODUCTION

Ectopic pregnancy is an obstetric emergency. Ectopic pregnancy means any pregnancy implanted outside the uterine cavity. It can have varied presentation and can prove fatal if undiagnosed and not managed in time. The possibility of an ectopic pregnancy should be kept as differential diagnosis in women presenting with unusual pain abdomen or syncope as many times history of amenorrhea may be missing. Though the presence of some of the risk factors increase the possibility of an ectopic pregnancy, but most of the times none of these may be present.

The factors which increase the risk for an ectopic pregnancy include:
- Previous history of tubal surgery or infection leading to tubal damage
- Failure of contraception
- Chronic pelvic inflammatory disease (PID)
- Progesterone only contraceptives
- In vitro fertilization (IVF)
- Smoking.

SITE OF AN ECTOPIC PREGNANCY

Tubal ectopic is the most common presentation. Rarely 3–5%, it can happen at other sites. Most common sites for ectopic is fallopian tube (mostly ampullary followed by isthmic, fimbrial, and cornual). Other sites where ectopic pregnancy has been reported include abdominal, ovarian or cervical.

CLINICAL PRESENTATION

Common presentation can be amenorrhea, irregular vaginal bleeding, and pain abdomen. But many times the classical presentation may not be there. There should be high clinical suspicion in women of reproductive age group even with nonspecific presentation should be offered pregnancy test. Sometimes the symptoms and signs of ectopic pregnancy can mimic other common pathologies like gastrointestinal tract (GIT) or urinary problems. Despite significant advances in diagnosis and treatment, ectopic pregnancy remains the leading cause of maternal death in the first trimester [Centers for Disease Control and Prevention (CDC) report on maternal mortality].[1]

DIAGNOSIS

Transvaginal sonography (TVS) is the preferred method for diagnosing ectopic pregnancy. It has sensitivity of 87–99% and specificity of 94–99.9% for the diagnosis of tubal ectopic pregnancy.[2]

In many cases, TVS alone can establish a definitive diagnosis in women with suspected ectopic pregnancies by clearly revealing an extrauterine gestational sac.

- While an extrauterine gestational sac containing a yolk sac and/or embryonic pole that may or may not have cardiac activity will be present in around 15–20% of cases.
- There is no specific endometrial appearance or thickness to support a diagnosis of tubal ectopic pregnancy.
- In up to 20% of cases, a collection of fluid may be seen within the uterine cavity, classically referred to as a "pseudosac".[3-6]
- The key is to distinguish this from an early intrauterine gestational sac. The intradecidual and double decidual signs can help to make a diagnosis of early intrauterine pregnancy. The intradecidual sign is described as a fluid collection with an echogenic rim located "within a markedly thickened decidua on one side of the uterine cavity".[7] The double decidual sign is presence of intrauterine fluid collection surrounded by two concentric echogenic rings.[8]
- Free fluid is often seen on ultrasound, but is not diagnostic of ectopic pregnancy. A small amount of anechoic fluid in the pouch of Douglas may be found in both intrauterine and ectopic pregnancies. Echogenic fluid has been reported in 28–56% of ectopic pregnancies.[9,10] It may indicate tubal rupture but most commonly is due to tubal abortion.

Serum Beta-Human Chorionic Gonadotropin Concentrations

In contrast to normal pregnancy, beta-human chorionic gonadotropin (β-hCG) levels are abnormally low for gestational age or rise at a slower than normal rate in most women with failing intrauterine and ectopic pregnancies.

In clinically stable women with a nondiagnostic ultrasound scan [pregnancy of unknown location (PUL)], hCG measurements taken 48 hours apart indicated that if rise was less than 66%, an ectopic pregnancy was more likely.

- Unfortunately, β-hCG levels also may rise normally, at least initially.
- Paired serum β-hCG determinations alone cannot reliably distinguish ectopic pregnancies from abnormal or even normal intrauterine pregnancies.[10]

In this strategy of using serial hCG, 13% of ectopic pregnancies would not have been diagnosed and 15% of normal intrauterine pregnancies will be falsely labeled as ectopic.

Serum Progesterone

Serum progesterone is not useful is predicting an ectopic pregnancy. Serum progesterone levels less than 5 ng/mL may indicate a nonviable pregnancy (intra- or extrauterine).[11,12]

Laparoscopy

No longer considered gold standard for diagnosis as diagnosis can be made with certainty in almost all the cases by TVS combined with sensitive serum β-hCG levels.

Chapter 5: Ectopic Pregnancy

But laparoscopy remains important treatment modality for ectopic pregnancy.

Majority of ectopic can be diagnosed on initial TVS, remaining few are classified as PUL. In case of PUL, follow-up with β-hCG after 48 hours and checking the increase in β-hCG levels helps to decide further fate of pregnancy **(Flowchart 1)**. Possibilities can be

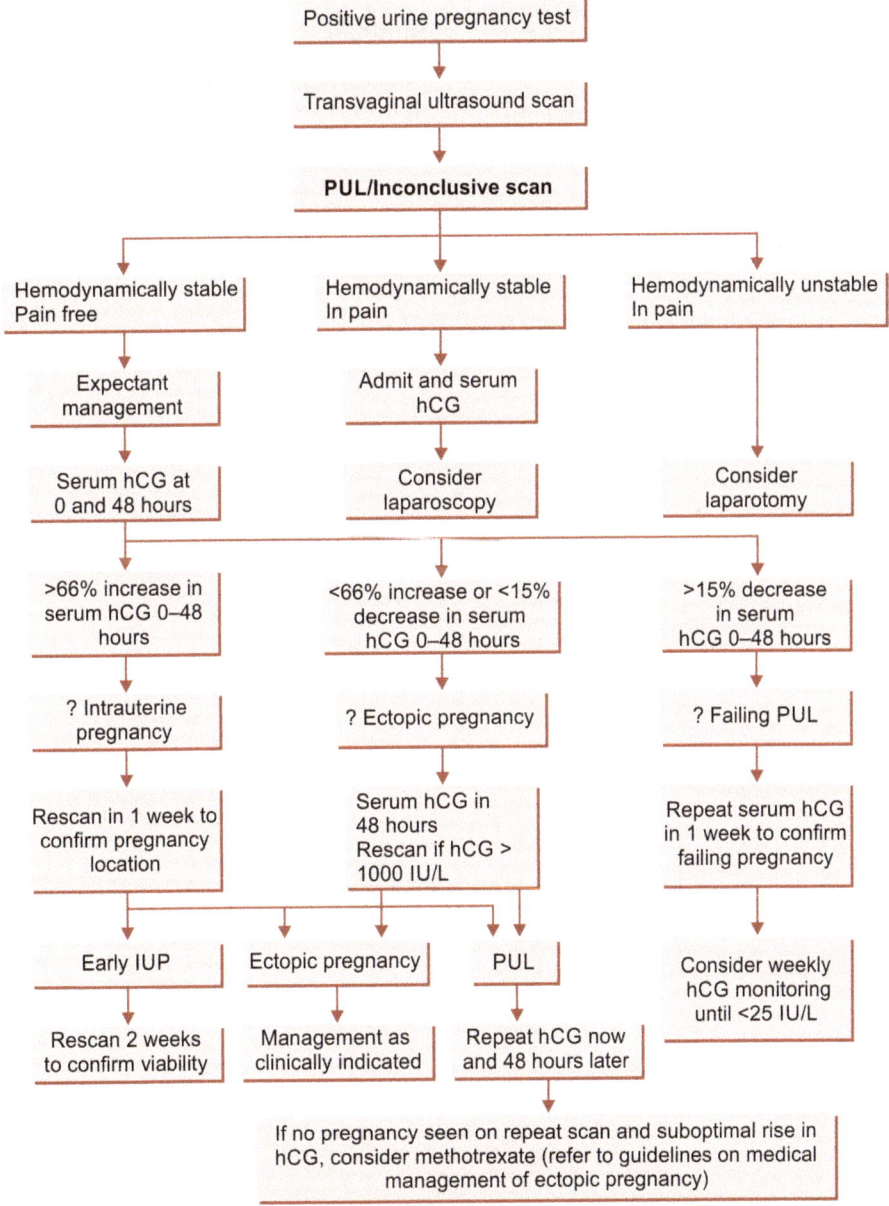

Flowchart 1: Guidelines on management of pregnancy of unknown location (PUL).

(hCG: human chorionic gonadotropin; IUP: intrauterine pregnancy) early intrauterine pregnancy, miscarriage or an ectopic pregnancy. Follow-up with serial serum β-hCG is recommended and once serum β-hCG crosses discriminatory zone, TVS is advisable.[13]

MANAGEMENT (FLOWCHART 2)

Expectant

Expectant management is an option for clinically stable women with an ultrasound diagnosis of ectopic pregnancy and a decreasing β-hCG level initially less than 1,500 IU/L. Proper selection and counseling of women is important and they must be willing to come for follow-up. Success rate of expected management vary from 57% to 100% and depend upon case selection.[14]

Medical

Methotrexate has been widely used as a medical treatment of ectopic pregnancy. Dose prescribed is 50 mg/m^2 single dose **(Table 1)**.[15]

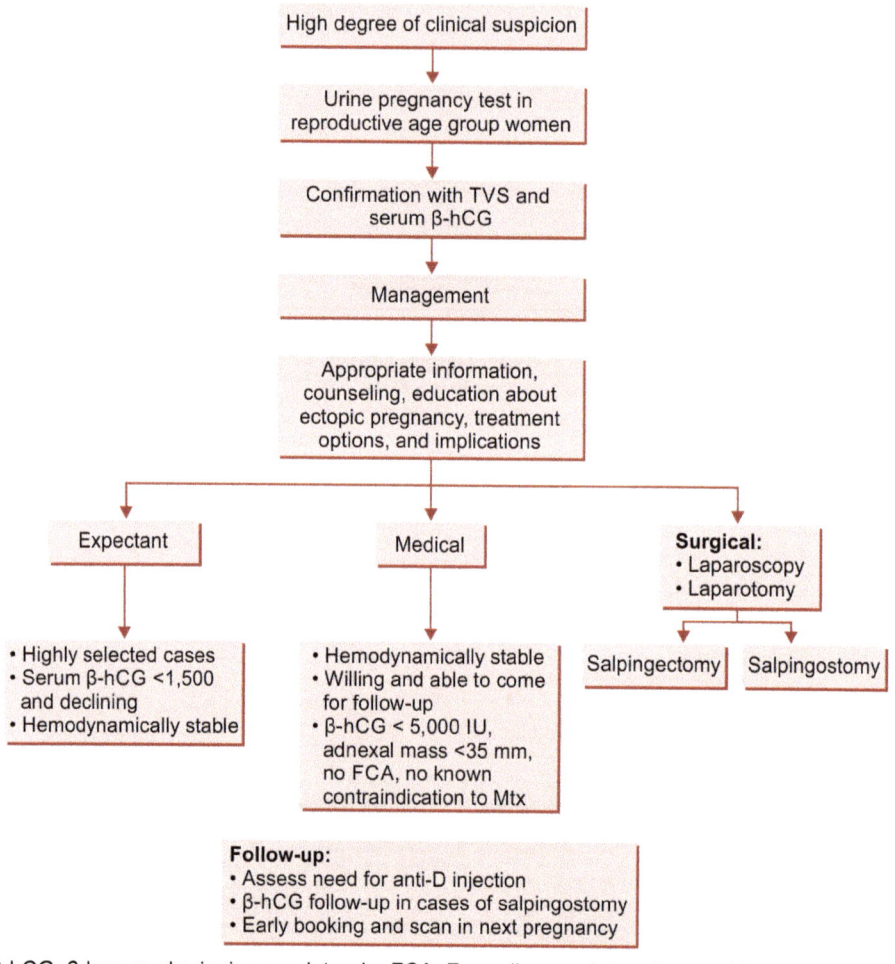

Flowchart 2: Management of an ectopic pregnancy.

(β-hCG: β-human chorionic gonadotropin; FCA: Freund's complete adjuvant; Mtx: methotrexate; TVS: transvaginal sonography)

TABLE 1: Single-dose protocol for intramuscular methotrexate.

Day	Therapy
1	Serum β-hCG, U&E, LFTs, FBC, blood group, 50 mg/m² intramuscular methotrexate
4	Serum β-hCG
7	Serum β-hCG • If β-hCG decrease less than 15% days 4–7, for repeat TVS and methotrexate 50 mg/m² if still fulfils criteria for medical management • If β-hCG decrease greater than 15% days 4–7, for repeat β-hCG weekly until levels less than 15 IU/L

(β-hCG: beta-human chorionic gonadotropin; FBC: full blood count; LFTs: liver function tests; TVS: transvaginal sonography; U&E: urea and electrolyte)

A good candidate for methotrexate has the following characteristics:
- Hemodynamic stability
- Low serum β-hCG (between 1,500 IU and 5,000 IU)
- No fetal cardiac activity
- Confirmation that there is no intrauterine pregnancy
- Willingness to attend for follow-up
- No known allergy to methotrexate.

Detailed counseling and consent and documentation are very important. Women need to understand importance of follow-up and provided with 24-hour contact in case of emergency and given full information.[16] 15% of patients may require a repeat injection and 7% of them may need surgery.

Contraindications to methotrexate:
- Hemodynamically unstable
- Intrauterine pregnancy seen on TVS
- Breastfeeding
- Unable to comply with follow-up
- Known allergy to methotrexate
- Chronic liver disease
- Pre-existing blood dyscrasias
- Active pulmonary disease
- Immunodeficiency
- Peptic ulcer disease.

Surgical

The majority of tubal ectopic pregnancies are managed surgically. Laparoscopy has many advantages over laparotomy such as shorter operation time, less blood loss, shorter hospital stay, lower requirements for pain killers, and less adhesion postoperatively. Evidence, however, suggests that there is no difference in terms of health benefits between laparoscopy and laparotomy, including the key outcome of subsequent successful pregnancy.[17]

In the presence of a healthy contralateral tube, salpingectomy should be performed in preference to salpingotomy. In women with a history compromised fertility (previous ectopic pregnancy, other side tubal damage, prior abdominal surgery, and PID), salpingotomy should be considered.[18,19]

In case of salpingotomy, women should be informed about the risk of persistent trophoblast and serial serum β-hCG level should be checked. Counseling should also include need for further treatment in the form of systemic methotrexate or salpingectomy.[20]

FOLLOW-UP

Follow-up early in future pregnancy is very important as one ectopic pregnancy increases the risk of future ectopic pregnancy. Overall chances of having another ectopic pregnancy is 7–10% compared to 1% in general population. Early scan in next pregnancy is recommended.

CONCLUSION

Ectopic pregnancy is an obstetric emergency and has to keep in mind as differential in any women of reproductive age group presenting with abdominal pain. Presence of amenorrhea or abnormal bleeding and syncope added further to diagnosis. Early diagnosis is key to timely management and avoid catastrophic rupture and bleeding.

REFERENCES

1. Centers for Disease Control and Prevention (CDC). Ectopic pregnancy—United States, 1990-1992. MMWR Morb Mortal Wkly Rep. 1995;44:46-8.
2. Kirk E, Papageorghiou AT, Condous G, et al. The diagnostic effectiveness of an initial transvaginal scan in detecting ectopic pregnancy. Hum Reprod. 2007;22:2824-8.
3. Condous G, Okaro E, Khalid A, et al. The accuracy of transvaginal ultrasonography for the diagnosis of ectopic pregnancy prior to surgery. Hum Reprod. 2005;20:1404-9.
4. Marks WM, Filly RA, Callen PW, et al. The decidual cast of ectopic pregnancy: a confusing ultrasonographic appearance. Radiology. 1979;133:451-4.
5. Frates MC, Laing FC. Sonographic evaluation of ectopic pregnancy: an update. Am J Roentgenol. 1995;165:251-9.
6. Benson CB, Doubilet PM, Peters HE, et al. Intrauterine fluid with ectopic pregnancy: a reappraisal. J Ultrasound Med. 2013;32:389-93.
7. Yeh HC, Goodman JD, Carr L, et al. Intradecidual sign: a US criterion of early intrauterine pregnancy. Radiology. 1986;161:463-7.
8. Bradley WG, Fiske CE, Filly RA. The double sac sign of early intrauterine pregnancy: use in exclusion of ectopic pregnancy. Radiology. 1982;143:223-6.
9. Fleischer AC, Pennell RG, McKee MS, et al. Ectopic pregnancy: features at transvaginal sonography. Radiology. 1990;174:375-8.
10. Nyberg DA, Hughes MP, Mack LA, et al. Extrauterine findings of ectopic pregnancy of transvaginal US: importance of echogenic fluid. Radiology. 1991;178:823-6.
11. Darai E, Benifla JL, Naouri M, et al. Transvaginal intratubal methotrexate treatment of ectopic pregnancy: Report of 100 cases. Hum Reprod. 1996;11:420-4.
12. Diagnosis and management of ectopic pregnancy: Green-top Guideline No. 21. BJOG. 2016;123(13):e15-e55.
13. Banerjee S, Aslam N, Zosmer N, et al. The expectant management of women with early pregnancy of unknown location. Ultrasound Obstet Gynecol. 1999;14:231-6.
14. Craig LB, Khan S. Expectant management of ectopic pregnancy. Clin Obstet Gynecol. 2012;55:461-70.
15. Ipscomb GH. Medical management of ectopic pregnancy. Clin Obstet Gynecol. 2012;55:424-32.
16. Stovall TG, Ling FW, Gray LA. Single-dose methotrexate for treatment of ectopic pregnancy. Obstet Gynecol. 1991;77:754-7.
17. Vermesh M, Silva PD, Rosen GF, et al. Management of unruptured ectopic gestation by linear salpingostomy: a prospective, randomized clinical trial of laparoscopy versus laparotomy. Obstet Gynecol. 1989;73:400-4.
18. Mol F, van Mello NM, Strandell A, et al. Salpingotomy versus salpingectomy in women with tubal pregnancy (ESEP study): an open-label, multicentre, randomised controlled trial. Lancet. 2014;383:1483-9.
19. Becker S, Solomayer E, Hornung R, et al. Optimal treatment for patients with ectopic pregnancies and a history of fertility-reducing factors. Arch Gynecol Obstet. 2011;283:41-5.
20. Lund CO, Nilas L, Bangsgaard N, et al. Persistent ectopic pregnancy after linear salpingotomy: a non-predictable complication to conservative surgery for tubal gestation. Acta Obstet Gynecol Scand. 2002;81:1053-9.

CHAPTER 6

Leiomyoma Uterus Presenting as Emergency

Arya Rajendran

■ INTRODUCTION

Fibroids are the most common pelvic tumors among women, worldwide.[1] They arise as a monoclonal expansion of smooth muscle cells, derived from myometrium.[2] Although, often asymptomatic and benign in nature, fibroids can cause a variety of symptoms such as dysmenorrhea, dyspareunia, menorrhagia, pressure effects on bowel and bladder, infertility, and obstetric complications. Nevertheless, they present occasionally as a case of acute abdomen with or without hemodynamic shock as well.

■ RED/CARNEOUS DEGENERATION/ NECROBIOSIS OF FIBROID

Pregnancy with coexisting fibroid uterus is on the rise due to advancement in maternal age in recent times. The incidence is estimated between 12% and 25%.[3] Most fibroids remain asymptomatic during pregnancy as well. However, fibroid can give rise to acute pain abdomen in pregnancy during red degeneration, torsion or impaction.

Occurrence of pain during pregnancy due to fibroid is seen with fibroids >5 cm in size and during the last two trimesters.[4]

Mechanism of Pain in Red Degeneration of Fibroid

Red/carneous degeneration of fibroid is a kind of hemorrhagic degeneration that happens during pregnancy. It results from venous thrombosis on the periphery of the fibroid or rupture in intramural arteries.[5]

Several theories exist to explain the pain during red degeneration of fibroid.
- Rapid growth of fibroid in pregnancy leads to mismatch between supply and demand of blood supply, causing tissue necrosis/infarction.

- Increase in size of uterus can lead to kinking of blood vessels, reducing the blood supply to the fibroid. This can lead to infarction/necrosis of fibroid, even when the fibroid has not grown during pregnancy.
- Cellular damage that results from either of above mechanisms leads to release of prostaglandins resulting in pain abdomen.[4,6]

Management

Red degeneration is diagnosed by the symptoms of pain abdomen and fever, after excluding other causes of pain abdomen during pregnancy such as preterm labor, abruptio placentae, etc. as well as other causes of acute abdomen like appendicitis.

Ultrasonography (USG) might show cystic degeneration of a pre-existing fibroid. T1-weighted magnetic resonance imaging (MRI) images can show peripheral or diffuse high-intensity signals due to protein content of collected blood.[7] Complete blood count (CBC) can show mild leukocytosis.

The condition is managed conservatively, with bed rest, analgesics [nonsteroidal anti-inflammatory drugs (NSAIDs), opioid narcotics, and epidural analgesia], and hydration. If not relieved by above measures, infrequently, surgical intervention like exploratory laparotomy will be needed.

Bhave et al. reported a case of red degeneration of fibroid arising from right lateral wall of uterus with superimposed infection that presented as a retroperitoneal abscess in a postpartum lady and necessitated an emergent exploratory laparotomy **(Figs. 1A and B)**.[8]

Singhal et al. reported the case of fibroid in pregnancy that presented as acute abdomen with hemoperitoneum. Exploratory laparotomy revealed a large fibroid with vascular degenerative changes and ruptured

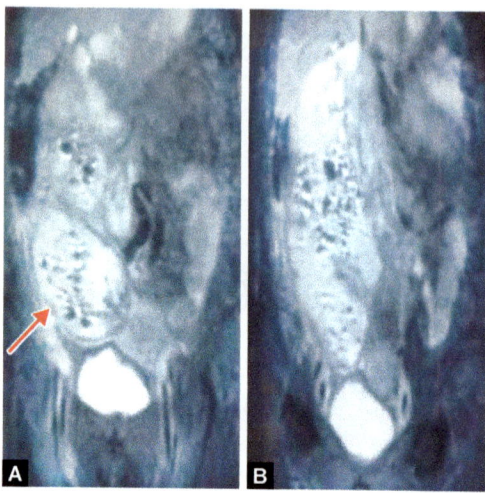

Figs. 1A and B: Red degeneration of fibroid with retroperitoneal abscess. MRI plates showing (A) Mass adherent to right side of uterus (marked by red arrow); (B) Collection in right posterior pararenal space.
Source: Bhave N, PK Shah, Chaudhari H. An unusual presentation of degenerating fibroid. Int J Reprod Contracept Obstet Gynecol. 2016;5(2):582-4.

peripheral vessels, building up a quick hemoperitoneum.

Histopathology of specimen revealed hemorrhagic degeneration of leiomyoma.[9]

■ TORSION OF FIBROID

Torsion of fibroid commonly occurs with pedunculated subserosal fibroids that get twisted around its pedicle. Rarely, a sessile leiomyoma can lead to torsion of uterus as a whole. Uterine torsion refers to rotation of uterus along the longitudinal axis, by more than 45°. Uterus is normally retained in its axial position by virtue of cardinal and uterosacral ligaments. When there is a heavy mass arising from the uterus or during gravid state, there is an impetus for the uterus to twist around its own axis, usually at the level of isthmus.[10,11] Fibroids are the most common cause of torsion of nongravid uterus and peristaltic movements of sigmoid colon helps in initiating the torsion.[12] Torsion can proceed to congestion and ultimately gangrene.

Clinical Presentation

Clinical features are vague and mostly presentation is as acute abdomen with pain, nausea, vomiting, and leukocytosis. On USG, torsion of myomatous uterus can be identified by change in the relative position of fibroids from a previous baseline scan **(Figs. 2A and B)**. Computed tomography (CT) can reveal a whorled structure at the lower segment of uterus, comprised of the twisted uterus/cervix **(Figs. 3A and B)**. Hemorrhagic infarction can give hyperintense signals.

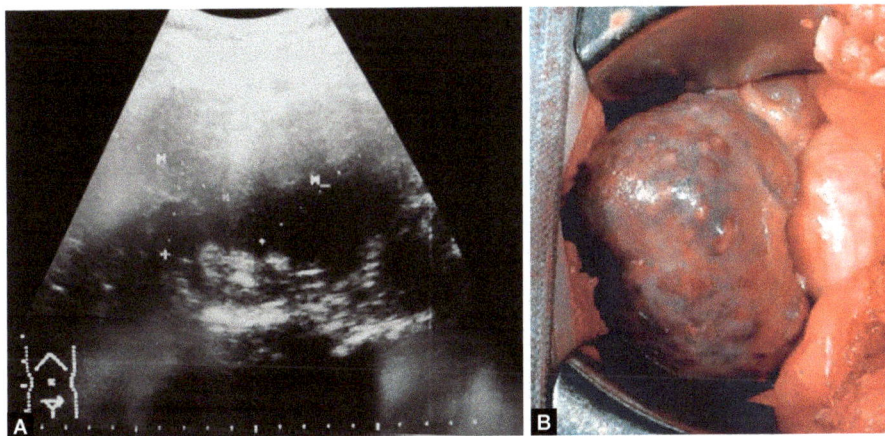

Figs. 2A and B: (A) Ultrasound shows a subserosal leiomyoma measuring 6.6 × 5.2 cm (left "M"); (B) Pedunculated leiomyoma (bluish mass on the left side) that had undergone torsion is seen at laparotomy.
Source: Tsai YJ, Yeat SK, Jeng CJ, et al. Torsion of a uterine leiomyoma. Taiwane J Obstet Gynecol. 2006;45(4):333-5.

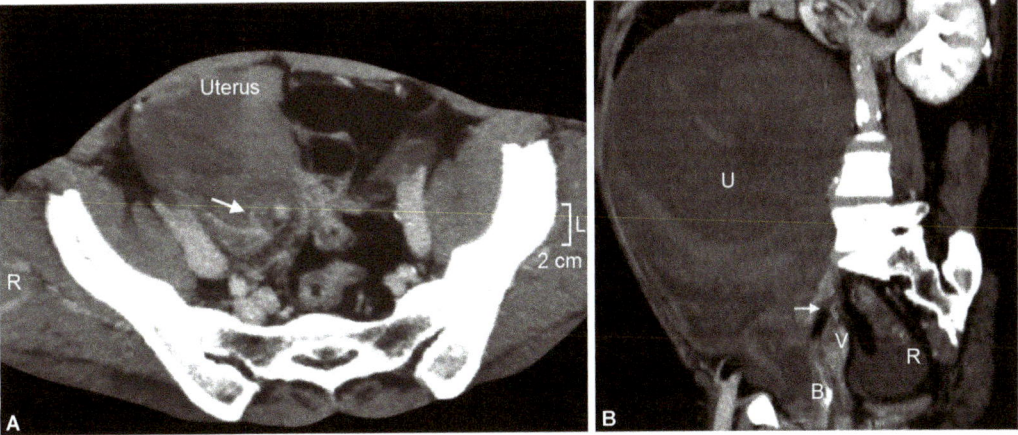

Figs. 3A and B: (A) Axial computed tomographic image after intravenous contrast showing the uterine cervix with a whorled appearance (arrow); (B) Oblique coronal CT image after intravenous contrast showing the uterine cervix with a whorled appearance (arrow). (U: uterus; B: bladder; V: vagina; R: rectum).
Source: Luk SY, Leung JL, Cheng ML, et al. Torsion of a nongravid myomatous uterus: radiological features and literature review. Hong Kong Med J. 2010;16:304-6.

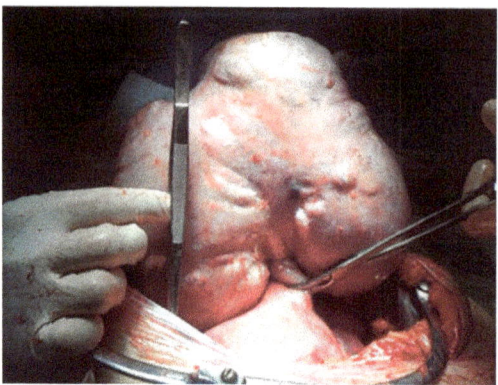

Fig. 4: Myoma of the uterine fundus with evidence of torsion of its pedicle.
Source: Basso A, Catalano MR, Lovero F, et al. Uterine fibroid torsion during pregnancy: A case of laparotomic myomectomy at 18 weeks' gestation with systematic review of the literature. Case Rep Obstet Gynecol. 2017;2017:4970802.

Management

Exploratory laparoscopy/laparotomy can clinch the final diagnosis of torsion of pedunculated fibroid/uterine torsion from sessile fibroid **(Fig. 4)**. Pedunculated fibroids can be removed by cutting and ligating the pedicle, without residual damage on uterus. Uterine torsion can be corrected by myomectomy and detorsion and watching for signs of reperfusion and viability **(Fig. 5)**. Plication of round ligaments, uterosacral ligaments can help in preventing a subsequent retorsion. Profound congestion and gangrenous changes will necessitate hysterectomy.[11]

■ IMPACTED FIBROID

Occasionally, fibroid can get impacted in pelvis, with/without an element of associated torsion. This can also present as acute pain abdomen or with pressure symptoms obstructing the bowel/bladder. A careful physical examination can reveal the presence of an impacted mass in vaginal fornices. Subserosal pedunculated fibroids can be removed by laparoscopy/laparotomy whereas intramural fibroids with severe clinical features will necessitate myomectomy, even during pregnancy, and is associated with morbidity and risk of abortions, blood loss, etc. The risks and benefits of the procedure must be carefully weighed before undertaking the challenge.[13]

■ SUMMARY

- Leiomyoma uterus can present as emergency with acute abdomen in three situations—Red degeneration, torsion, impaction.
- Red degeneration often occurs in pregnancy and is managed conservatively with analgesics, fluids and rest.
- Torsion uterus is a rare occurrence and needs prompt surgical intervention to prevent advancing necrosis.
- Impacted fibroid also requires urgent resuscitation and myomectomy.

■ CONCLUSION

Leiomyoma complicating pregnancy is a common entity in present time obstetric practice, owing both to advancing maternal age as well as slow rise in prevalence of fibroids among women. Such a pregnancy warrants watchful expectancy as most women get through with no severe consequences. However, acute presentations like red degeneration, torsion and impaction are possible and needs to be ruled out in a symptomatic patient, during pregnancy and not.

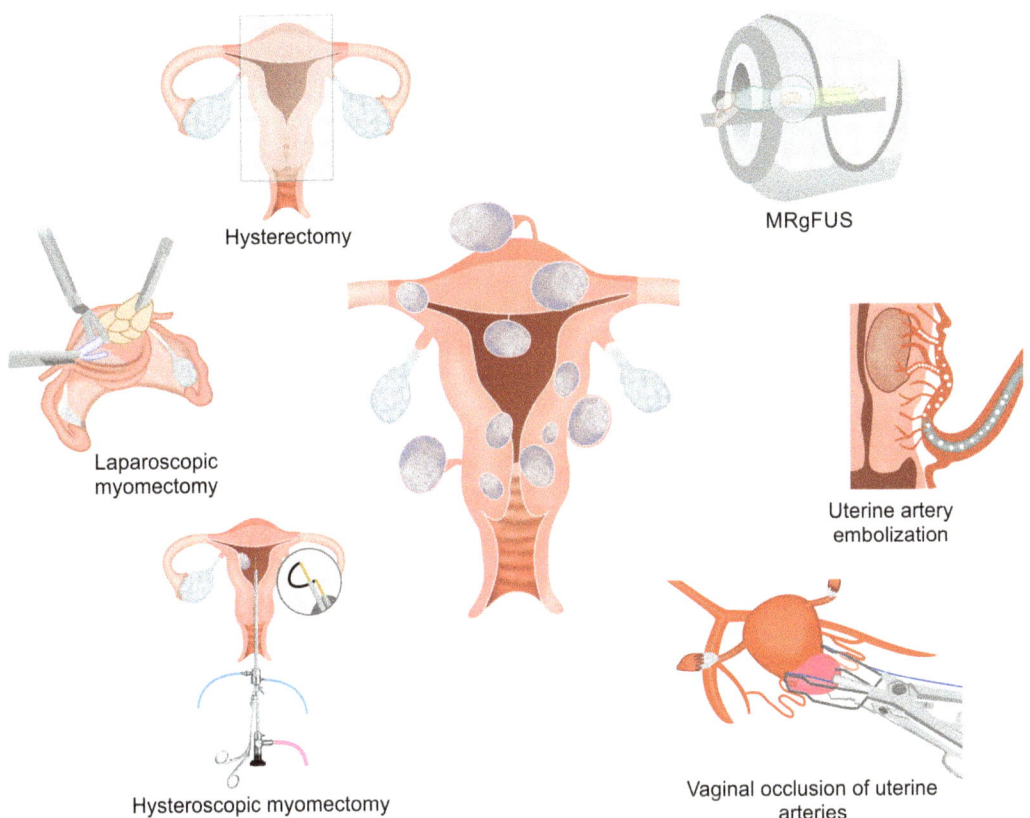

Fig. 5: Current surgical and nonsurgical management strategies of myomas. Left panel: Hysterectomy, laparoscopic myomectomy, and hysteroscopic myomectomy are the most widely used surgical interventions for myomas. Right panel: Alternatives to surgical interventions include uterine artery embolization (UAE), high-frequency magnetic resonance-guided focused ultrasound surgery (MRgFUS), and vaginal occlusion of uterine arteries.
Source: Donnez J, Dolmans MM. Uterine fibroid management: from the present to the future. Hum Reprod Update. 2016;22(6):665-86.

■ REFERENCES

1. Stewart EA. Uterine fibroids. Lancet. 2001;357:293-8.
2. Kim J, Sefton EC. The role of progesterone signaling in the pathogenesis of uterine leiomyoma. Mol Cell Endocrinol. 2012;358: 223-31.
3. Klatsky PC, Tran ND, Caughey AB, et al. Fibroids and reproductive outcomes: a systematic literature review from conception to delivery. Am J Obstet Gynecol. 2008;198:357-66.
4. Katz VL, Dotters DJ, Droegemueller W. Complications of uterine leiomyomas in pregnancy. Obstet Gynecol. 1989;73:593-6.
5. Murase E, Siegelman ES, Outwater EK, et al. Uterine leiomyomas: histopathologic features, MR imaging findings, differential diagnosis, and treatment. Radiographics. 1999;19(5):1179-97.
6. Parker WH. Etiology, symptomatology, and diagnosis of uterine myomas. Fertil Steril. 2007;87:725-36.
7. Kawakami S, Togashi K, Konishi I, et al. Red degeneration of uterine leiomyoma:

MR appearance. J Comput Assist Tomogr. 1994;18(6):925-8.
8. Bhave N, PK Shah, Chaudhari H. An unusual presentation of degenerating fibroid. Int J Reprod Contracept Obstet Gynecol. 2016;5(2):582-4.
9. Singhal B, Kohli S, Singh A, et al. Uterine leiomyoma presenting as acute emergency. IJBAMR. 2014;4(1):380-3.
10. Jeong YY, Kang HK, Park JG, et al. CT features of uterine torsion. Eur Radiol. 2003;13 (Suppl 6):L249-50.
11. Hawes CH. Acute axial torsion of the uterus. Ann Surg. 1935;102:37-40.
12. Nicholson W, Colson CC, McCoy MC, et al. Pelvic magnetic resonance imaging in the evaluation of uterine torsion. Obstet Gynecol. 1995;855:888-90.
13. Dobrowolska-Redo A, Teliga-Czajkowska J, Romejko-Wolniewicz E, et al. Impacted uterine myoma in a 14 week pregnant patient. MEDtube Science. 2015;3(3):8-10.

CHAPTER 7

Dysmenorrhea

Arveen Vohra

INTRODUCTION

Dysmenorrhea is one of the most common causes of pelvic pain. It negatively affects a woman's quality of life and often results in activity restriction.

DEFINITION

"Dysmenorrhea" is derived from a Greek root translating to difficult menstrual flow. Dysmenorrhea, one of the most frequently encountered gynecologic disorders, refers to painful menstruation. It is defined as pain related to menstruation that may occur just before or during menses.

PATHOGENESIS

It is thought to be due to a release of prostaglandins (PGs) and leukotrienes in the menstrual fluid, which in turn produces vasoconstriction in the uterine vessels, causing the uterine contractions which produce the pain. The PG release may also be responsible for gastrointestinal disturbance, which may occur in association with dysmenorrhea.

CLASSIFICATION

There are different types including:
- Primary (spasmodic) dysmenorrhea
- Secondary (congestive) dysmenorrhea
- Membranous dysmenorrhea
- Ovarian dysmenorrhea
  - Ovulatory pain
  - Premenstrual tension syndrome.

Primary Dysmenorrhea (Fig. 1)

Primary dysmenorrhea occurs in young females with no pelvic pathology. Primary dysmenorrhea is a very common gynecologic problem in menstruating women. It is often debilitating and affects between 45% and 95% of menstruating women.[1]

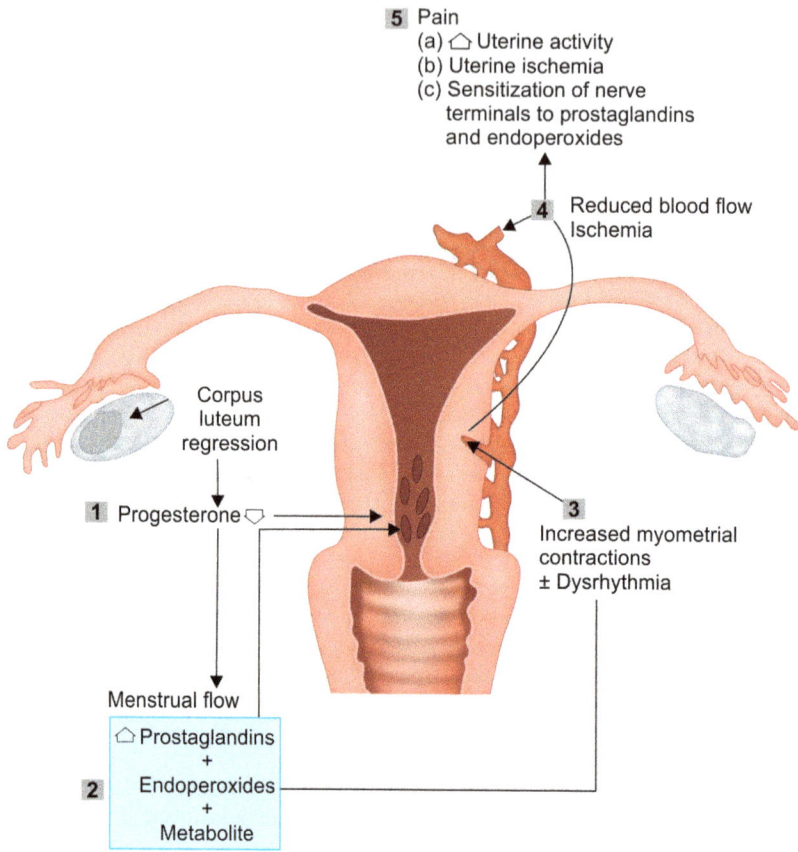

Fig. 1: Mechanism of pain generation from the pelvic structure in primary dysmenorrhea.
Source: Dawood MY. Hormones, prostaglandins, and dysmenorrhea. In: Dawood MY (Ed). Dysmenorrhea. Baltimore: Williams & Wilkins; 1981. p. 21.

Primary dysmenorrhea is defined as painful menstrual cramps without any evident pathology to account for them. It refers to any degree of perceived cramping pain during menstruation.

Primary dysmenorrhea usually begins a few hours before or just after the onset of menstruation. The cramps are most severe on the 1st or 2nd day of menstruation.

Characteristically, the pains are spasmodic in nature and strongest over the lower abdomen, but they may also radiate to the back and the inner aspects of the thigh, and they are often described as labor-like pains.

The cramp is commonly accompanied by one or more systemic symptoms, including nausea and vomiting (89%), fatigue (85%), diarrhea (60%), lower backache (60%), and headache (45%). Nervousness, dizziness, and in some severe cases, syncope and collapse can be associated with primary dysmenorrhea.

- It often begins with the onset of ovulatory cycles 6 months to 2 years after the menarche.
- The pain begins with the onset of the period and may last for 24–72 hours.
- There is some evidence to suggest that it may occur more frequently, or be more

Chapter 7: Dysmenorrhea

Flowchart 1: The arachidonic acid cascade displaying the cyclooxygenase (COX) pathway, the biosynthesis of cyclic endoperoxides (PGG2 and PGH2), and finally the synthesis of PGs (PGF2a and PGE2). PGF2a and PGE2 mediate myometrial contractions, vasoconstriction, hypersensitization of pain nerve fibers and, ultimately, pain. Enzymes are shown in italics.

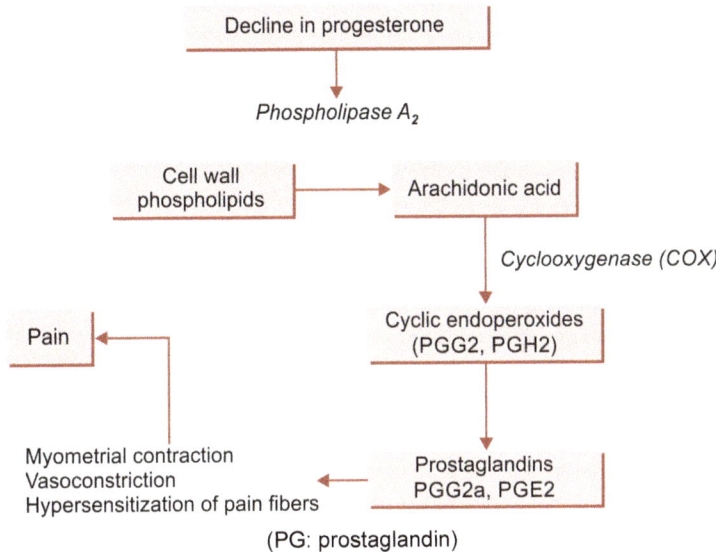

(PG: prostaglandin)

severe in young women whose periods start at an early age.[2]

All women have increased levels of PGs during the luteal phase compared with the follicular phase of ovulatory cycles. However, dysmenorrheic women have higher levels of PGs, compared with eumenorrheic women, as measured in luteal phase endometrial biopsies and menstrual fluids **(Flowchart 1)**.[1]

Along with their elevated PG levels, dysmenorrheic women have higher levels of uterine activity during menstruation compared with asymptomatic women. The basal or resting uterine tone (>10 mm Hg), active intrauterine pressure (>120 mm Hg), frequency of uterine contractions, and uncoordinated uterine contractions all are greater in these women. Vasopressin has also been implicated in the etiology of primary dysmenorrhea, although the involvement of vasopressin remains controversial.[3]

A schematic representation of the proposed (dotted lines) and known (solid lines) effects of recurrent dysmenorrhea, as well as the interrelationships of these effects is highlighted in **Flowchart 2**. Women with dysmenorrhea have reduced sleep quality, quality of life, physical activity, and poorer mood when in pain, as well as increased comorbidity with chronic pelvic pain (CPP) conditions. Throughout the menstrual cycle, women with dysmenorrhea have an increased sensitivity to painful stimuli. It is however unknown whether the increased sensitivity to pain is the cause or effect of recurrent menstrual pain. Unknown genetic or environmental factors and underlying differences in the pain processing of the central nervous system (CNS) may also play a role in predisposing these women to greater pain sensitivity and consequently recurrent menstrual pain.[1]

Women with primary dysmenorrhea exhibit a shift in the balance between

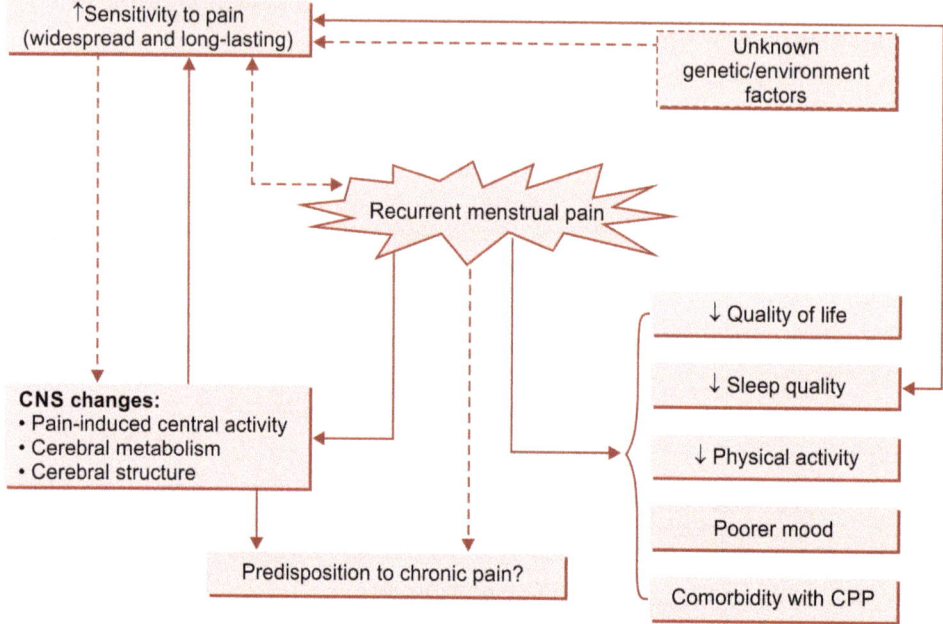

Flowchart 2: A schematic representation of the proposed (dotted lines) and known (solid lines) effects of recurrent dysmenorrhea, as well as the inter-relationships of these effects.

(CNS: central nervous system; CPP: chronic pelvic pain)

expression patterns of proinflammatory cytokines and transforming growth factor-beta family member genes related to anti-inflammatory responses, with upregulation of genes coding for proinflammatory cytokines and downregulation of genes related to anti-inflammatory responses.[1]

Secondary Dysmenorrhea

Secondary dysmenorrhea occurs in association with some form of pelvic pathology.
- The pain typically precedes the start of the period by several days and may last throughout the period.
- There may be associated dyspareunia.

Causes of Secondary Dysmenorrhea

Table 1 presents causes of secondary dysmenorrhea.

TABLE 1: Causes of secondary dysmenorrhea.

Uterine causes	Extrauterine causes
Adenomyosis	Endometriosis
Pelvic inflammatory disease	Inflammation and scarring (adhesions)
Cervical stenosis and polyps	Functional ovarian cysts
Fibroids (intracavitary or intramural)	Benign or malignant tumors of ovary, bowel or bladder, or other site
Intrauterine contraceptive devices	Inflammatory bowel disease

Source: Smith RP. Gynecology in Primary Care. Baltimore: Williams & Wilkins; 1997. pp. 389-404.

Membranous Dysmenorrhea

It is a rare condition that resembles spasmodic dysmenorrhea and in addition the endometrium is shed in form of big membranous casts due to an abnormality in its separation.

Ovarian Dysmenorrhea

It is premenstrual dull aching pain occurring in one or both iliac fossae in patient with pelvic congestion leading to ovarian congestion.

Ovulatory Pain

It is midcycle pain in one iliac fossa due to increased tension in mature follicle or rupture of the follicle at ovulation causing irritation of the peritoneum.

Premenstrual Tension Syndrome

It is premenstrual irritability, depression and pain in breasts, and sensation of fullness in the abdomen which occurs few days before menstruation and is relieved by menstruation. It is due to salt retention or increase estrogen and deficient progesterone.

EPIDEMIOLOGY

- Dysmenorrhea is very common although the precise incidence is not known as it frequently goes unreported.
- Approximately 50% of women will at some stage complain of moderately painful periods.
- Primary dysmenorrhea is the most commonly given reason for absence from school amongst adolescent girls and approximately 15% will complain of severe dysmenorrhea.[4]
- Nulliparity, early menarche, smoking, and lengthy periods are all risk factors associated with dysmenorrhea.[2]
- Females who are depressed and/or have poor social support networks are also more likely to experience pain.[5]

DIFFERENTIAL DIAGNOSIS OF DYSMENORRHEA

- Primary dysmenorrhea
- Secondary dysmenorrhea
  - Endometriosis
  - Adenomyosis
  - Uterine myomas
  - Endometrial polyps
  - Cervical stenosis
  - Obstructive malformations of the genital tract
- Sudden onset of dysmenorrhea
  - Pelvic inflammatory disease
  - Unrecognized ectopic pregnancy or spontaneous abortion
- Other causes of pain
  - Chronic pelvic inflammatory disease
  - Pelvic adhesions
  - Irritable bowel syndrome
  - Inflammatory bowel disease
  - Interstitial cystitis.

RISK FACTORS FOR DYSMENORRHEA

Table 2 presents risk factors for dysmenorrhea.

ASSESSMENT

A presumptive diagnosis of primary dysmenorrhea may be made on history with or without

TABLE 2: Risk factors for dysmenorrhea.

Risk factor	Odds ratio
Heavy menstrual loss	4.7
Premenstrual symptoms	2.4
Irregular menstrual cycles	2.0
Age younger than 30 years	1.9
Clinically suspected pelvic inflammatory disease	1.6
Sexual abuse	1.6
Menarche before 12 years of age	1.5
Low body mass index	1.4
Sterilization	1.4

Section 2: Reproductive Age Group

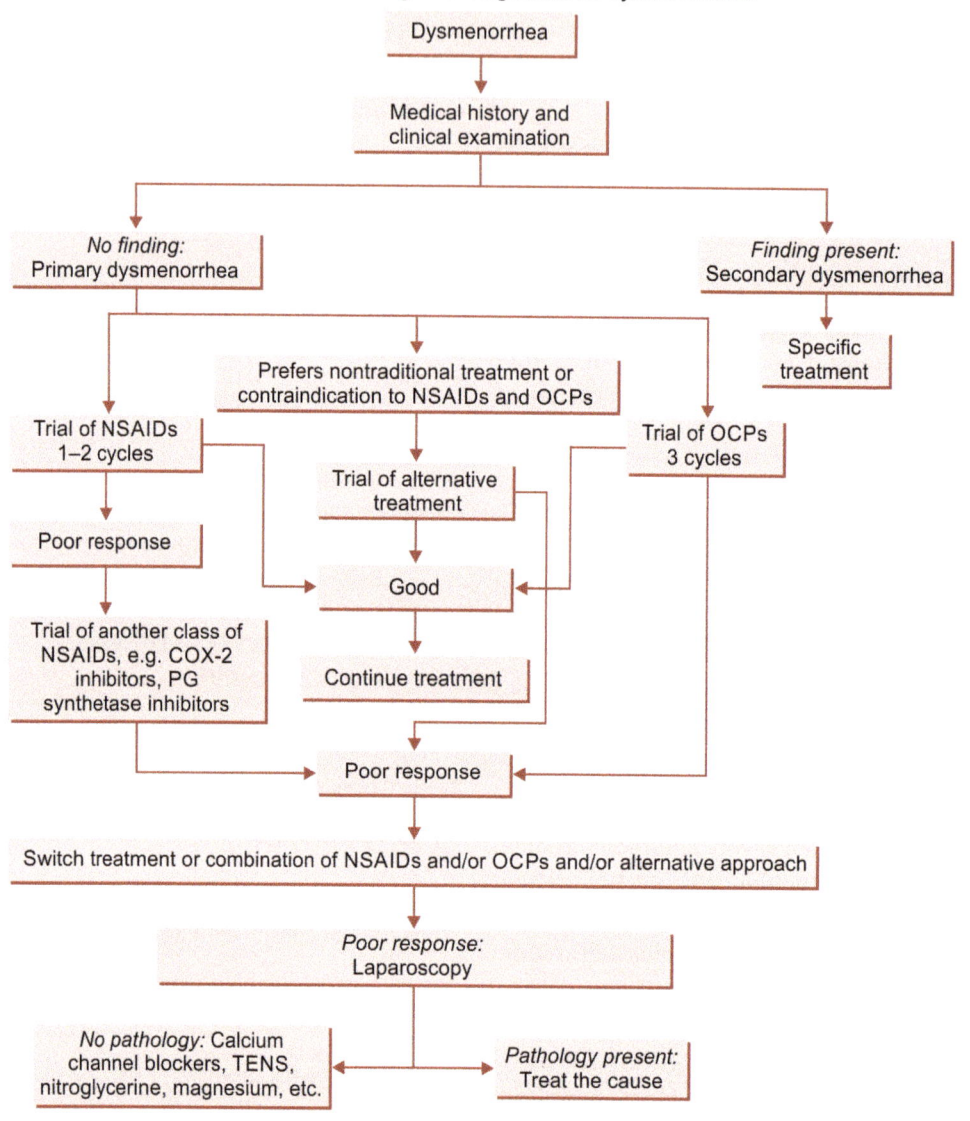

Flowchart 3: Management algorithm for dysmenorrhea.

(COX-2: cyclooxygenase-2; NSAIDs: nonsteroidal anti-inflammatory drugs; OCPs: oral contraceptive pills; PG: prostaglandin; TENS: transcutaneous electrical nerve stimulation)

abdominal examination alone in young patients who are not sexually active; vaginal examination is not normally required in this group of patients. Investigation of dysmenorrhea is primarily aimed at ruling out underlying pathology and may include any or all of the following as appropriate to the individual **(Flowchart 3)**.

History

- Age at menarche
- Cycle length

- Whether the cycle is regular
- Duration of bleeding
- Timing of pain in relation to period
- Smoking history
- Whether the patient is sexually active
- Obstetric history
- Contraceptive history
- Any features suggestive of underlying pathology (e.g. vaginal discharge, intermenstrual or postcoital bleeding, and dyspareunia).

Examination

Abdominal/vaginal examinations are indicated if sexually active:
- *Adenomyosis*: Uterus may be enlarged and tender with a typical "boggy" feel
- *Endometriosis*: Generalized tenderness in pelvic area. Uterus may be fixed and/or retroverted due to adhesions, nodules may be palpable in the uterosacral ligaments
- Partially imperforate hymen and vaginal septum (rarely).

Investigations

- Vaginal examination—if sexually active
- High vaginal swab and chlamydial swabs
- Cervical smear
- Pelvic ultrasound—if uterine enlargement or adnexal mass present
- Transvaginal ultrasound
- MRI scan
- Laparoscopy
- Laparotomy with biopsy.

MANAGEMENT

General Measures

Patients may be concerned about the possibility of underlying pathology and, when appropriate, reassurance and an explanation of the mechanism of menstrual pain may be helpful.

- *Lifestyle changes*: Various studies have looked at risk factors for dysmenorrhea and have found a clear association between smoking and dysmenorrhea,[6] patients should therefore be informed of this relationship and assisted in any attempts to stop smoking.[7] There also appears to be a link between obesity and dysmenorrhea, although this link is inconsistent, and there is some evidence to suggest that dysmenorrhea is independent of body mass index (BMI) but rather is linked to attempts to loose weight.[8] Previous studies had suggested that there may be a link between alcohol consumption and exercise levels and dysmenorrhea; however, once again, the evidence for this is inconsistent.[6]
- *Self-help techniques*: Anecdotally, many women find the following measures to be helpful in relieving the symptoms of dysmenorrhea:
  - Tea, regular, chamomile or mint
  - A warm bath
  - Abdominal and/or back massage
  - Lying in the supine position.
- *Complementary and alternative medicines*: Several dietary supplements and herbal remedies have been shown to be more effective than placebo in a study group.[9] These include:
  - Calcium and magnesium[10]
  - Thiamine
  - Ginger[11]
  - Fish oil supplements[12]
  - Toki-shakuyaku-san (TSS)—a Japanese herbal remedy
  - Transcutaneous electrical nerve stimulation (TENS)
  - Acupuncture
  - Acupressure

Pharmacological

- *Nonsteroidal anti-inflammatory drugs (NSAIDs)*: These are the most commonly used drugs for the treatment of dysmenorrhea due to their inhibition of PG synthesis. This is a class effect and all NSAIDs appear equally effective.[13] Evidence-based data support the efficacy of COX inhibitors, such as ibuprofen, naproxen sodium, and ketoprofen, and estrogen-progestin oral contraceptive pills (OCPs). Ibuprofen is most often used due to its low incidence of side-effects. COX inhibitors reduce the amount of menstrual prostanoids released, with concomitant reduction in uterine hypercontractility, while OCPs inhibit endometrial development and decrease menstrual prostanoids. Adolescents and young adults with symptoms that do not respond to treatment with NSAIDs for three menstrual periods should be offered pills for three menstrual cycles.[14] American College of Obstetricians and Gynecologists (ACOG) practice bulletin, 2010 recommends the following as first-line treatments based on effectiveness and tolerability as follows, though all NSAIDs are proven effective:
    - Ibuprofen (loading dose: 400–800 mg, subsequent dose: 400–800 mg every 6-8 hours)
    - Mefenamic acid (loading dose: 500 mg, subsequent dose every 250 mg every 6-8 hours)
    - Naproxen sodium (loading dose: 440 mg, subsequent dose 220–440 mg every 12 hours).
- *Oral contraceptive pills*: The mechanism of action is reduced PG release during menstruation. OCPs may be given by the oral or vaginal route for the treatment of dysmenorrhea; the vaginal route having fewer systemic side effects and greater analgesic effect.[15] Despite the common use of OCPs in the treatment of dysmenorrhea (and guidance from the Faculty of Family Planning stating it can be used for this purpose from the menarche),[16] recent Cochrane reviews have been inconclusive, due to a lack of evidence from randomized controlled trials.[17] OCPs can also be used to increase cycle length and therefore reduce the frequency of the symptoms. Adolescents and young adults who do not respond to this treatment should be evaluated for secondary causes of dysmenorrhea.[14] This is likely in approximately 10% of patients. Intravaginal NuvaRing, injectable Depo-Provera, subdermal implant—Implanon, Mirena (levonorgestrel-releasing intrauterine system), and transdermal Ortho Evra are various hormonal devices recommended by ACOG.
- *Depo-Provera*: Depo-medroxyprogesterone acetate (Depo-Provera) is also sometimes used as many women become amenorrheic within a year of starting treatment. Due to the potential risk of osteoporosis in women using Depo-Provera at an early age, this treatment should only be considered if other therapies have been unsuccessful.
- *Mirena*: There is some evidence to suggest that use of the levonorgestrel intrauterine device (Mirena) may be of use in some women.
- *Danazol*: Danazol may be used occasionally, with specialist supervision, in the treatment of severe refractory cases.
- *Leuprolide acetate*: May be used in rare cases to suppress the menstrual cycle, but has a significant side effect profile.
- *Nonhormonal pharmacologic therapy* includes terbutaline, nifedipine, and verapamil.

Surgery

Laparoscopic uterine nerve ablation (LUNA) is sometimes used for the treatment of severe refractory cases, however a Cochrane meta-analysis has recently concluded that there is insufficient evidence of its effectiveness to recommend the procedure.[18,19]
- Presacral neurectomy[3]
- *Hysterectomy*: In severe refractory cases, particularly in women who feel they have completed their families, hysterectomy may be considered.

KEY RECOMMENDATIONS FOR PRACTICE[20]

- A pelvic examination should be performed in all sexually active patients with dysmenorrhea and in those in whom endometriosis is suspected. (Level of evidence C)
- Nonsteroidal anti-inflammatory drugs should be used as first-line treatment for primary dysmenorrhea. (Level of evidence A)
- Oral contraceptives may be effective for relieving symptoms of primary dysmenorrhea, but evidence is limited. (Level of evidence B)
- Combined hormonal contraceptives and intramuscular, intrauterine, and subcutaneous progestin-only contraceptives are effective treatments for dysmenorrhea caused by endometriosis. (Level of evidence B)
[Strength of Recommendation Taxonomy (SORT) levels of evidence: A = consistent, good-quality patient-oriented evidence; B = inconsistent or limited-quality patient-oriented evidence; C = consensus, disease-oriented evidence, usual practice, expert opinion, or case series.]

CONCLUSION

Primary dysmenorrhea is underdiagnosed and undertreated. It generally affects adolescents and young women; usually in the absence of any underlying gynecological pathology. The initial treatment for primary dysmenorrhea is either with NSAIDs or OCPs, depending on the woman's symptoms and contraceptive needs. If one approach fails, combination of various medical modalities is tried. When combination therapy is unsuitable or ineffective, a trial of transcutaneous electrical nerve stimulation may be warranted.

Thorough history, relevant examination and timely investigation of women who fail to respond to these approaches will usually reveal the underlying cause of secondary dysmenorrhea. The long-term effects of newer techniques as presacral neurectomy and laser ablation of uterosacral ligaments have not yet been established, although their use for intractable, debilitating pain cases is increasing.

When no cause is found to explain dysmenorrhea and conventional therapies fail to provide relief, hysterectomy may be considered in women who have completed childbearing.

REFERENCES

1. Iacovides S, Avidon I, Baker FC. What we know about primary dysmenorrhea today: a critical review. Hum Reprod Update. 2015;21(6):762-78.
2. Sundell G, Milsom I, Andersch B. Factors influencing the prevalence and severity of dysmenorrhoea in young women. Br J Obstet Gynaecol. 1990;97(7):588-94.
3. Yusoff Dawood M. Primary Dysmenorrhea. Advances in Pathogenesis and Management. Obstet Gynecol. 2006;108:428-4.
4. Andersch B, Milsom I. An epidemiologic study of young women with dysmenorrhea. Am J Obstet Gynecol. 1982;144(6):655-60.

5. Alonso C, Coe CL. Disruptions of social relationships accentuate the association between emotional distress and menstrual pain in young women. Health Psychol. 2001;20(6):411-6.
6. Harlow SD, Park M. A longitudinal study of risk factors for the occurrence, duration and severity of menstrual cramps in a cohort of college women. Br J Obstet Gynaecol. 1996;103(11):1134-42.
7. Dorn LD, Negriff S, Huang B, et al. Menstrual symptoms in adolescent girls: association with smoking, depressive symptoms, and anxiety. J Adolesc Health. 2009;44(3):237-43.
8. Montero P, Bernis C, Fernandez V, et al. Influence of body mass index and slimming habits on menstrual pain and cycle irregularity. J Biosoc Sci. 1996;28(3):315-23.
9. Wilson ML, Murphy PA. Herbal and dietary therapies for primary and secondary dysmenorrhoea. Cochrane Database Syst Rev. 2001;(3):CD002124.
10. Penland JG, Johnson PE. Dietary calcium and manganese effects on menstrual cycle symptoms. Am J Obstet Gynecol. 1993;168(5):1417-23.
11. Ozgoli G, Goli M, Moattar F. Comparison of Effects of Ginger, Mefenamic Acid, and Ibuprofen on Pain in Women with Primary Dysmenorrhea. J Altern Complement Med. 2009;15:129-32.
12. Harel Z, Biro FM, Kottenhahn RK, et al. Supplementation with omega-3 polyunsaturated fatty acids in the management of dysmenorrhea in adolescents. Am J Obstet Gynecol. 1996;174(4):1335-8.
13. Marjoribanks J, Proctor ML, Farquhar C. Nonsteroidal anti-inflammatory drugs for primary dysmenorrhoea. Cochrane Database Syst Rev. 2003;(4):CD001751.
14. Harel Z. Dysmenorrhea in adolescents and young adults: etiology and management. J Pediatr Adolesc Gynecol. 2006;19(6):363-71.
15. Ziaei S, Rajaei L, Faghihzadeh S, et al. Comparative study and evaluation of side effects of low-dose contraceptive pills administered by the oral and vaginal route. Contraception. 2002;65(5):329-31.
16. Faculty of Family Planning and Reproductive Health Care (FSRH) Clinical Effectiveness Unit. First prescription of combined oral contraception. London: FSRH; 2006.
17. Proctor ML, Roberts H, Farquhar CM. Combined oral contraceptive pill (OCP) as treatment for primary dysmenorrhoea. Cochrane Database Syst Rev. 2001;(4):CD002120.
18. Latthe PM, Proctor ML, Farquhar CM, et al. Surgical interruption of pelvic nerve pathways in dysmenorrhea: a systematic review of effectiveness. Acta Obstet Gynecol Scand. 2007;86(1):4-15.
19. Proctor ML, Latthe PM, Farquhar CM, et al. Surgical interruption of pelvic nerve pathways for primary and secondary dysmenorrhoea. Cochrane Database Syst Rev. 2005;(4):CD001896.
20. Osayande AS, Mehulic S. Diagnosis and Initial Management of Dysmenorrhea. Am Fam Physician. 2014;89(5):341-46.

CHAPTER 8

Abnormal Uterine Bleeding

Mekhala B Dwarakanath, Jahnavi Esanakula

INTRODUCTION

Abnormal uterine bleeding (AUB) is described as any deviation from the regularity, frequency, heaviness, and duration of flow.[1] It is difficult to describe AUB as there exist considerable variations in normal menses of different women and in same women during various stages of life.

Presence of AUB impairs the quality of life of the women.[2] It is debilitating disorder physically, socially, and mentally. If not corrected, women will tend to suffer in the prime years of life with AUB. It is, therefore, prudent to improve the quality of life rather than just focusing on blood loss.

The one of the common presenting complaints in women attending gynecological outpatient is AUB. The incidence of AUB is 14–25% in women of reproductive age group.[3,4] In combination with existing nutritional anemia in developing countries this poses a high risk to women of developing countries like India.

Fertility preservation is essential, especially in young women. As newer medical and surgical options that offer relief from symptoms of AUB are now available, the decision of hysterectomy should be taken with due consideration.

TERMINOLOGY

Understanding the terminology of AUB has been the key component of describing the various symptoms of AUB. Old terminology leads to confusion and hence new acceptable terminology was derived **(Table 1)**. The terms like menorrhagia, metrorrhagia, polymenorrhea, oligomenorrhea, hypomenorrhea, and dysfunctional uterine bleeding are to be discarded.[5]

CLASSIFICATION

Depending on duration of symptoms:
- *Acute*: Episode of abnormal bleeding sufficient to need immediate intervention in the opinion of clinician.

TABLE 1: Acceptable terminology.[6]

Disturbances in regularity:	
Irregular menstrual bleeding	A range of varying lengths of bleeding-free intervals >17 days within a 90-day reference period
Amenorrhea	No bleeding for a 90-day period
Disturbances in frequency:	
Infrequent cycles	One or two episodes of bleeding in a 90-day period
Frequent cycles	Four or more episodes of bleeding in a 90-day period
Disturbances in amount of flow:	
AUB (abnormal uterine bleeding)	The overarching term that covers all the deviation in normal menstruation
HMB (heavy menstrual bleeding)	Excessive menstrual blood loss which interferes with woman's physical, emotional, social, and material quality of life
HPMB (heavy and prolonged menstrual bleeding)	Bleeding pattern described above for longer than 8 days
IMB (intermenstrual bleeding)	Bleeding between the cycles
PMB (postmenopausal bleeding)	Bleeding after 1 year of no bleeding
Disturbances in duration of flow:	
Prolonged menstrual bleeding	Bleeding for more than 8 days
Shortened menstrual bleeding	Bleeding for no longer than 2 days

- *Chronic*: Abnormal bleeding from uterine corpus has been present for more than 6 months.
- *Intermenstrual*: Bleeding between two menstrual cycles.

Depending on the age of the female:
- Pubertal
- Reproductive age women
- Postmenopausal women.

PALM COEIN system was proposed to classify AUB according to causes in reproductive age group women. PALM represents the structural causes and COEIN the nonstructural causes **(Fig. 1)**.[7]

All the causes which can cause AUB that cannot be clearly defined into other categories, like chronic endometritis, myometrial hypertrophy, and arteriovenous malformation can be grouped under N—not yet classified **(Table 2)**.

The categories have scope for further subcategories in each category. The notation also allows allocating multiple causes for one person with AUB.

■ DIAGNOSIS[2]

History

The importance of proper history about the symptoms cannot be over emphasized. Proper history of nature of problem along with associated symptoms like pain, pressure symptoms, impact on qualities of living, and comorbidities which might change the treatment are needed.

Chapter 8: Abnormal Uterine Bleeding

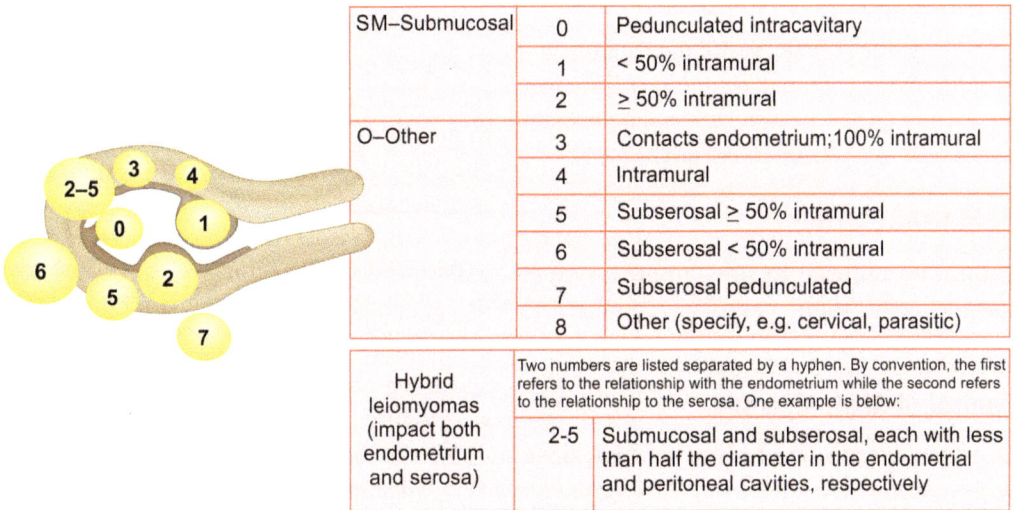

SM–Submucosal	0	Pedunculated intracavitary
	1	< 50% intramural
	2	≥ 50% intramural
O–Other	3	Contacts endometrium; 100% intramural
	4	Intramural
	5	Subserosal ≥ 50% intramural
	6	Subserosal < 50% intramural
	7	Subserosal pedunculated
	8	Other (specify, e.g. cervical, parasitic)
Hybrid leiomyomas (impact both endometrium and serosa)	Two numbers are listed separated by a hyphen. By convention, the first refers to the relationship with the endometrium while the second refers to the relationship to the serosa. One example is below:	
	2-5	Submucosal and subserosal, each with less than half the diameter in the endometrial and peritoneal cavities, respectively

Fig 1: Leiomyoma subclassification system.

Physical Examination

- *Signs of underlying pathology*: Bruising, typical hypothyroid features, features of polycystic ovary syndrome (PCOS) (hirsutism, acne, and overweight), pallor, and koilonychia.
- *Abdominal examination*: Tenderness and palpable masses (uterine and ovarian).
- *Pelvic examination*: Vulval inspection, speculum examination, and bimanual palpation for masses.
- *Cervical smear*: As and when appropriate to screen for carcinoma cervix.
- *Infection screening*: High vaginal and endocervical swabs as appropriate.

Investigations[2]

- Complete blood picture
- Pregnancy test to rule out pregnancy-related complications
- Coagulation disorders if there is clinical suspicion
- Thyroid hormone testing if thyroid disease symptoms are noticed

TABLE 2: PALM COEIN system.

P-Polyp	C-coagulopathy
A-adenomyosis	O-ovulatory dysfunction
L-leiomyoma	E-endometrial
M-malignancy and hyperplasia	I-iatrogenic
	N-not yet classified

- *Ultrasonography:* As a preliminary investigation of cause of AUB, especially in suspicion of:
  - Large fibroids
  - Pelvic mass
  - Inconclusive or difficult examination
  - Adenomyosis
- Outpatient hysteroscopy if history is suggestive of submucosal fibroids, polyps or endometrial pathology
- *Endometrial biopsy*: Hysteroscopy and endometrial biopsy should be chosen over blind biopsy:
  - Persistent intermenstrual or persistent irregular bleeding
  - Obese or women with history of PCOS

- Women taking tamoxifen
- Previous unsuccessful treatment.
- *Magnetic resonance imaging (MRI)*: Not to be used as a routine, but can be used in women with suspicion of adenomyosis.

MANAGEMENT

Should be tailored to the symptoms, age, socioeconomic status, pathology, compliance, and preference of the women.

Control of Acute Episode

In an acute episode of bleeding high-dose progesterone preferably norethisterone can be used. In patients with prolonged history of bleeding, combined oral contraceptives or equine estrogen along with progesterones will be more effective. In cases not controlled with the agents above, therapeutic curettage of uterine cavity will be effective.

Treatment

Correction of anemia with blood product transfusion if severe and hematinics in mild to moderate cases is needed. Anemia correction should be done parallel to regulation of menstruation.

Treatment of the Cause

The management algorithm of AUB in women of reproductive age group and perimenopausal age group has been depicted in **Flowchart 1**.

- Medical:
    - *Nonhormonal:* These are the first-line agents in most of the women
        - Tranexamic acid
        - Nonsteroidal anti-inflammatory drugs (NSAIDs)
        - Ethamsylate
    - *Hormonal:*
        - Progestogens

Flowchart 1: The management algorithm of AUB in women of reproductive age group and perimenopausal age group.

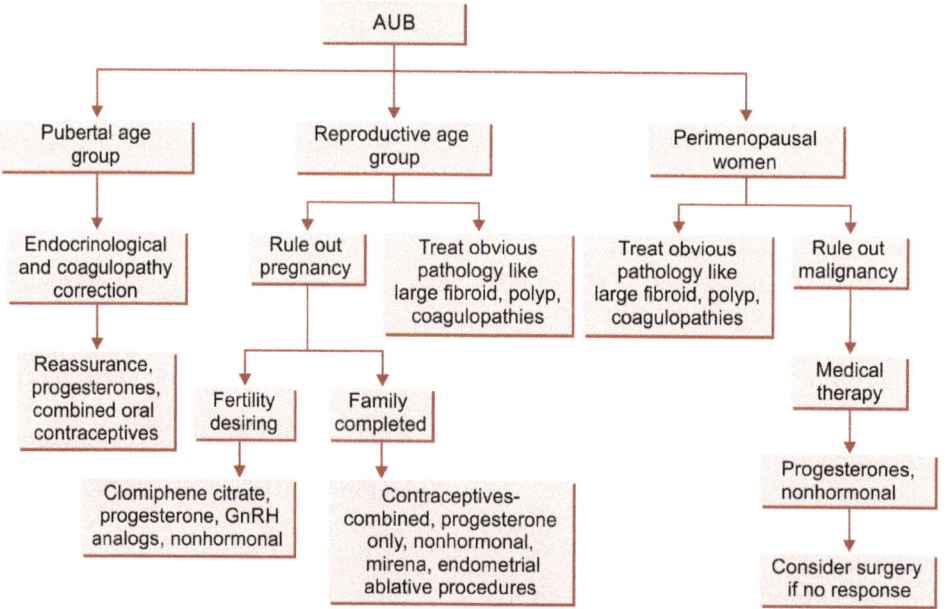

(AUB: abnormal uterine bleeding; GnRH: gonadotropin-releasing hormone)

- Combined hormonal contraceptives
- Conjugated equine estrogen
- Danazol
- Clomiphene citrate
- Ormeloxifene
- Gonadotropin-releasing hormone (GnRH) agonists.

Tranexamic acid: It is an antifibrinolytic. Used as dose 1–2 g orally per day in three to four divided doses during menstruation. It is effective in 50% of cases. 10 mg/kg intravenous dose is advisable in acute conditions. It should be used with caution in patients with risk of thromboembolic disorders and in concomitant treatment with combined oral contraception. It should be avoided in women with acute impairment of color vision and current thromboembolic episode.[8]

Ethamsylate: It is a drug that reduces capillary fragility. It can be used in combination with tranexamic acid in three to four divided doses.

Nonsteroidal anti-inflammatory drugs:[8] One of the proposed mechanisms of action for heavy menstrual bleeding is production of inflammatory mediators. Hence, NSAIDs most commonly mefenamic acid were used in AUB. Mefenamic acid will cause reduction of blood loss by 25–50%. Side effects are gastrointestinal and it should be avoided in women with peptic ulcer. NSAIDs and antifibrinolytics can be used together, but should be stopped after 3 months if there is no symptomatic improvement.

Progestogens: They are the main stay of treatment in AUB.[9] Progesterone causes increase in activity of 17-beta-dehydrogenase causing conversion of estradiol to weaker estrogen and causes endometrial atrophy. Various progesterones used for AUB are medroxyprogesterone, norethisterone, Duphaston, and gestrinone (vaginal). Various protocols are discussed below:

- *Cyclical oral progesterones:* Can be used cyclically from day 5 to day 25 or from day 15 to day 25 for 3–6 months. Contraindications are previous history of vascular thrombosis, current or past breast cancer, and impaired liver function. Duphaston can be used in women desiring pregnancy.
- *Levonorgestrel intrauterine device:*[10] Levonorgestrel intrauterine device causes slow release of levonorgestrel preventing proliferation of endometrium. Side effects include unscheduled bleeding, infection, perforation, and expulsion of intrauterine system (IUS). It should be used with care in women with distorted endometrial cavity.
- *Injectable progesterones:* Intramuscular or subcutaneous injections of medroxyprogesterone can induce amenorrhea in 50% of patients. Depot injections can be given every 12 weeks. It has an added benefit of contraception and reduction in dysmenorrhea. Side effects include weight gain, acne, bloating, irregular bleeding patterns, and decrease in bone mineral density with long-term use.[11]

Combined oral contraceptives: They are to be given in 3 weeks doses followed by 1 week pill-free interval. The estimated blood loss reduction was 50%.[12] To be used in caution in women with risk of thromboembolism, cerebrovascular disease, ischemic heart disease, migraine, hypertension, severe liver disease, breast cancer, diabetes with vascular complications, and heart disease.

Conjugated equine estrogen: Can be used in acute AUB in a dose of 25 mg intravenous every 4–6 hours for 24 hours. These have been recently replaced with progesterones.

Danazol: Limited role due to androgenic side effects. Should be used in a dose of 200 mg daily if there is no response to oral contraceptives or progesterones.

Gonadotropin-releasing hormone agonists: Reduces estrogen and progesterone. To be given as depot injections 3.6 mg monthly, for 4–6 months. It is not useful in acute episodes because of its long onset of action. It causes menopausal symptoms and osteoporosis. Hence, it should not be given for greater than 6 months. Osteoporosis should be counteracted with add back therapy by giving norethisterone or tibolone.

Clomiphene citrate: It is given in a dose of 50–150 mg for 5 days starting from day 2 or day 3. In women desiring pregnancy this will help development of follicles.

Ormeloxifene: It is a selective estrogen receptor modulator. It has to be given in dose of 60 mg twice per week for 12 weeks followed by weekly doses. It is also effective in fibroid uterus. It causes functional cyst and headaches.

Minimally invasive methods: Endometrial ablation is best if performed if the endometrial thickness is less than 4 mm. It is not advised in women desiring children. It can be done by curettage or hormone replacement therapy. About 23–60% of the treated women have postprocedural amenorrhea.[13]

There are two kinds of ablative procedures:
1. *Hysteroscopic procedure:* Using hysteroscope ablation can be done with hydrothermal laser, radio frequency, electrical energy or electrodes.
2. *Nonhysteroscopic procedure:* Devices that ablate the endometrium by delivering energy in uniform manner.[13]

   Hydrothermal ablation involves insertion of 3 mm hysteroscope. Heated saline is instilled and maintained at 90°F for 10 minutes pressure of <45 mm Hg.

Uterine artery embolization: Can be done if the cause of AUB if fibroid of >3 cm. It is not to be used in women desiring fertility. Symptoms of heavy menorrhagia, pressure symptoms, and volume of fibroid were found to be reduced. Symptoms were relieved in 70–80% of women. The drawback is that the procedure requires expertise and cannot be performed at all places.

Myomectomy: Submucosal fibroids are to be removed by hysteroscopic removal. Intramural and subserosal fibroids are to be removed if they are causing heavy menstrual bleeding, pressure symptoms or infertility. Care must be taken to avoid hemorrhage which may ultimately lead to hysterectomy. Using GnRH agonists can be used to reduce the size of fibroids, but surgical difficulty may be experienced due to thinning of capsule.

Newer techniques like MRI-guided focus ultrasound and laparoscopic myolysis have been introduced to manage fibroids.

Hysterectomy: Can be done in laparoscopic, abdominal, and vaginal route. Though hysterectomy is the most effective treatment for AUB, this has to be considered after thorough evaluation of cause, optimum trial of medical treatment, and discussion with the patient because of high risk of adverse effects like hemorrhage, surgical complications, wound-related complications, and thromboembolic events.[14]

SUMMARY

- Abnormal uterine bleeding is any deviation from normal pattern of bleeding. It impairs the quality of life of the women. The incidence of AUB is about 14–25%.
- Archaic and confusing terminologies of menorrhagia, metrorrhagia, polymenorrhea, oligomenorrhea and hypomenorrhea terminologies have been replaced by newer and well-defined terminologies

recommended by International Federation of Gynecology and Obstetrics (FIGO).
- PALM COEIN system was introduced for easy clinical classification of AUB. FIGO introduced sub-classification of fibroid.
- Meticulous history taking and examination is of prime importance for diagnosis. Pregnancy-related complications have to be ruled out in women of reproductive age group. Ultrasonography, hormonal analysis and rarely MRI also aid in diagnosis.
- Various hormonal, nonhormonal and surgical methods are available for treatment of AUB. Treatment depends on the age of the patient, symptoms and severity of AUB.
- Progesterone in the form of oral, injectable or intrauterine system has been the mainstay of treatment in AUB after excluding any obvious cause.

CONCLUSION

Abnormal uterine bleeding is one of the most common compliant with which women present to a gynecologist. Several treatment modalities are available for treatment of AUB. In a country like India, it falls upon the attending gynecologist to choose the best for the women. Recently there has been paradigm shift from towards conserving the uterus.

REFERENCES

1. Fraser IS, Inceboz US. Defining disturbances of the menstrual cycle. In: O'Brien PNS, Cameron IT, MacLean AB (Eds). Disorders of the Menstrual Cycle. London, UK: RCOG Press; 2000. pp. 151-2.
2. NICE guidelines. Heavy menstrual bleeding: assessment and management; 2018.
3. Fraser IS, Langham S, Uhl-Hochgraeber K. Health-related quality of life and economic burden of abnormal uterine bleeding. Expert Rev Obstet Gynecol. 2009;4:179-89.
4. Shapley M, Jordan K, Croft PR. An epidemiological survey of symptoms of menstrual loss in the community. Br J Gen Pract. 2004;54:359-63.
5. Woolcock JG, Critchley HOD, Munro MG, et al. Review of the confusion in current and historical terminology and definitions for disturbances of menstrual bleeding. Fertil Steril. 2008;90(6):2269-80.
6. Fraser IS, Critchley HO, Broder M, et al. The FIGO recommendations on terminologies and definitions for normal and abnormal uterine bleeding. Semin Reprod Med. 2011;29:383-90.
7. Munro MG, Critchley HO, Broder MS, et al. FIGO classification system (PALM-COEIN) for causes of abnormal uterine bleeding in nongravid women of reproductive age. Int J Gynecol Obstet. 2011;113:3-13.
8. Cameron IT, Haining R, Lumsden MA, et al. The effects of mefenamic acid and norethisterone on measured menstrual blood loss. Obstet Gynecol. 1990;76(1):85-8.
9. Maybin JA, Critchley HO. Medical management of heavy menstrual bleeding. Womens Health. 2016;12(1):27-34.
10. Andersson K, Odlind V, Rybo G. Levonorgestrel-releasing and copper-releasing (Nova T) IUDs during five years of use: a randomized comparative trial. Contraception. 1994;49(1):56-72.
11. Said S, Omar K, Koetsawang S, et al. A multicentered Phase III comparative clinical trial of depot medroxyprogesterone acetate given three-monthly at doses of 100 mg or 150 mg: II. The comparison of bleeding patterns. World Health Organization. Task Force on Long-Acting Systemic Agents for Fertility Regulation Special Programme of Research, Development and Research Training in Human Reproduction. Contraception. 1987;35(6):591-610.
12. Fraser IS, Kovacs GT. The efficacy of non-contraceptive uses for hormonal contraceptives. Med J Aust. 2003;178(12):621-3.
13. The Practice Committee of the American Society for Reproductive Medicine. Indications and options for endometrial ablation. Fertil Steril. 2008;90:S236-40.
14. Matteson KA, Abed H, Wheeler TL, et al. A systematic review comparing hysterectomy to less invasive treatments for abnormal uterine bleeding. J Minim Invasive Gynecol. 2012;19(1):13-28.

CHAPTER 9

Postcoital Bleeding

Sowmya Davuluri

■ INTRODUCTION

Postcoital bleeding refers to spotting or bleeding per vagina that occurs after intercourse and is not related to menstruation. The incidence ranges between 0.75% and 9% of menstruating women.[1] Postcoital is mostly cervical in origin and is mostly attributed to the benign process. In 50% cases, spontaneous resolution occurs within 2 years.[1] Postcoital bleeding is usually associated with abnormal uterine bleeding in 30% of cases and 15% in dyspareunia cases.[2,3]

■ ETIOLOGY

Postcoital bleeding is primarily due to the surface lesions of the genital tract like cervicitis, cervical polyps, ectropion, cervical intraepithelial neoplasia (CIN) or carcinomas.[4] The causes with which a woman can present are broad of which the prevalence of cervical cancer is 3–5% and CIN is 6.8–17.8% **(Fig. 1)**.[1]

Risk of cervical cancer according to the age groups is shown in **Table 1**.[5]

■ MANAGEMENT

No established guidelines or recommendations or evidence on the diagnosis or treatment of postcoital bleeding. The following considerations can be taken into account while approaching a postcoital bleeding patient.

History plays an important role in the diagnosis of postcoital bleeding.

History
- Age
- *Menstrual history*: Helps to identify if the source of the bleeding is from cervix or uterus
- *Duration of menstruation*:
  – History of menorrhagia
  – Presence of intermenstrual bleeding
  – Regular/irregular bleeding

Chapter 9: Postcoital Bleeding

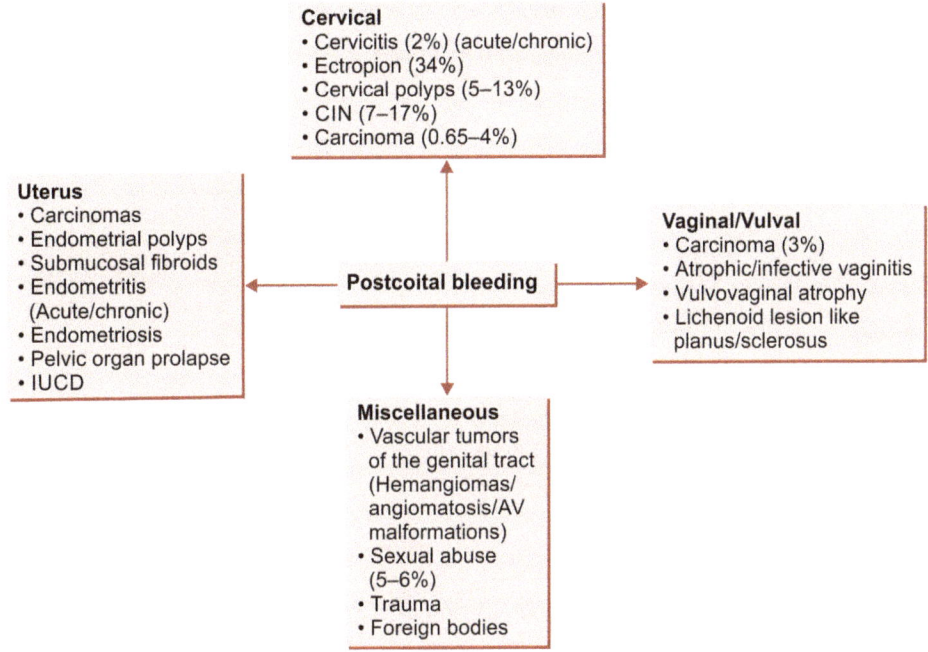

Fig. 1: Etiology of postcoital bleeding. (AV: arteriovenous; CIN: cervical intraepithelial neoplasia; IUCD: intrauterine contraceptive device)

TABLE 1: Risk of cervical cancer according to age.	
20–24 years	1:44,000
25–34 years	1:5,600
35–44 years	1:2,800
45–54 years	1:2,400

- Differentiate if it is true postcoital bleeding or secondary to irregular menstrual bleeding
- *Past medical history*: History of any bleeding disorders
- *Sexual history*: Number of partners/new partners, history of sexually transmitted diseases (STDs) for patient or the partners
- History of sexual abuse/genital trauma
- History of dyspareunia
- History of vaginal discharge, color, consistency, odor, and the frequency
- History of prolapse
- Rule out pregnancy.

Examination

Examination of women with postcoital bleeding is shown in **Flowchart 1**.

Ultrasonography

- *To rule out*: Bulky uterus/pyometra/hydrometra/endometrial thickness >12 mm.
- If the endometrial thickness >12 mm, an endometrial biopsy is to be done send for histopathological examination followed by an MRI pelvis.[6,7]

Important Point to Note!!

Normal Pap smear *does not rule out* malignancy in women presenting with postcoital bleeding, but the incidence of cervical cancer in women

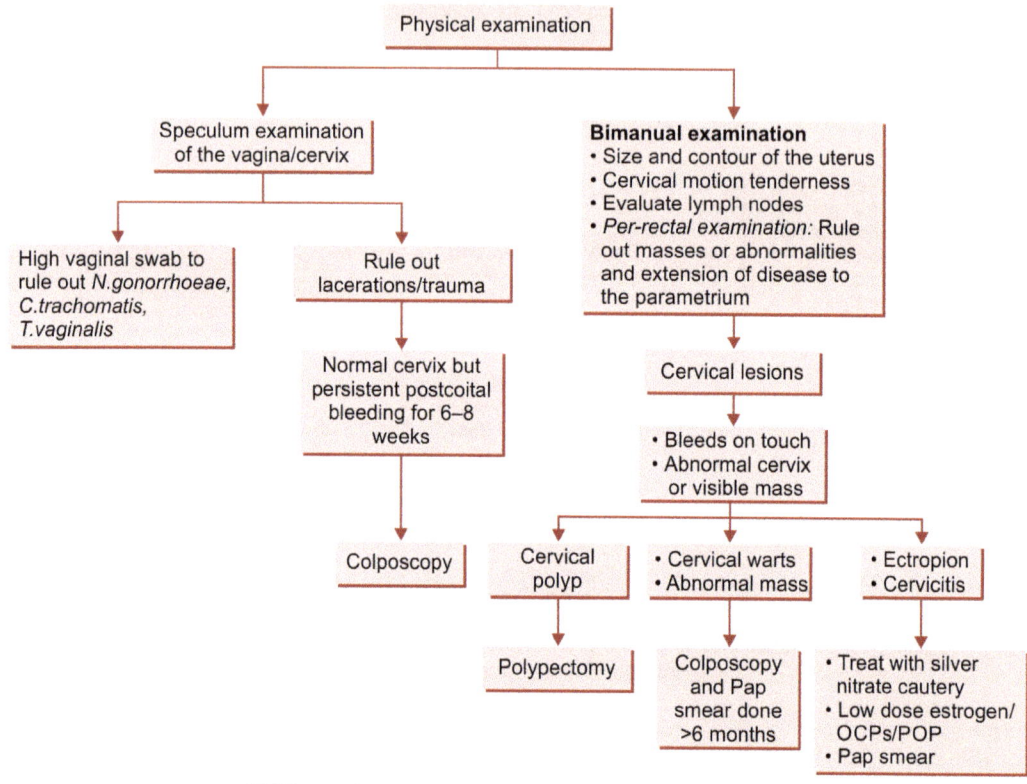

Flowchart 1: Examination of women with postcoital bleeding.

(OCPs: oral contraceptive pills; POP: progestin-only pill)

who had a recent normal Pap smear is as low as 0.6%.

Role of colposcopy in the diagnosis and management

There is limited evidence for the role of colposcopy in women with negative Pap smears and in patients with no cervical lesions. According to American College of Obstetricians and Gynecologists (ACOG), colposcopy should be done on all visible lesions.

How many biopsies?

Studies have shown that detection of CIN-2 and higher lesions are more in four quadrant biopsies than single direct biopsy.[8,9]

When is colposcopy indicated?

Indications for colposcopy is described in Figure 2.

Referral to a tertiary center

Urgent referral to a tertiary center is required if:[10,11]

- The woman is >35 years with persistent postcoital bleeding >4 weeks
- Clinical features suggestive of cervical cancer on examination (previous negative Pap smear should not delay the referral)
- Unexplained lump in the vulval region/vulval ulcers
- On hormone replacement therapy (HRT) with persistent or unexplained

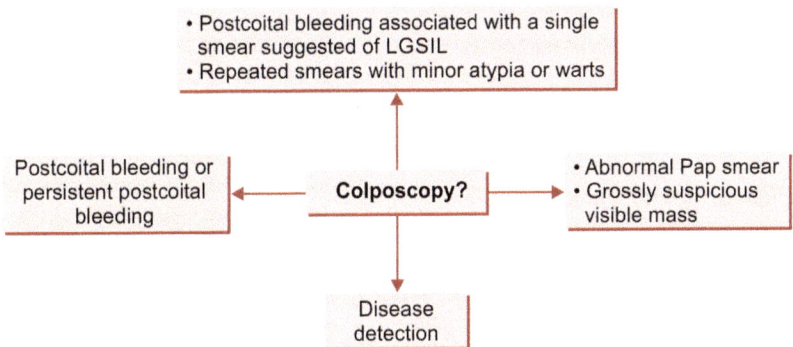

Fig. 2: Indications for colposcopy.

postmenopausal bleeding after cessation of treatment for 6 weeks
- Women with friable cervix.

Primary principle of management is to exclude malignancy.

SUMMARY

- Postcoital bleeding refers to spotting or bleeding per vagina that occurs after intercourse and is not related to menstruation.
- The causes for postcoital bleeding includes cervical, uterine, vaginal/vulval and miscellaneous reasons. Cervical causes contribute to the majority of cases with post-coital bleeding.
- Detailed history and physical examination play a major role in the diagnosis.
- There is no evidence for role of colposcopy in patients with negative Pap smear or absent cervical lesions.
- Management includes treating the underlying cause.

CONCLUSION

Postcoital bleeding is a worrying symptom due to increased risk of malignancy. The etiology varies widely from common cervicitis to carcinomas. A detailed history and physical examination are the most important things to get to a differential diagnosis and planning the further plan of management. There are no specific recommendations on the management of postcoital bleeding.

REFERENCES

1. Tarney CM, Han J. Postcoital bleeding: a review on etiology, diagnosis and management. Obstet Gynecol Int. 2014;2014:192087.
2. Tehranian A, Rezaii N, Mohit M, et al. Evaluation of women presenting with postcoital bleeding by cytology and colposcopy. Int J Gynecol Obstet. 2009;105(1):18-20.
3. Selo-Ojeme DO, Dayoub N, Patel A, et al. A clinico-pathological study of postcoital bleeding. Arch Gynecol Obstet. 2004;270(1):34-6.
4. Fraser IS, Petrucco OM. Management of intermenstrual and postcoital bleeding, and an appreciation of the issues arising out of the recent case of O'Shea versus Sullivan and Macquarie pathology. Aust NZJ Obstet Gynaecol. 1996;36(1):67-73.
5. Anorlu RI, Abdul-Kareem FB, Abudu OO, et al. Cervical cytology in an urban population in Lagos, Nigeria. J Obstet Gynaecol. 2003;23(3):285-8.
6. NHS. (2010). Practice guidance for the assessment of young women aged 20-24 with abnormal vaginal bleeding. [online] Available from https://assets.publishing.service.gov.uk/government/uploads/system/uploads/

attachment_data/file/436924/doh-guidelines-young-women.pdf [Last accessed September, 2019].

7. American College of Obstetricians and Gynecologists. ACOG Committee Opinion No. 440: The Role of Transvaginal Ultrasound in the Evaluation of Postmenopausal Bleeding. Obstet Gynaecol. 2009;114:409-11.

8. Cuzik J, Szarewski A, Cubie H, et al. Management of women who test positive for high-risk types of human papillomavirus: the HART study. Lancet. 2003;362(9399):1871-6.

9. Kjaer SK, van der Brule AJ, Paull G, et al. Type specific persistence of high risk human papillomavirus (HPV) as an indicator of high grade cervical squamous intraepithelial lesion in young women: population based prospective follow up study. BMJ. 2002;325(7364):572.

10. Mulka O. NICE suspected cancer guidelines. Br J Gen Pract. 2005;55(517):580-1.

11. Luesley D, Leeson S. Colposcopy and Programme Management Guidelines for the NHS Cervical Screening Programme, 2nd edition. Sheffield: NHS Cancer Screening Programmes; 2010.

CHAPTER 10

Infections

Karthigayeni R

■ INTRODUCTION

Genitourinary infections are one of the most common disorders for which women seek gynecologist. By having an insight about the pathophysiology of these disorders and with effective strategies for diagnosis, most appropriate treatment approach can be implemented with reduction in further long-term sequelae.

■ INFECTIONS OF THE VULVA

Vulva is resistant to infections mostly however it presence of atrophy or degenerative changes infections are more likely to occur. The following are the causes of vulval infection as mentioned in **Table 1**.

Pyogenic Infection

Furunculosis
- Causative organism is *Staphylococcus aureus* affecting the hair follicle of the labia majora and mons leading to folliculitis followed by furunculitis
- Rule out diabetes, if it is recurrent
- Treat with systemic or local antibiotics and to maintain cleanliness.

Impetigo
- Causative organism is *S. aureus* or *Streptococcus*
- Pustular infection confined to vulva or might spread to other body parts.

Vulvar Abscess

Due to presence of loose areolar tissue in the subcutaneous layers, it has potential for significant expansion unlike other superficial abscess.

Causative organism:
- Includes *Staphylococcus*, *Enterococcus* species, group B *Streptococcus*, and *Escherichia coli* (*E. coli*)

TABLE 1: Causes of vulval infections.

Bacterial	Viral	Fungal	Parasitic
Pyogenic (nongonococcal) Tuberculosis Sexually transmitted disease (STD) • Syphilis • Gonorrhea • Lymphogranuloma venereum • Chancroid • Granuloma inguinale	Herpes genitalis Herpes zoster Molluscum contagiosum Condylomata acuminata	Ringworm Moniliasis	Threadworm Scabies Pediculosis pubis

- *Methicillin-resistant S. aureus (MRSA)* was responsible in 40–60% of cases.[1]

Management:
- Early stage present with cellulitis without abscess. Treat with oral antibiotic and sitz bath.
- *Smaller abscess*: Incision and drainage is recommended along with oral broad spectrum antibiotic covering MRSA in uncomplicated cases. However in women with diabetes or immunosuppression, intravenous antibiotic is preferred as there is a higher risk of necrotizing fasciitis.
- *Large abscess*: Admission in the hospital is required for incision and drainage under anesthesia. Adequate pain control and intravenous antibiotic are necessary.

Ring Worm

- Causative organism is tinea cruris
- Present as well circumscribed and bright red lesions
- Microscopic examination of the scrapings of the lesion shows presence of fungi
- Imidazole (miconazole or clotrimazole) creams are very effective. Some might respond to oral griseofulvin.

Thread Worm

- Causative organism is *Oxyuris vermicularis* and more common in children
- Present with nocturnal itching with perianal excoriation and parasite is found in stools
- Treated with antihelmintic drugs like mebendazole.

■ INFECTIONS OF THE BARTHOLIN'S GLAND

Bartholin's glands are a pair of small gland (2 cm) located at 5 o'clock and 7 o'clock position of the vagina between hymen and the labia minora.

Causative organism: Staphylococcus, E. coli, Streptococcus, Chlamydia or missed types. *Neisseria gonorrhoeae* and *Chlamydia trachomatis* might also be a cause.[2]

Pathology: Both the gland and the duct are involved. Duct lumen will be either blocked or open. The end result of acute infection is either complete resolution, cyst formation, abscess formation or recurrence.

Clinical features: Present with localized pain and discomfort. Palpation reveals induration and tenderness over the posterior half of the labia. Duct opening is congested with secretions coming out on pressing the gland.

Treatment: Hot compresses, analgesic, and systemic antibiotic are effective treatment methods.

Recurrent bartholinitis: Occur in 5–10% of the women with painful attack periodically. In quiescent phase excision of the duct and gland is performed.

Bartholin's Abscess

It occurs as result of acute bartholinitis. It might rupture into lower vaginal wall if left untreated and sinus tract will be open with periodic discharge of the abscess contents.

Clinical features: Intense pain and discomfort associated with fever. Tender swelling unilaterally in posterior part of labia majora extending up to labia minora. Skin over swelling is edematous and red.

Treatment: Daily sitz bath, analgesic, antipyretic, and systemic antibiotics are effective. Abscess has to be drained early before spontaneous rupture. In case of recurrence, in quiescent phase excision should be done.

■ INFECTIONS OF THE VAGINA

Normal Vagina

- Normal vaginal discharge includes the secretions from vulva (sebaceous, bartholin, and skene gland), vaginal transudate, exfoliated cervical and vaginal cells, cervical mucus, and oviductal and endometrial fluid.
- The physiological reasons for increase in vaginal discharge include combined oral contraceptive pills, pregnancy and during midcycle result of progesterone effect.
- Vaginal epithelial cells include superficial cells (predominant under estrogen stimulation), intermediate cells (predominant under progesterone stimulation), and parabasal cells (seen in postmenopausal women).
- The normal vaginal flora is aerobic with hydrogen peroxide producing lactobacilli being the predominant organism.
- Normal vaginal potential of hydrogen (pH) is less than 4.5 due to presence of lactic acid produced by lactobacilli.
- In young female, the vaginal pH is neutral, lined by simple cuboidal epithelium, colonized organism are same as skin commensals.
- At pubertal age due to estrogen effect, pH is between 3.5 and 4.5 lined by stratified squamous epithelium and colonized by lactobacilli predominantly.
- Once after menopause is attained the pH of the vagina rises to 7 with atrophic changes and again colonized organism are same as skin commensals.[3]
- Vaginitis includes the conditions associated with vulvovaginal symptoms.
- Common causes include bacterial vaginosis (BV) (40–45%), vulvovaginal candidiasis (20–25%) and trichomoniasis (15–25%).

Bacterial Vaginosis

- Also referred as *Gardnerella vaginitis* or nonspecific vaginitis.
- Most frequent cause causing vaginitis.
- Associated with changes in vaginal flora with increase in *Gardnerella vaginalis*, *Ureaplasma urealyticum*, *Mobiluncus* species, and *Mycoplasma hominis* along with reduction in lactobacilli.
- *Risk factors*:
  - Douching
  - Black race
  - Sexual intercourse at early age
  - Oral sex
  - Multiple sex partners
  - Sex during menses
  - Cigarette smoking.

- This is not an STD;[4] however, in case of recurrent BV possibility of sexual transmission may be considered.[5]
- *Clinical features*:
  - Asymptomatic in 50% of cases
  - Vaginal discharge which is creamy or grayish white with fishy odor
  - Neither associated with itching nor inflammation
  - Mostly occur during or immediately after menses.
- *Diagnosis*:
  - Wet mount:
    - Secretion from posterior fornix is taken
    - pH will be more than 4.5
    - Microscopy reveals lot of clue cells (epithelial cells covered with bacteria) in absence of leukocytes and they are the most reliable evidence suggesting BV
    - *Whiff test:* Mixture of KOH with vaginal discharge reveals a fishy odor due to amines
  - Amsel's criteria:
    - At least three among the four following features should be present to make diagnosis:
      1. pH of the vaginal secretion being more than 4.5
      2. Homogeneous, creamy or grayish white vaginal discharge
      3. Wet mount showing clue cells
      4. Positive whiff test
  - Nugent criteria:
    - Scored according to the microscopic examination of vaginal discharge using Gram stain
    - Scored as per the proportion of anaerobic species
    - Score of presence of bacterial vaginosis

TABLE 2: Treatment regimen for bacterial vaginosis.[4]

Main regimens	Metronidazole	500 mg two times a day for 7 days orally
	Metronidazole gel 0.75%	5 g once a day for 5 days intravaginally
	Clindamycin cream 2%	5 g at bedtime for 7 days intravaginally
Alternative regimens	Tinidazole	2 g daily for 3 days orally
	Clindamycin	300 mg two times a day for 7 days orally

- *Treatment*: The following are the treatment regimens for BV **(Table 2)**:
  - Cure rate with this regimen in 1 week is about 80–90%, but 30% reported recurrence with 3 months.
  - Not recommended to treat the male partner since it was not shown to improve the response to the treatment.

Vulvovaginal Candidiasis

- Accounts as a cause in about one-third of the cases of vaginitis.
- Rarely occur before menarche and in postmenopausal women. However, 50% of the female would have acquired by the age of 25 years.
- About 75% of women in premenopausal age group would have had at least one episode.
- *Candida albicans* is the most common organism causing infection. Other non-*albicans Candida* species includes *C. tropicalis, C. glabrata,* and *C. krusei.*
- May be sexually transmitted, orogenital sex and candidiasis was found to be associated.

- *Predisposing factors*:
  - Immunosuppression
  - Underlying dermatosis, e.g. eczema
  - On immunosuppressive drugs, e.g. steroids
  - Human immunodeficiency virus (HIV)
  - On broad-spectrum antibiotics
  - Using oral contraceptive pill in high doses
  - Pregnancy
  - Vaginal douching
- *Diagnosis*:
  - Clinical features:
    - Pruritus of the vulva and vagina
    - Burning sensation externally when they void due to exposure of inflammatory epithelium to urine
    - Whitish vaginal discharge described as cottage cheese-like
    - Vulval edema and erythema
    - Dyspareunia
  - Wet mount:
    - pH is normal (4–4.5)
    - Microscopic examination with saline or with 10% KOH shows presence of yeast buds or spore or hyphae
    - Sensitivity of KOH preparation is about 70% with negative result in 50% of the culture proven cases
- The vulvovaginal candidiasis is classified in **Table 3**.

TABLE 3: Classification of vulvovaginal candidiasis.[4]

Uncomplicated	Complicated
Sporadic occurrence	Recurrent infection
Candida albicans most likely cause	Non-*albicans Candida*
Mild to moderate type	Severe type
Occur in nonimmuno-compromised women	Occur in women with uncontrolled diabetes, pregnancy or with immunosuppression

- *Management*:
  - Improvement is noted within 2 days of starting the treatment
  - The clinical cure rate with treatment is more than 80%
  - There is no difference in outcome between different routes of administration of treatment
  - Uncomplicated cases:
    - Oral imidazole's includes:
      - Fluconazole 150 mg given as single dose
      - Itraconazole 200 mg taken as two times in a day
    - Topical application includes:
      - Clotrimazole given as single dose 500 mg or 100 mg pessary given as a course over 6 days
  - Complicated cases:
    - In cases with severe infection, treatment might be continued for 14 days to notice an improvement
  - Recurrent cases:
    - Infection is said to be recurrent if per year four episodes of infection occur or microscopy reveals moderate to heavy growth
    - Includes induction regimen and maintenance regimen
    - In induction regimen—Fluconazole 150 mg orally given as three doses 72 hours apart
    - In maintenance regimen—Fluconazole 150 mg given weekly once for 6 months.

Trichomonas Vaginitis

- It is sexually transmitted by flagellated protozoan parasite *Trichomonas vaginalis*
- Third most common cause of vaginitis
- Infects vagina, urethra, and paraurethral gland

- Often found along with BV in about 60% of cases
- Diagnosis:
  - Clinical features:
    - Presentation may vary from milder form to severe form[6]
    - Pruritus, soreness of vulva
    - Dysuria, dyspareunia
    - Thin frothy malodorous purulent vaginal discharge
    - Strawberry cervix (patchy erythema)
  - Wet mount:
    - Trichomonads is observed in only 50–70% of cases
    - Vaginal discharge pH is more than 5
    - Increased leukocytes along with motile trichomonads is seen on microscopy
- Treatment:
  - Metronidazole is the drug of choice to be prescribed and has a greater cure rate of about 95%
  - Primary therapy:[4]
    - Metronidazole 2 g single dose orally or
    - Tinidazole 2 g single dose orally
  - Alternative therapy:[4]
    - Metronidazole 500 mg two times a day for 7 days orally
    - Metronidazole gel is not preferred in treatment of this infection
    - Male partner should be treated
    - If no response to repeated treatment, should be referred for expert opinion.

Toxic Shock Syndrome

- Commonly seen in women of age group 15–30 years.
- Most common cause is due to usage of tampons and may be also be associated with use of diaphragm (female barrier contraceptive).
- The pathology occurs due to infection with *S. aureus* which liberates exotoxin causing the clinical features.
- Diagnostic criteria of toxic shock syndrome (TTS):
  - Major criteria:
    - Temperature (>38.8°C)
    - Hypotension
    - Diffuse macular erythroderma
    - Skin desquamation (hand, palm, and soles)
  - Minor criteria:
    - Low platelet count (<100,000 mm^3)
    - Acute respiratory distress
    - Deranged renal function test/liver function test
    - Hyperemia of mucous membrane
    - Diarrhea and vomiting
    - Altered consciousness.
- Main mode of treatment is supportive in intensive care unit.
- Remove the tampons, cotton tampons are safer.
- Intravenous fluid and dopamine infusion is used to correct hypotension and hypovolemia.
- Check serum electrolytes and blood coagulation parameters and correct accordingly.
- Treat with beta-lactamase resistant antistaphylococcal penicillin (clindamycin, oxacillin, and cloxacillin) for 10–14 days.
- Toxic shock syndrome mortality rate is about 6–10%.

INFECTIONS OF THE CERVIX

- Cervix is made up of squamous epithelium and glandular epithelium.
- Trichomonas, herpes simplex virus (HSV), and *Candida* causes ectocervical inflammation.

- *Chlamydia trachomatis* and *N. gonorrhoeae* infects only the endocervix (glandular epithelium).[7]
- Can be acute or chronic.

Neisseria Gonorrhoeae

- It is a gram-negative diplococcic
- Primary site of infection are endocervix, Bartholin gland, Skene gland, and urethra
- One-third of the women have associated chlamydial infection and they are at high risk for acquiring syphilis infection and other sexually transmitted infection (STI)
- Almost half of women are asymptomatic
- *Risk factors*:
  - Age < 25 years
  - Multiple sex partner
  - Drug user
  - Associated with other STI
  - Previous gonococcal infection
  - No barrier protection.
- *Clinical features*:
  - Present with lower reproductive tract symptoms either as vaginitis or cervicitis or with urinary symptoms like dysuria
  - Cervicitis present with odorless profuse white to yellow vaginal discharge
  - May ascend to endometrium and fallopian tube causing pelvic inflammatory disease (PID)
  - May present with features of perihepatitis.
- *Diagnosis*:
  - Nucleic acid amplification testing (NAAT) of endocervical discharge or urine is preferred method with sensitivity and specificity of 95%.
    - Presumptive diagnosis can be done initially by detection of gram-negative intracellular diplococcic following staining; further confirmation is done with growth of organism in Thayer-Martin medium.
- *Treatment*:
  - For women with uncomplicated gonococcal infection single dose treatment is recommended as following:[8]
    - Ceftriaxone 250 mg intramuscular with azithromycin 1 g once or
    - Doxycycline 100 mg orally two times a day for 7 days
  - If women has been treated with above, test of cure is not advised if it is uncomplicated gonococcal infection
  - Retesting after 3 months after initial treatment might be considered
  - Male partner should be treated simultaneously
  - To use barrier contraceptive until both partners are free from disease.

Chlamydial Infections

- The causative organism is *C. trachomatis*, it is an intracellular, obligate, gram-negative bacteria.
- Sexually transmitted infection with higher prevalence in developed countries compared to gonorrhea.
- Incubation period is longer (6–14 days) compared to gonorrhea (3–7 days).
- Infects the transitional and columnar epithelium of the genitourinary tract.
- *Clinical features*:
  - Mostly asymptomatic in about 75% of the cases as the lesions are superficial
  - Present with features of cervicitis like mucopurulent cervical discharge and urethral discharge.
- *Complications*:
  - Like gonorrhea, this can ascend to upper genital tract causing PID

- Tubal scarring leading to ectopic pregnancy and infertility
- Common cause of perihepatitis (Fitz-Hugh–Curtis syndrome).
- *Diagnosis*:
  - Sample for testing are taken from endocervical canal and urethra.
  - Nucleic acid amplification test and polymerase chain reaction (PCR) are more sensitive and specific (95%) to detect chlamydial infection. Preferred is first void urine sample.
  - Enzyme-linked immunosorbent assay (ELISA) technique is used to detect chlamydia antigen (lipopolysaccharide), but the sensitivity and specificity is less compared to NAAT.
  - Tissue culture (McCoy cell monolayers) can be used to detect chlamydia. This method has 100% specificity to detect bacteria.
- *Treatment*: The following treatment is recommended by oral route **(Table 4)**:[4]
  - Treat the sexual partner
  - If symptoms resolve after treatment, retesting is not required.

TABLE 4: Treatment regimen for chlamydial infections.

Primary treatment	Azithromycin	1 g single dose (or)
	Doxycycline	100 mg two times a day for 7 days
Alternative regimens	Erythromycin base	500 mg four times a day for 7 days (or)
	Erythromycin ethylsuccinate	800 mg four times a day for 7 days (or)
	Ofloxacin	300 mg two times a day for 7 days (or)
	Levofloxacin	500 mg once a day for 7 days

INFECTIONS OF THE UPPER GENITAL TRACT

Pelvic Inflammatory Disease or Disorders

- Spectrum of infections involving the upper female genital organs involving the fallopian tubes, ovaries, uterus, pelvic peritoneum, and the parametrium.
- Pelvic inflammatory disease is considered to be clinically significant disease due to following reasons:
  - Varied clinical presentation
  - Higher risk in young women
  - Long-term sequel.

Epidemiology

- Every year about more than 1 million women experience PID
- About 85% occur in sexually active women as spontaneous infection
- Remaining 15% occur following surgical procedures
- Two-thirds of the infections occur in age group of less than 25 years
- Teenage group females have a reduced hormonal defense to infections and are more prone to acquire the disease.

Risk Factors

- Previous acute PID
- Multiple sexual partners
- Teenage group
- Copper intrauterine device (IUD) users
- Not using contraception
- Lower socioeconomic status.

Microbiology

- Pelvic inflammatory disease occur mainly due to ascending infection from lower genital tract.
- The predominant organism causing PID are *N. gonorrhoeae* and *C. trachomatis*.
- However, the organism detected in acute PID cases are declining with about <50% cases showing the presence of either of the two organisms.
- Other causative organisms of PID are *Haemophilus influenzae, Gardnerella vaginalis, Mycoplasma hominis, Ureaplasma urealyticum, Cytomegalovirus*, and anaerobes such as *Bacteroides* and *Peptococcus* species.
- In 30–40% of the cases PID cause are detected to be polymicrobial.
- *Mycobacterium genitalium* was also detected to cause PID as per newer data.

Pathology

- Mostly there is bilateral tubal involvement
- Endosalpinx is primarily involved
- In severe cases all layers of tube might be involved and tube becomes hyperemic and edematous
- Exudate along with exfoliated cells may cause tubal blockage
- According to the virulence of the organism, the exudate can be watery (hydrosalpinx) or it can be purulent (pyosalpinx)
- The infection may resolve within 2–3 weeks and the resulting adhesions are not so dense since there is only little involvement of serous layer
- Exudate might pour into peritoneal cavity and might lead to pelvic abscess and tubo-ovarian abscess as well if ovary is involved
- According to severity of involvement of upper genital structures, acute PID can be graded as following:
    - Grade 1—uncomplicated—disease limited to fallopian tube ± peritonitis
    - Grade 2—complicated—presence of inflammatory mass ± peritonitis
    - Grade 3—distant spread beyond pelvis.

Clinical Presentation

Symptoms:
- Lower abdominal pain and pelvic pain
- Nausea, vomiting, fever, headache, and lassitude
- Purulent vaginal discharge
- Irregular vaginal bleeding if associated endometritis
- Dyspareunia
- In 5–10% of cases, right hypochondrial pain or discomfort is associated due to perihepatitis (Fitz-Hugh–Curtis syndrome)

Signs:
- Fever (temperature > 38.3°C)
- Lower abdominal tenderness (bilateral)
- Abnormal vaginal discharge
- Congested cervix with purulent discharge
- On bimanual examination—adnexal and cervical motion tenderness.

Diagnostic criteria for PID[4] are shown in **Table 5**.

Diagnosis

- *Detection of organism*: Material like discharge from cervical canal, Bartholin's gland, urethra or pus from fallopian tube detected during laparoscopy can be collected for diagnosis. They are subjected to Gram stain and culture (both anaerobe and aerobe), look for presence of organism.
- *Blood*: Look for leukocytosis and increased erythrocyte sedimentation rate (ESR) and C-reactive protein (CRP). Syphilis serology test to be done for both partners.
- *Sonology*: Fluid in pouch of Douglas, dilated fluid filled tubes, thickened tube

TABLE 5: Diagnostic criteria for pelvic inflammatory disease (PID).

Minimum criteria	• Tenderness in lower abdomen • Cervical motion tenderness • Tenderness in the adnexa
Additional criteria	• Febrile (temperature measured in oral cavity >38.3°C) • Microscopy of the discharge shows abundant white blood cells • Mucopurulent vaginal or cervical discharge • Increased erythrocyte sedimentation rate (ESR) and C-reactive protein • Detection of chlamydial or gonorrheal cervical infection in the laboratory
Definitive criteria	• Tubo-ovarian complex ± thickened fluid filled tube in imaging studies (ultrasound or MRI) • Evidence of endometritis on histopathological examination of the biopsy • Evidence of PID on laparoscopy

with incomplete septations, cogwheel appearance in cross section,[9] adnexal mass are the suggestive features of PID, but is of limited value. Might be helpful in obese women or in conditions where clinical examination is difficult.
- *Laparoscopy*: It is the most reliable method to diagnose PID, but not applicable in all women. The following are the laparoscopic finding correlating with severity of PID:
  - *Milder form*: Mobile edematous tubes without exudate
  - *Moderate form*: Tubes are not mobile with fimbrial end showing purulent exudate
  - *Severe form*: Tubo-ovarian mass/abscess and pyosalpinx
  - Violin string like adhesions around the liver and in the pelvis indicates chlamydial infection.
- *Endometrial biopsy*: In case of acute endometritis, polymorphonuclear leukocytes are detected whereas in women with chronic endometritis, plasma cells are detected. However, in the presence of mucopurulent discharge biopsy has no diagnostic value.[10]
- *Culdocentesis*: Peritoneal fluid aspiration shows white blood cell (WBC) >30,000/mL, it is suggestive feature of PID. Culture of the fluid might not be of much use since vaginal contamination is more likely.
- Investigation should be done in male partner such as smear and culture of the urethral secretion.

Differential Diagnosis

- Appendicitis
- Torsion ovarian cyst
- Ruptured ectopic pregnancy
- Diverticulitis
- Endometriosis
- Urinary tract infection.

Complications

- *Immediate*:
  - Peritonitis (generalized or localized to pelvis)
  - Septicemia
- *Late*:
  - Chronic pelvic pain (15–20%)
  - Pelvic adhesive disease
  - Infertility occurrence after one episode is 15%, two episodes is 35%, and following three episodes is 75%[11]
  - Increased risk of ectopic pregnancy of about 6- to 10-fold.

Management

- The main principle of the treatment is to control the spread of infection, to prevent reinfection, and late complications.

Chapter 10: Infections

- In mild to moderate cases, compared to inpatient therapy outpatient therapy has similar clinical outcomes.

Outpatient therapy:
- Advice adequate rest and analgesic.
- Prescribe combination of antibiotic as the infection is mostly polymicrobial and start them even before getting the microbiological reports.
- Treated outpatient patients should be reviewed 48 hours later. Look for signs of clinical improvement, if not hospitalize the patient. The treatment regimen for PID as outpatient care is given in **Box 1**.
- As part of outpatient treatment, initial dose of parental antibiotic might be helpful.[12]

Inpatient therapy: Indication for hospitalization is as follows:
- Severe illness with fever (temperature >38°C) and vomiting
- Suspected tubo-ovarian abscess
- Intolerant to oral antibiotic
- No response to outpatient treatment for 48 hours
- If surgical emergencies cannot be ruled out
- Coexisting with HIV infection or pregnancy

- Advice bed rest, restrict the oral intake, and correct dehydration and acidosis.

The recommended inpatient antibiotic therapy is as follows in **Table 6**.

After commencement continue the intravenous antibiotic therapy for at least 48 hours, but might be continued up to 4 days according to the clinical improvement.

Indications for Surgery

Surgery is considered in following conditions:
- Tubo-ovarian abscess
- Pelvic abscess
- Generalized peritonitis.

Precautions to Prevent Reinfection

- Advised to use barrier contraceptive
- Avoid multiple sex partners
- Sexual partner should be investigated and treated. In presence of nongonococcal urethritis, doxycycline 100 mg twice daily or tetracycline 500 mg 6th hourly given for total of 7 days.

BOX 1: Treatment regimen used in outpatient care.

- Ceftriaxone 250 mg intramuscular (IM) once daily (plus)
- Doxycycline 100 mg two times a day orally for 14 days (with/without)
- Metronidazole 500 mg two times a day for 14 days
- Cefoxitin 2 g IM with 1 g probenecid orally once day (plus)
- Doxycycline 100 mg same dose as above (with/without)
- Metronidazole 500 mg same dose as above
- Other third-generation cephalosporin given as single dose intramuscularly (plus)
- Doxycycline 100 mg same as above dose (with/without)
- Metronidazole same as above dose

TABLE 6: Treatment regimen used in inpatient care.

Regimen A	• Cefotetan 2 g every 12 hours by intravenous (IV) route (or) • Cefoxitin 2 g every 6 hours by IV route (plus) • Doxycycline 100 mg IV or orally every 12 hours
Regimen B	• Clindamycin 900 mg every 8 hours by IV route (plus) • Gentamycin loading dose 2 mg/kg IV/IM (intramuscular) followed by 1.5 mg/kg every 8 hours as maintenance dose (3–5 mg/kg per day given as single dose may be given)
Alternative regimen	• Ampicillin/sulbactam 3 g every 6 hours given by IV route (plus) • Doxycycline given same as above

Follow-up

- After full course of treatment repeat smear and culture are done after 7 days after discharge.
- Until three consecutive negative reports the test should be performed after every menstrual cycle
- Advised to avoid intercourse until patient and the partner is treated.

Genital Tuberculosis

It is recognized as clinical entity in 1000 BC. Discovered first by Morgagni 1744 following postmortem examination of a young woman whose tubes and uterus were studded with caseous material.

Incidence

In infertility clinic worldwide the incidence is 5% and in India it is about 19%. About 5–13% women with pulmonary tuberculosis (TB) develop into genital TB. About 80–90% of the cases occur in age group of 20–40 years. Genital TB in women with surgically removed adnexa 2–20%.

Causative Organism

Mycobacterium tuberculosis and occasionally *Mycobacterium bovis*. It is a gram-positive *Bacillus* which is both acid and alcohol fast due to presence of mycolic acid in cell wall. It is an obligate aerobe nonsparing, nonmotile, and with no capsule. It has a slow generation time of about 17–24 hours.

Pathogenesis

The disease occurs almost always secondary. Usually pulmonary infections are the primary site to be involved. Almost all organs are susceptible to TB infection. If close to menarche primary infection occurs then there is higher chance of genital TB.[13] In early stage if the primary infections are not eradicated there is chance that it is more likely to get reactivated later in case of immunocompromised state.

Mode of Spread

- *Hematogenous*: Fallopian tube is the most common site to be affected and earliest lesions are found in the mucosa. From tubes dissemination of the infection occurs to other genital organs and the peritoneum.
- *Lymphatic*: Mainly happens if primary lesions are present in abdominal cavity.
- Direct spread occurs from tuberculosis abdominal viscera, such as the bladder and rectum.

Genital Organs

Frequency of genital organ involvement is as follows: Fallopian tubes 90–100%, endometrium 50–60%, ovaries 20–30%, cervix 5–15%, and vulva and vagina 1%.[14]

Tuberculosis of pelvis: Pelvic TB and genital TB are not the same. May present as tuberculosis adenitis involving either pelvic or mesenteric lymph node. May also present as generalized miliary peritoneal TB.

Tuberculosis of fallopian tube: TB salpingitis can present in any of these forms. The most common is endosalpingitis. Other forms are exosalpingitis, salpingitis isthmica nodosa, and interstitial salpingitis. The earliest and most commonly affected part is ampulla. The fimbrial end might become swollen and tubal ostia might remain open or closed. Gross appearance may show like tobacco pouch appearance or present as productive adhesive form.

Tuberculosis of the endometrium: Uterus size and shape are not affected. Fundus is extensively involved. There is no involvement of myometrium. During menstruation the infected issue is shed off, but gets reinfected from tubes. Cases with extensive involvement present as secondary amenorrhea due to intrauterine adhesions[15] or present as pyometra with occluded internal os. Noncaseating granulomas are the classic lesion of tuberculosis endometritis. Lesions are best detected within 12 hours of menses onset or on day 24–26.[16]

Tuberculosis of the ovary: Can present as two forms either as perioophoritis and oophoritis.

Clinical Presentation

Symptoms: Menstrual disturbances (menorrhagia, oligomenorrhea, and amenorrhea), infertility, abdominal pain, abdominal swelling, vaginal discharge, postcoital bleeding, and dyspareunia.

Signs: In about 30–50% of cases no signs are found. May present with abdominal/pelvic mass with tenderness, ascites, excessive vaginal discharge, genital ulcer, enlarged uterus (pyometra), and fistula (between the genital tract and the bowel, bladder, or cutaneous area).[17]

Diagnosis

Suspect TB in following situations:[18]
- Women with unexplained infertility along with personal or family history of TB
- Lower abdominal discomfort along with persistent ill health or low grade fever over a period of time and also associated with weight loss
- Abdominal pain, ascites, and low grade fever in an adolescent female
- Tense, tender, enlarged uterus (pyometra) in menopausal women
- Recurrent PID not responding to antibiotic therapy.

Investigations

Investigation include following:
- *Imaging modalities*: Ultrasonography (USG) and hysterosalpingogram (HSG)
- *Microbiology*: Mantoux, QuantiFERON-TB Gold, microscopy, culture, molecular tests—Gen-probe/PCR
- *Surgical diagnosis*: Laparoscopy and hysteroscopy
- Nonspecific—X-ray and hematology
- Active disease can be detected in following ways such as clinical suspicion and response to treatment, acid-fast bacillus (AFB) staining, culture, histopathology, nucleic acid amplification test, USG, CT scan, laparoscopy, and hysteroscopy
- Test to detect latent TB includes Mantoux Tuberculin skin test and QuantiFERON-TB Gold.

Hysterosalpingogram: It should not be performed in presence of active infection. Presentation of tubal involvement presents as tubal occlusion, tubal dilatation, hydrosalpinx, diverticular outpouching, peritubal adhesions, and they appear as pipestem tube, beaded tube, tobacco pouch, cobblestone tube, corkscrew appearance, peritubal halo.[19]

Presentation of uterine involvement appears with T-shaped uterus, pseudo-unicornuate uterus, obliteration of uterine cavity, distorted uterine contour, and venous and lymphatic intravasation.[20]

Ultrasound: Tubes appear with clear fluid or thick material with dilatation and thickened wall.[21] Heterogeneous endometrium with hyperechoic areas, intrauterine adhesions and persistently thin endometrium are features present when uterus is affected.

Laparoscopy and hysteroscopy: Combined procedure aids in diagnosis as well as therapeutic interventions if necessary in case of endometrial involvement presenting with intrauterine adhesions and pale endometrium.[22] Finding usually found in laparoscopy are tubercles on tubal surface, tubal beading, fimbrial phimosis or block, periovarian or peritubal adhesions, tubo-ovarian mass, rigid tubes, and hydrosalpinx.

Histopathology: Granulomatous caseous lesions are typical features of TB. In early stage, occasional noncaseating granulomas are present and in late stage multiple epithelioid granulomas in lamina propria are seen. Specimen should be taken from multiple sites.[23] Late secretory phase of the menstrual cycle is the ideal time to take endometrial sample.[24]

Bacteriological Evaluation

Acid-fast Bacillus staining and culture:
- Isolation of TB bacilli makes a definitive diagnosis of TB.
- Usually used stains are acid-fast or fluorescent stains. Ziehl-Neelsen (ZN) and Kinyoun are the acid-fast stains. Fluorescent stains are auramine and rhodamine. 10^4–10^6 bacilli/mL is required for staining result to become positive.
- Culture test is more sensitive and requires 10–100 bacilli/mL to make diagnosis.[24] On day 1 of menstruation, menstrual blood can be collected and used to make diagnosis.[25]

Culture methods:
- Egg-based Löwenstein-Jensen (LJ) medium and Middlebrook 7H10 medium agar based are the solid culture media used.
- BACTEC Mycobacterial Growth Indicator Tube 960 (MGIT 960) automated liquid culture media based on oxygen sensitive fluorescence in Middlebrook 7H9 broth.[26]
- Longer time is required to make a diagnosis with positive result using liquid culture media. It takes about 9–10 days and about 4–8 weeks to get positive result with solid media.[24]

Molecular methods: PCR assays detect both live and dead bacilli, can detect <10 bacilli/mL. Testing time of PCR is 8–12 hours.[27] PCR has higher sensitivity and specificity is about 100%.[28] PCR has high false positivity, so antituberculous treatment (ATT) should not be initiated based on positive PCR alone.[29]

Nucleic acid amplification test (NAAT) has high specificity and detects TB by amplifying target nucleic acid sequences. Two direct NAAT are available such as Gen-Probe *M. tuberculosis* Direct (MTD) test and Roche Amplicor *M. Tuberculosis* test. Amplicor test is a PCR-based test that amplifies *M. tuberculosis* deoxyribonucleic acid (DNA). Gen-Probe MTD amplifies *M. tuberculosis* ribosomal ribonucleic acid (rRNA). The Gen-Probe MTD test takes only 3 hours to perform.

GeneXpert is a real-time PCR-based molecular testing. It is an automated diagnostic test that can detect MTB and resistance to rifampicin (RIF) within 2 hours time frame.[30]

Mantoux test: It is a test based on delayed hypersensitivity reaction. A standard dose of five tuberculin units (TU) (0.1 mL) is injected intradermally (into the skin) and read 48–72 hours later. A discrete, pale elevation of the skin (a wheal) 6–10 mm in diameter should be produced when the injection is given correctly. The volar aspect of the left forearm is the preferred site of test. Sensitivity and specificity of the test in cases with laparoscopically proven diagnosis is about 55–80%.[31]

QuantiFERON-TB Gold (QFT-G): It is a type of interferon-gamma (IFN-gamma) release assay. Whole blood is incubated with antigens and then this test is performed on sensitized white cells. Value more than 0.35 IU/mL is considered positive.

In cases of latent genital TB, QFT-G along with PCR can be used to diagnose as well as monitor the therapeutic response to ATT in women. A negative result predicts the response after therapy.[32]

Nonspecific Tests

- Complete hemogram may show anemia, leukocytosis with lymphocytosis, and raised ESR.
- Chest X-ray (posteroanterior film) should be performed to exclude or confirm coexisting respiratory TB or old stigmata of previous pulmonary TB.

Complications

Subfertility and infertility: Residual damage of the fallopian tubes is often irreversible even following medical regimens, unless genital TB is diagnosed and treated early in its course.

Ectopic pregnancy: Risk following medical treatment is estimated to be 33–72%.

Congenital TB: Rare but potentially serious complication. Overwhelming systemic infection in the newborn has considerable morbidity and mortality.

Management

Once diagnosed must consider following points, such as:
- Rule out active TB at any other site.
- Know the extent of genital lesion.
- Will medical management cure the lesion?
- Is pregnancy possible following treatment?

Medical treatment:
- It is easier to treat these cases because they are paucibacillary
- Three basic principles for chemotherapy for TB are as follows:
  1. Regimen must contain multiple drugs to which organism is susceptible
  2. Drugs are to be taken regularly
  3. Drugs should continue for a sufficient period of time
- TB patients are classified into two groups based on the history of previous treatment such as "New" or "Previously Treated"
- New patients are with no prior history treatment for TB or anti-TB drugs was taken for less than 1 month (regardless of whether their smear or culture result)
- The anti-TB drugs used are tabulated in Table 7.

Fixed dose combination (FDC) of drug was equally effective as compared to single pills and was more accepted by patients.[33]

The FDC kits are available as AKT-4 (isoniazid, rifampicin, pyrazinamide, and ethambutol), AKT-3 (isoniazid, rifampicin, and ethambutol), and AKT-2 (isoniazid and rifampicin).

New patient:
- Treatment given for total of 6 months
- Intensive phase therapy for 2 months with HRZE

TABLE 7: Antituberculosis drugs.

Drugs	Category	Dose (mg/kg body weight/day)	Side effects
Isoniazid (H)	B	5	Hepatitis, peripheral neuropathy
Rifampicin (R)	C	10	Hepatitis, flu-like syndrome, rashes, orange colored urine
Pyrazinamide (Z)	C	25	Hepatitis, hyperuricemia
Ethambutol (E)	B	15	Optic neuritis
Streptomycin (S)	D	15	Ototoxicity, renal toxicity

- Continuation phase therapy for 6 months with HR
- Can be used each drug three times a week or as fixed dosage kits

Treated patient (either with relapse or failure):
- Treatment given for total of 8 months
- Intensive phase therapy for 2 months with HRZE + S and 1 month with HRZE
- Continuation phase therapy for 5 months with HRE
- Can be used each drug three times a week or as fixed dosage kits.

Surgical treatment: The following are the indications:
- Persistent and recurrent disease/pelvic masses or pain despite adequate treatment
- Persistent nonhealing fistula
- Multidrug-resistant disease
- Concomitant neoplasia of genital tract.

Chemotherapy should precede surgery by 1–2 weeks. Surgery should be done at midcycle in premenopausal women. Chemotherapy should be continued for 6–12 months in the postoperative period. In premenopausal women save ovaries if normal, otherwise total hysterectomy with bilateral salpingo-oophorectomy should be done followed by hormone replacement therapy (HRT).

Failure to conceive even after 6 months of ATT, laparoscopy and hysteroscopy may be repeated to see any remaining disease. After ATT, tuboplasty is of not much help however associated with chances of flare-up and increased risk of ectopic pregnancy.[34]

SEXUALLY TRANSMITTED INFECTIONS

Sexually transmitted diseases include variety of clinical infections and syndromes caused the pathogens that are transmitted by sexual activity. The following infections are sexually transmitted:
- Gonorrhea
- Chlamydial infections
- Bacterial vaginosis
- Syphilis
- Herpes genitalis
- Human immunodeficiency virus
- Chancroid
- Lymphogranuloma venereum (LGV)
- Granuloma inguinale (donovanosis)
- Molluscum contagiosum
- Condyloma acuminate
- Scabies.

Clinical prevention guidance for STD are:[35]
- Assess the risk and educate the person at risk to avoid STDs to modify the sexual behaviors and use prevention services
- For preventable STDs advice to have pre-exposure vaccination for at risk persons
- Identifying both symptomatic and asymptomatic women with infections
- Effective counseling, treatment, and follow-up of women with STD
- Evaluate and treat the sex partners.

Syphilis

Systemic disease caused by spirocheta and *Treponema pallidum*
- Presents at various stages based on clinical presentation
- Primary syphilis presents with chancre or ulcer at the site of infection
- Secondary syphilis occurs within 6 weeks to 6 months after onset of primary infection. Includes mucocutaneous lesions, skin rashes, and lymphadenopathy
- Latent syphilis is a quiescence phase with no clinical manifestation, can be detected only by serology test
- Tertiary syphilis includes gummatous and cardiac lesions, aortic aneurysm, tabes dorsalis, and general paresis due to neurologic involvement.

Diagnosis

- The definitive method to detect the organism is by darkfield microscopy, sample for examination taken from lesion exudate or tissue.[36]
- For presumptive diagnosis two serologic tests are required such as a nontreponemal test and a treponemal test.
- Nontreponemal test includes venereal disease research laboratory (VDRL) or rapid plasma reagin (RPR).
- Treponemal test includes fluorescent treponemal antibody-absorbed (FTA-ABS) tests, various enzyme immunoassays (EIAs) and *T. pallidum* passive particle agglutination (TP-PA) assay.
- Venereal disease research laboratory is positive after 6 weeks of primary infection. Various medical conditions, autoimmune conditions, pregnancy, immunizations, and injection drug use are associated with false-positive nontreponemal test.[37]
- Women with reactive treponemal tests for remaining life will have reactive test. However, 15–25% treated might revert to being nonreactive after 2–3 years.[38]
- Treponemal EIA tests have high quantitative index values which correlate with TP-PA positivity; however, the clinical benefit of this finding needs further investigation.[39,40]
- Neurosyphilis diagnosis depends on a combination of cerebrospinal fluid (CSF) tests (reactive CSF-VDRL and CSF cell count or protein), reactive serologic test, and along with clinical features suggesting neurologic involvement.

Treatment

Parenterally administered penicillin G is the drug recommended in all stages of syphilis. The preparation used, length and dosage of treatment varies according to clinical manifestations and stage of the disease.[4] The treatment regimen are given in **Table 8**.

Penicillin allergy:
- Doxycycline 100 mg orally twice daily and tetracycline 500 mg four times daily for 14 days are used widely.[41]
- For primary and secondary syphilis, azithromycin 2 g as a single oral dose has been recommended.[42]
- In women with latent syphilis the only recommended regimen is doxycycline or tetracycline given for 28 days as same previous mentioned dosage.

Follow-up

- After treatment of early syphilis serologic test should be done at 1, 3, and 12 months.
- In women with late stages, annual serologic tests are done lifelong.

Human Immunodeficiency Virus and Acquired Immunodeficiency Syndrome

Virus

Human immunodeficiency virus belongs to retrovirus family. It is double-stranded RNA virus. Two strains are there; HIV-1 and HIV-2. It has reverse transcriptase enzyme which gets viral RNA to transcribe into DNA and it gets into host cell genome causing chronic infection. Has core protein (p24) and glycoprotein envelope (gp120 and gp41). Acquired immunodeficiency syndrome (AIDS) occurs at later stage and it develops over months to years with approximately over 11-year period.[43]

Incidence

Acquired immunodeficiency syndrome diagnoses made at or within 12 months of their HIV diagnosis is about 32%.[44] Only 45%

TABLE 8: Treatment regimen for syphilis.

Stage of disease	Without HIV	With HIV
Primary and secondary	Benzathine penicillin G 2.4 million units as single dose by intramuscular route	Benzathine penicillin G 2.4 million units as single dose by intramuscular route
Early latent	Benzathine penicillin G 2.4 million units as single dose by intramuscular route	Benzathine penicillin G 2.4 million units as single dose by intramuscular route
Late latent	Benzathine penicillin G 7.2 million units given as weekly once 2.4 million units as three doses by intramuscular route	Benzathine penicillin G 7.2 million units given as weekly once 2.4 million units as three doses by intramuscular route
Tertiary	With normal CSF test: • Benzathine penicillin G 7.2 million units given as weekly once 2.4 million units as three doses by intramuscular route Neurosyphilis: • Aqueous crystalline penicillin G 18–24 million units daily given as 3–4 million units 4 hours once by IV or for 10–14 days as continuous infusion • Procaine penicillin G 2.4 million units IM once daily plus probenecid 500 mg orally four times a day, both for 10–14 days	Same as non-HIV infected

(HIV: human immunodeficiency virus; IM: intramuscular; IV: intravenous)

of adults between the age group of 18–64 years had been tested.[45] Approximately 41% of newly diagnosed cases had never been tested previously.[46]

Route of Transmission

- Sexual intercourse—male to female transmission is high
- Transfusion of infected blood products
- Intravenous drug users
- Needlestick injury with contaminated needle
- Perinatal transmission
- Breastfeeding.

Pathogenesis and Clinical Presentation

Human immunodeficiency virus targets the CD4 receptor molecules present on cells of immune system. As $CD4^+$ lymphocytes are depleted, there occurs profound immunosuppression. Count of 200–500 cells/mm^3 have symptoms and <200 cells/mm^3 have AIDS defining criteria.

Antibodies are developed within 8–12 weeks of infection. Present with flu-like syndrome. In 50–90% of persons with infection, acute retroviral syndrome occurs within few weeks.[47] Highly infectious during this period, the concentration of virus is very high in plasma and genital secretions.[48] Takes about 8–10 years to develop AIDS. AIDS-related complex (ARC) patients present nonspecific features like fever, diarrhea, weight loss, orogenital candidiasis, ulcers in oral or genital area, thrombocytopenia and tubo-ovarian abscess.

Chapter 10: Infections

Diagnosis of Human Immunodeficiency Virus

Serologic tests to detect antibodies against HIV-1 and HIV-2 are used; however, most often used are HIV type 1 antibody test. IgG antibody to gp120 is commonly used to detect the infection. Begins with screening test such as ELISA or rapid assay. Confirmed with western blot. HIV-1/HIV-2 antigen-antibody immunoassay if reactive should be followed by an HIV-1/HIV-2 antibody differentiation assay to confirm the diagnosis.[49] However, HIV RNA by PCR is the gold standard method used for diagnosis. Women diagnosed with any STD in particular genital ulcer should be offered HIV testing.[50]

Preventive Measures

- Health education regarding safe sex practices
- Male circumcision reduces half of the transmission
- Levonorgestrel intrauterine system (LNG-IUS) with condom
- Blunt stick needles to avoid injury
- Screening the donor and to transfuse HIV-negative blood
- In cases with artificial donor insemination use HIV-negative frozen semen
- Avoid breastfeeding
- Postexposure prophylaxis (PEP)
- Strict protocol to handle the body fluids.

Treatment

- Initiate antiretroviral therapy (ART) after considering clinical condition, HIV RNA viral load and CD4$^+$ T cell count.
- Primary goal is to maximize the viral load suppression, restore the immune function, and restore HIV-related mortality and morbidity.
- Treatment should be offered if plasma HIV RNA level is more than 100,000 copies/mL or CD4$^+$ T cells less than 350. And also women with symptoms, those with 6 months of seroconversion and with acute retroviral syndrome should be offered treatment.[51]
- Antiretroviral drugs are grouped as:
  - Nucleoside reverse transcriptase inhibitors (NRTIs)—zidovudine, lamivudine, abacavir, zalcitabine
  - Non-nucleoside reverse transcriptase inhibitors (NNRTIs)—nevirapine, efavirenz, and delavirdine
  - Protease inhibitor (PI)—indinavir, ritonavir, and saquinavir
  - Entry inhibitor—enfuvirtide
  - Integrase inhibitor—raltegravir.
- Antiretroviral drugs preferred are two nucleoside regimen with either non-nucleoside reverse transcriptase inhibitor or protease inhibitor.
- Combination therapy is preferred over monotherapy and known as highly active antiretroviral therapy (HAART).
- Women with CD4$^+$ count of less than 200 must receive prophylaxis for opportunistic infections.[51]
- With treatment the viral load decreases to less than 50 copies/mL and CD4$^+$ count rises.
- *Pre-exposure prophylaxis (PrEP):* Combination of tenofovir and emtricitabine is used. Observed reduction in HIV transmission of up to 92% reduction in high risk cases.[52]
- *Postexposure prophylaxis (PEP):* It is used in emergency situations. Started as soon as possible, always within 72 hours after an exposure. The first dose preferably should be taken within 2 hours to be more effective. Medicines are taken every day

for 28 days. Preferred regimen includes tenofovir + emtricitabine plus raltegravir. Zidovudine and lamivudine can be used but zidovudine is no longer recommended as preferred regimen.

Herpes Genitalis

It is a lifelong chronic viral infection. It is caused by two types of HSV: HSV-1 and HSV-2. Recurrent infections are mostly due to HSV-2 and approximately 50 million are affected with this type of virus,[53] but anogenital herpes are mostly affected by HSV-1 infection.[54]

Clinical Features

About 2–14 days is the incubation period. Inflamed painful areas appear in the genitals initially. Subsequently multiple vesicles appear which progress into ulcers, which are multiple and shallow and heal with crusting. Multiple vesicles are associated with constitutional symptoms and inguinal lymphadenopathy. Subclinical shedding and recurrences are more common with HSV-2 infection.[55]

Diagnosis

Prognosis of the patient and counseling depends on the type of infection either by HSV-1 or HSV-2, henceforth clinical diagnosis should be confirmed by laboratory testing of type specific causing genital herpes.[56] Tissue culture and isolation of virus is more specific. ELISA or immunofluorescent method can be used to detect the virus. At low index values HerpeSelect HSV-2 might be falsely positive,[57] should be confirmed by western blot.[58] But the more sensitive and specific test is PCR to identify HSV DNA.[59] Sensitivity of direct immunofluorescence (IF) assay is less in spite of its availability to detect HSV antigen.[60]

Treatment (Table 9)

Antiviral chemotherapy is the mainstay of treatment. Three drugs have been shown to be effective such as acyclovir, famciclovir, and valacyclovir.[61]

In cases with severe disease, intravenous acyclovir is recommended followed by oral ART up to 10 days. Intravenous acyclovir is continued for 21 days in case of HSV encephalitis.

Granuloma Inguinale (Donovanosis)

It is a ulcerative genital disease caused by *Klebsiella granulomatis* (also known as *Calymmatobacterium granulomatis*).

Clinical Features

Present with slowly progressive painless ulcer on genital or perineum. Pseudobuboes may occur. They are highly vascular lesions might develop secondary bacterial infection. Extragenital infections might coexist.

Diagnosis

Direct visualization of dark-staining Donovan bodies within mononuclear cells is required to make a diagnosis. No molecular tests for the detection of infection DNA exist.

Treatment (Table 10)

With the treatment the ulcer heals, but prolonged treatment is recommended. Relapse will occur 6–12 months after treatment.

If no improvement, addition of antibiotic might be helpful. Examination and treatment of sex partner is recommended.

Lymphogranuloma Venereum

Caused by *C. trachomatis* L serovars L1, L2, and L3.[62]

Chapter 10: Infections

TABLE 9: Treatment of herpes genitalis.

Initial therapy	Suppressive therapy	Recurrent therapy
Acyclovir 400 mg for 7–10 days given as thrice a day orally OR Acyclovir 200 mg for 7–10 days given as five times a day orally OR Valacyclovir 1 g two times a day orally for 7–10 days OR Famciclovir 250 mg for 7–10 days orally thrice a day	Acyclovir 400 mg two times a day orally OR Valacyclovir 500 mg once a day orally OR Valacyclovir 1 g once a day orally OR Famciclovir 250 mg two times a day orally	Acyclovir 400 mg for 5 days thrice a day orally OR Acyclovir 800 mg for 5 days orally OR Acyclovir 800 mg for 2 days thrice a day orally OR Valacyclovir 500 mg for 3 days two times a day OR Valacyclovir 1 g for 5 days once a day orally OR Famciclovir 125 mg for 5 days twice a day orally OR Famciclovir 1 g for 1 day two times a day orally OR Famciclovir 500 mg once, followed by 250 mg twice daily for 2 days
In case with incomplete healing extend the treatment after 10 days	Compared to other dosing regimens, valacyclovir 500 mg once a day has lower efficacy in recurrent patients	

TABLE 10: Treatment of granuloma inguinale.

Recommended treatment	Azithromycin 1 g weekly once orally or 500 mg given once a day for 3 weeks, continued till lesions are completely healed
Alternative treatment	Doxycycline 100 mg given for at least 3 weeks as twice a day orally, continued till lesions are completely healed OR Ciprofloxacin 750 mg given for at least 3 weeks as twice a day orally, continued till lesions are completely healed OR Erythromycin base 500 mg given for at least 3 weeks as four times a day orally, continued till lesions are completely healed OR Trimethoprim-sulfamethoxazole one double-strength (160 mg/800 mg) tablet given for at least 3 weeks as twice a day orally, continued till lesions are completely healed

Clinical Features

Initially present with painless papule or ulcer in vulva, cervix, urethra or rectum. Unilateral inguinofemoral lymph nodes are involved. Present as acute adenitis, bubo formation might occur. Painful lymphadenopathy occurs later. Groove sign, a depression between the lymph node groups is the classical feature.

TABLE 11: Treatment of lymphogranuloma venereum.	
Recommended treatment	Doxycycline 100 mg for 21 days, twice a day
Alternate treatment	Erythromycin base 500 mg for 21 days, four times a day

Diagnosis

Based on clinical features and by excluding other etiology for signs diagnosis is made. Confirmatory diagnosis is by culture and isolation of LGV. Detect the LGV antigens by IF assay or ELISA examining the specimen from rectum, genital lesions or bubo aspirates.[63] NAAT done with rectal specimens is the preferred. Intradermal Frei test is nonspecific. *C. trachomatis* serologic tests are not recommended.

Treatment

Tissue damage is prevented by treatment. Buboes are aspirated. The following treatment is recommended as presented in **Table 11**.

The partner should be examined and should be presumptively treated.

Chancroid

Caused by *Haemophilus ducreyi* and gram-negative *Streptobacillus*. It is a risk factor for HIV transmission and acquisition.[64]

Clinical Features

Initially present as tender multiple vesiculo-pustular lesions and later forms an ulcer. It is associated with unilateral inguinal lympha-denitis.

Diagnosis

First rule out syphilis before making diagnosis. Painful genital ulcer with tender inguinal adenopathy suggests chancroid.[65] However, confirmatory diagnosis is by demonstration of bacteria in specialized culture media.

Treatment

Successful treatment cures the infection and prevents transmission. In advanced cases, scarring can result. Recommended regimens are azithromycin 1 g orally in a single dose or ceftriaxone 250 mg IM in a single dose or ciprofloxacin 500 mg orally twice a day for 3 days or erythromycin base 500 mg orally three times a day for 7 days.

Genital Warts (Condyloma Acuminata)

Although 100 types of human papilloma virus (HPV) has been identifies, only 40 affects genital area.[66] Caused by low risk and nononcogenic HPV type 6 and 11. Appear as multiple papillary lesions, can be transmitted by sexual route. Lesions have a cauliflower appearance. May be associated with other oncogenic high risk HPV types such as 16, 18, 45, and 56.

Diagnosis

About 3–5% acetic acid will cause affected areas to turn white, but the routine use of this to detect mucosal changes is not recommended.

Prevention

Cervarix and Gardasil are the two vaccines available. Cervarix is bivalent that prevent HVP type 16 and 18 infection. Gardasil is quadrivalent vaccine that prevents infection with HPV type 6, 11, 16, and 18. Given as three doses over a period of 6 months. Recommended age group to vaccinate is 11–12 years, but can be administered from 9 years.[67] Vaccine can prevent 90% of genital warts.

Treatment

Cryotherapy with liquid nitrogen, topical use of trichloroacetic acid, imiquimod cream, photodynamic therapy or laser therapy are recommended.

Molluscum Contagiosum

It is caused by pox virus. Appear as small multiple pearly white, dome-shaped, and umbilicated lesions affecting genitals and other areas in the skin. On Giemsa stain molluscum bodies, inclusion bodies in the cytoplasm of affected cell are seen under microscopy.

Treatment

Under local anesthesia evacuate the content from the nodule and treat the floor of the nodule with 85% trichloroacetic acid solution or ferric subsulfate. Cryotherapy can be applied on the lesion.

Scabies

It is caused by Sarcoptes scabiei. It is associated with intense itching and excoriation of the skin. Apply below neck all over the body 5% permethrin cream or 0.5% malathion aguan solution and washed after 12–14 hours. Can also apply 25% benzyl benzoate emulsion. Treat the family members also simultaneously.

URINARY TRACT INFECTIONS

Acute Cystitis

- Presents with onset of dysuria, urgency, frequency associated with low back ache or suprapubic pain with suprapubic tenderness.
- Risk factors include use of diaphragm and spermicide, sexual intercourse, history of recent urinary tract infection, and delayed postcoital micturition.[68]
- Urinalysis reveals pyuria detected by microscopy or leukocyte esterase test and in some cases hematuria. Almost in 80% of cases *E. coli* is isolated and in about 5–15% of women *Staphylococcus saprophyticus* is isolated.
- In uncomplicated cystitis, nitrofurantoin 100 mg two times a day orally for 7 days or ciprofloxacin 250 mg two times a day orally for 3 days are recommended.[69]
- The resistance to trimethoprim and trimethoprim-sulfamethoxazole is on increasing trend.
- No follow-up or urine culture is required unless the symptoms recur or persist.

Recurrent Cystitis

- Twenty percent have recurrent infection in premenopausal age group and about more than 90% are due to exogenous reinfection.
- Urine culture is mandatory to rule out resistant organism.
- Can manage with the following treatment:
  - Postcoital prophylaxis
  - Continuous prophylaxis
  - At the starting of symptoms only initiate the treatment.
- In postmenopausal women hormonal therapy along with antimicrobial prophylaxis is helpful.

Urethritis

- Present with gradual onset dysuria along with abnormal vaginal discharge, lower abdominal pain if associated cervicitis.
- Examination reveals mucopurulent cervicitis or vulvovaginitis.
- Caused mainly by *C. trachomatis* and *N. gonorrhoeae*.

- Treat with regimen for chlamydial or gonococcal infection.

Acute Pyelonephritis

- Presentation might vary from cystitis like illness to gram-negative septicemia.
- In more than 80% of cases the causative organism is *E. coli*.[70]
- In all cases urine culture is mandatory and blood culture can be considered in hospitalized patients.
- If milder illness with no nausea or vomiting, outpatient oral therapy is recommended.
- In women with severe illness or pregnancy, women should be hospitalized.
- Trimethoprim-sulfamethoxazole or quinolones are given for 10–14 days as outpatient treatment.
- In case of severe illness parental ceftriaxone, ampicillin, and gentamycin are recommended. If flank pain or fever persists after 72 hours, do computed tomography (CT) or USG to rule out renal abscess or obstruction in urethra.
- After treatment completion follow-up culture done after 2 weeks.[70]

■ CONCLUSION

- Most appropriate treatment approach for genitourinary infections can be implemented with aim to reduce further long-term sequelae.
- Vulval abscess mainly caused by *Staphylococcus*, *Enterococcus* species, group B *Streptococcus*, and *E. coli*.
- The end result of acute infection involving the Bartholin gland includes either complete resolution, cyst formation, abscess formation or recurrence.
- Bartholin abscess presents as tender swelling unilaterally in posterior part of labia majora extending up to labia minora.
- Bacterial vaginosis is not an STD. However, in recurrent cases possibility of sexual transmission may be considered.
- *Trichomonas vaginitis* often found along with BV in about 60% of cases.
- About 75% of women in premenopausal age group would have had at least one episode of vulvovaginitis and *C. albicans* is the most common organism causing this infection.
- The most common cause of TTS is due to tampons usage and might be also associated with use of diaphragm (female barrier contraceptive).
- About 75% of chlamydial infections are asymptomatic as the lesions are superficial.
- One-third of the women with *N. gonorrhoeae* have associated chlamydial infection and also they are at high risk for acquiring syphilis infection and other STI.
- Pelvic inflammatory disease includes spectrum of infections involving the upper female genital organs involving the fallopian tubes, ovaries, uterus, pelvic peritoneum, and the parametrium.
- Genital TB occurs almost always secondary. Almost all organs are susceptible to TB infection. If close to menarche primary infection occurs then there is higher chance of genital TB.
- Tuberculosis patients are classified into two groups based on the history of previous treatment such as "New" or "Previously Treated".
- Syphilis is systemic disease caused by spirocheta and *T. pallidum*. The definitive method to detect the organism causing syphilis is by darkfield microscopy, sample for examination taken from lesion exudate or tissue.
- Human immunodeficiency virus targets the CD4 receptor molecules present on cells of immune system. As CD4$^+$

lymphocytes are depleted there occurs profound immunosuppression. Count of 200–500 cells/mm^3 have symptoms and <200 cells/mm^3 have AIDS defining criteria.
- Primary goal of ART is to maximize the viral load suppression, restore the immune function, and restore HIV-related mortality and morbidity. Treatment should be offered if plasma HIV RNA level is more than 100,000 copies/mL or CD4$^+$ T cells less than 350.
- Herpes genitalis is a lifelong chronic viral infection. Caused by two types of HSV: HSV-1 and HSV-2.
- Granuloma inguinale present with slowly progressive painless ulcer on genital or perineum. Pseudobuboes may occur in some cases.
- Lymphogranuloma venereum caused by *C. trachomatis* L serovars L1, L2, and L3. Initially present with painless papule or ulcer in vulva, cervix, urethra or rectum. Unilateral inguniofemoral lymph nodes are mostly involved.
- Chancroid is caused by *Haemophilus ducreyi* and gram-negative *Streptobacillus*. It is a risk factor for HIV transmission and acquisition.
- Molluscum contagiosum is caused by low risk, nononcogenic HPV type 6 and 11.
- In uncomplicated cystitis, nitrofurantoin 100 mg two times a day orally for 7 days or ciprofloxacin 250 mg two times a day orally for 3 days are recommended.
- About 20% have recurrent cystitis in premenopausal age group and about more than 90% are due to exogenous reinfection.
- The presentation of acute pyelonephritis might vary from cystitis-like illness to gram-negative septicemia. In more than 80% of cases the causative organism is *E. coli*.

REFERENCES

1. Tae-Hee Kim, Bel Seap, Soo Ah Kim, et al. Vulvar Abscess Caused by Methicillin-resistant *Staphylococcus aureus* (MRSA) in a Postmenopausal Woman. J Menopausal Med. 2016;22(2):118-21.
2. Pundir J, Auld BJ. A review of the management of diseases of the Bartholin's gland. J Obstet Gynaecol. 2008;28(2):161-5.
3. Caillouette JC, Sharp CF Jr, Zimmerman GJ, et al. Vaginal pH as a marker for bacterial pathogens and menopausal status. Am J Obstet Gynecol. 1997;176(6):1270-5.
4. Workowski KA, Berman S; Centers for Disease Control And Prevention. Sexually Transmitted Diseases Treatment Guidelines, 2010. MMWR Recomm Rep. 2010;59(RR-12):1-110.
5. Bradshaw CS, Morton AN, Hocking J, et al. High recurrence rates of bacterial vaginosis over the course of 12 months after oral metronidazole therapy and factors associated with recurrence. J Infect Dis. 2006;193(11):1478-86.
6. Wølner-Hanssen P, Krieger JN, Stevens CE, et al. Clinical manifestations of vaginal trichomoniasis. JAMA. 1989;261(4):571-6.
7. Kiviat NB, Paavonen JA, Wølner-Hanssen P, et al. Histopathology of endocervical infection caused by *Chlamydia trachomatis*, herpes simplex virus, *Trichomonas vaginalis*, and *Neisseria gonorrhoeae*. Hum Pathol. 1990;21(8):831-7.
8. Centers for Disease Control and Prevention. Sexually Transmitted Disease Surveillance, 2009. Atlanta, US: Department of Health and Human Services; 2009.
9. Timor-Tritsch IE, Lerner JP, Monteagudo A, et al. Transvaginal sonographic markers of tubal inflammatory disease. Ultrasound Obstet Gynecol. 1998;12(1):56-66.
10. Achilles SL, Amortegui AJ, Wiesenfeld HC. Endometrial plasma cells: do they indicate subclinical pelvic inflammatory disease? Sex Transm Dis. 2005;32(3):185-8.
11. Weström L. Effect of acute pelvic inflammatory disease on fertility. Am J Obstet Gynecol. 1975;121(5):707-13.
12. Dunbar-Jacob J, Sereika SM, Foley SM, et al. Adherence to oral therapies in pelvic inflammatory disease. J Womens Health (Larchmt). 2004;13(3):285-91.

13. BURNE JC. The age of onset of genital tuberculosis in women. J Obstet Gynaecol Br Emp. 1956;63(1):96-9.
14. Schaefer G. Female genital tuberculosis. Clin Obstet Gynecol. 1976;19(1):223-39.
15. Frantzen C, Schlösser HW. Microsurgery and postinfectious tubal infertility. Fertil Steril. 1982;38:397-420.
16. Czernobilsky B. Endometritis and infertility. Fertil Steril. 1978;30(2):119-30.
17. Harvey B Simon, Allan J Weinstein, Mark S Pasternak, et al. Genitourinary tuberculosis. AM J Med. 1977;63(3):410-20.
18. Varma TR. Tuberculosis of the female genital tract. Glob Libr Women's Med; 2008.
19. Ahmadi F, Zafarani F, Shahrzad G. Hysterosalpingographic appearances of female genital tract tuberculosis: Part I. Fallopian tube. Int J Fertil Steril. 2014;7(4):245-52.
20. Ahmadi F, Zafarani F, Shahrzad GS. Hysterosalpingographic appearances of female genital tract tuberculosis: Part II: Uterus. Int J Fertil Steril. 2014;8(1):13-20.
21. Shah HU, Sannananja B, Baheti AD, et al. Hysterosalpingography and ultrasonography findings of female genital tuberculosis. Diagn Interv Radiol. 2015;21(1):10-5.
22. Schaaf HS, Zumla A. Tuberculosis: A Comprehensive Clinical Reference. St Louis (MO): Elsevier Health Sciences; 2009.
23. Norbis L, Alagna R, Tortoli E, et al. Challenges and perspectives in the diagnosis of extrapulmonary tuberculosis. Expert Rev Anti Infect Ther. 2014;12(5):633-47.
24. Das P, Ahuja A, Gupta SD. Incidence, etiopathogenesis and pathological aspects of genitourinary tuberculosis in India: A journey revisited. Indian J Urol. 2008;24(3):356-61.
25. Simon HB, Weinstein AJ, Pasternak MS, et al. Genitourinary tuberculosis. Clinical features in a general hospital population. Am J Med. 1977;63(3):410-20.
26. Tortoli E, Cichero P, Piersimoni C, et al. Use of BACTEC MGIT 960 for recovery of mycobacteria from clinical specimens: multicenter study. J Clin Microbiol. 1999;37(11):3578-82.
27. Arora S, Merchant R, Allahbadia GN. Reproductive Medicine: Challenges, Solutions and Breakthroughs. New Delhi: Jaypee Brothers Medical Publishers (P) Ltd.; 2014.
28. Bhanu NV, Singh UB, Chakraborty M, et al. Improved diagnostic value of PCR in the diagnosis of female genital tuberculosis leading to infertility. J Med Microbiol. 2005;54(Pt 10):927-31.
29. Arora R, Sharma JB. Female genital tuberculosis—a diagnostic and therapeutic challenge. Indian J Tuberc. 2014;61(2):98-102.
30. Raj A, Singh N, Mehta PK. Gene Xpert MTB/RIF assay: A new hope for extrapulmonary tuberculosis. IOSR J Pharm. 2012;2(1):83-9.
31. Mahashur AA, Sheth SS, Raut VS. The Mantoux test in the diagnosis of genital tuberculosis in women. Int J Gynaecol Obstet. 2001;72(2):165-9.
32. Mori T, Sakatani M, Yamagishi F, et al. Specific detection of tuberculosis infection: an interferon-gamma-based assay using new antigens. Am J Respir Crit Care Med. 2004;170(1):59-64.
33. Bartacek A, Schütt D, Panosch B, et al. Comparison of a four-drug fixed-dose combination regimen with a single tablet regimen in smear-positive pulmonary tuberculosis. Int J of Tuberc Lung Dis. 2009;13(6):760-6.
34. Sharma JB. Tuberculosis and obstetric and gynecological practice. In: Studd J, Tan SL, Chervenak FA (Eds). Progress in Obstetric and Gynecology. Philadelphia: Elsevier; 2008. pp. 395-427.
35. CDC. (2011). A guide to taking a sexual history. [online] Available from https://npin.cdc.gov/publication/guide-taking-sexual-history [Last accessed September, 2019].
36. CDC, Association of Public Health Laboratories. Laboratory diagnostic testing for Treponema pallidum. Atlanta, GA: Expert Consultation Meeting Summary Report; 2009.
37. Nandwani R, Evans DT. Are you sure it's syphilis? A review of false positive serology. Int J STD AIDS. 1995;6(4):241-8.
38. Romanowski B, Sutherland R, Fick GH, et al. Serologic response to treatment of infectious syphilis. Ann Intern Med. 1991;114(12):1005-9.
39. Park IU, Chow JM, Bolan G, et al. Screening for syphilis with the treponemal immunoassay: analysis of discordant serology results and implications for clinical management. J Infect Dis. 2011;204(9):1297-304.

40. Wong EH, Klausner JD, Caguin-Grygiel G, et al. Evaluation of an IgM/IgG sensitive enzyme immunoassay and the utility of index values for the screening of syphilis infection in a high-risk population. Sex Transm Dis. 2011;38(6):528-32.
41. Ghanem KG, Erbelding EJ, Cheng WW, et al. Doxycycline compared with benzathine penicillin for the treatment of early syphilis. Clin Infect Dis. 2006;42(6):e45-9.
42. Riedner G, Rusizoka M, Todd J, et al. Single-dose azithromycin versus penicillin G benzathine for the treatment of early syphilis. N Engl J Med. 2005;353(12):1236-44.
43. Smit C, Geskus R, Walker S, et al. Effective therapy has altered the spectrum of cause-specific mortality following HIV seroconversion. AIDS. 2006;20(5):741-9.
44. CDC. HIV/AIDS Surveillance Report. Atlanta, GA: US Department of Health and Human Services; 2011.
45. CDC. Vital signs: HIV testing and diagnosis among adults—United States, 2001-2009. MMWR Morbid Mortal Wkly Rep. 2010;59:1550-5.
46. CDC. Previous HIV testing among adults and adolescents newly diagnosed with HIV infection—National HIV Surveillance System, 18 jurisdictions, United States, 2006-2009. MMWR Morbid Mortal Wkly Rep. 2012;61:441-5.
47. Schacker T, Collier AC, Hughes J, et al. Clinical and epidemiologic features of primary HIV infection. Ann Intern Med. 1996;125(4):257-64.
48. Wawer MJ, Gray RH, Sewankambo NK, et al. Rates of HIV-1 transmission per coital act, by stage of HIV-1 infection, in Rakai, Uganda. J Infect Dis. 2005;191(9):1403-9.
49. CDC. (2014). Laboratory testing for the diagnosis of HIV infection: updated recommendations. [online] Available from https://stacks.cdc.gov/view/cdc/23447 [Last accessed September, 2019].
50. Schmid GP. Approach to the patient with genital ulcer disease. Med Clin North Am. 1990;74(6):1559-72.
51. CDC. (2005). Guidelines for the use of antiretroviral agents in HIV-infected adults and adolescents. [online] Available from https://wonder.cdc.gov/wonder/prevguid/m0054080/m0054080.asp [last accessed September, 2019].
52. Grohskopf LA, Chillag KL, Gvetadze R, et al. Randomized trial of clinical safety of daily oral tenofovir disoproxil fumarate among HIV-uninfected men who have sex with men in the United States. J Acquir Immune Defic Syndr. 2013;64(1):79-86.
53. Bradley H, Markowitz LE, Gibson T, et al. Seroprevalence of herpes simplex virus types 1 and 2—United States, 1999-2010. J Infect Dis. 2014;209(3):325-33.
54. Ryder N, Jin F, McNulty AM, et al. Increasing role of herpes simplex virus type 1 in first-episode anogenital herpes in heterosexual women and younger men who have sex with men, 1992-2006. Sex Transm Infect. 2009;85(6):416-9.
55. Benedetti J, Corey L, Ashley R. Recurrence rates in genital herpes after symptomatic first-episode infection. Ann Intern Med. 1994;121(11):847-54.
56. Bernstein DI, Bellamy AR, Hook EW, 3rd, et al. Epidemiology, clinical presentation, and antibody response to primary infection with herpes simplex virus type 1 and type 2 in young women. Clin Infect Dis. 2013;56(3):344-51.
57. Golden MR, Ashley-Morrow R, Swenson P, et al. Herpes simplex virus type 2 (HSV-2) Western blot confirmatory testing among men testing positive for HSV-2 using the focus enzyme-linked immunosorbent assay in a sexually transmitted disease clinic. Sex Transm Dis. 2005;32(12):771-7.
58. Morrow R, Friedrich D. Performance of a novel test for IgM and IgG antibodies in subjects with culture-documented genital herpes simplex virus-1 or -2 infection. Clin Microbiol Infect. 2006;12:463-9.
59. Scoular A, Gillespie G, Carman WF. Polymerase chain reaction for diagnosis of genital herpes in a genitourinary medicine clinic. Sex Transm Infect. 2002;78(1):21-5.
60. Caviness AC, Oelze LL, Saz UE, et al. Direct immunofluorescence assay compared to cell culture for the diagnosis of mucocutaneous herpes simplex virus infections in children. J Clin Virol. 2010;49(1):58-60.
61. Leone PA, Trottier S, Miller JM. Valacyclovir for episodic treatment of genital herpes: a shorter

3-day treatment course compared with 5-day treatment. Clin Infect Dis. 2002;34(7):958-62.
62. Mabey D, Peeling RW. Lymphogranuloma venereum. Sex Transm Infect. 2002;78:90-2.
63. Papp JR, Schachter J, Gaydos C, et al. Recommendations for the laboratory-based detection of *Chlamydia trachomatis* and *Neisseria gonorrhoeae*—2014. MMWR Recomm Rep. 2014;63(RR-02):1-19.
64. Fleming DT, Wasserheit JN. From epidemiological synergy to public health policy and practice: the contribution of other sexually transmitted diseases to sexual transmission of HIV infection. Sex Transm Infect. 1999;75(1):3-17.
65. Lewis DA. Chancroid: clinical manifestations, diagnosis, and management. Sex Transm Infect. 2003;79(1):68-71.
66. de Villiers EM, Fauquet C, Broker TR, et al. Classification of papillomaviruses. Virology. 2004;324(1):17-27.
67. Markowitz LE, Dunne EF, Saraiya M, et al. Human papillomavirus vaccination: recommendations of the Advisory Committee on Immunization Practices (ACIP). MMWR Recomm Rep. 2014;63 (RR-05):1-30.
68. Remis RS, Gurwith MJ, Gurwith D, et al. Risk factors for urinary tract infection. Am J Epidemiol. 1987;126(4):685-94.
69. Gupta K, Scholes D, Stamm WE. Increasing prevalence of antimicrobial resistance among uropathogens causing acute uncomplicated cystitis in women. JAMA. 1999;281(8):736-8.
70. Ramakrishnan K, Scheid DC. Diagnosis and management of acute pyelonephritis in adults. 2005;71(5):933-42.

CHAPTER 11

Pelvic Mass

Ravishankar P, Tejaswi K

INTRODUCTION

Pelvic mass may present as abdominal or vaginal mass. Woman of any age can present with a mass abdomen. It is important to identify a potentially life-threatening disease. The prevalence of gynecological mass in postmenopausal women is 2.5–10%.[1,2]

Among the abdominal masses, uterine fibroids are the most common pelvic tumors of women. Being a major cause of abnormal uterine bleeding (AUB) they are the most commonly cited reason for hysterectomy.[3-5] Japan and Asian countries have rates of 2–6.5 new ovarian cancer cases per 100,000 women per year. Ovarian carcinoma represents the sixth most common female cancer and the fourth leading cause of death due to cancers in women and is seen predominantly after third decade. Lifetime risk of dying of ovarian cancer is 1 in 95.[6]

ETIOLOGY

The causes of mass abdomen could be either gynecological or surgical.

Gynecological Causes

- *Pregnancy-related*:
  - Normal intrauterine pregnancy
  - Old ruptured extrauterine pregnancy (abdominal and tubal pregnancy)
  - Molar pregnancy
- *Uterine origin*:
  - Uterine fibroids
  - Advanced uterine carcinoma or sarcoma
  - Hematometra/pyometra
- *Tubal origin*:
  - Hydrosalpinx/pyosalpinx
  - Tubo-ovarian abscess
  - Advanced cancer of the tube

- *Ovarian origin*:
  - Ovarian torsion
  - Benign cyst
  - Endometrioma
  - Benign tumor (dermoid, fibroma, and cystadenoma)
  - Borderline tumor
  - Malignant tumor (carcinoma, granulosa cell or germ cell tumor).

Surgical Causes

- Appendicular abscess
- Obstructed hernia
- Intussusception
- Colorectal carcinoma
- Subacute intestinal obstruction
- Diverticular abscess
- Large bowel tumor/mesenteric tumor
- Abdominal aortic aneurism
- *Renal tumor*: Pelvic kidney, bladder carcinoma, and urinary retention
- Neurological causes
- Neuroblastoma
- Hematological causes
- Hodgkin's and non-Hodgkin's lymphoma, and pelvic spleen.

SYMPTOMS

Pain abdomen, vomiting, changes in bowel habits, abdominal heaviness, distension, frequent urination, dysuria, polyuria, and mass abdomen are some of the symptoms a woman can present with in mass abdomen. Heavy menstrual bleeding and dysmenorrhea could be the symptoms of a fibroid. Women can often be asymptomatic where the mass is detected on physical examination incidentlly. The difference can be made out with clinical examination and an ultrasonography (USG).

INVESTIGATIONS

Pregnancy Test

To rule out pregnancy-related complications.

Ultrasonography

High frequency transvaginal or transabdominal USG can help in diagnosis by producing high resolution images. No other imaging technique has been found to be superior to Doppler USG for overall accuracy of adnexal masses.[7]

Uterine Origin

Differentiating features between adenomyosis and myoma are shown in **Table 1**.

TABLE 1: Differentiating features between adenomyosis and myoma.

	Myoma	Adenomyosis
Uterine size	Variable to markedly enlarged	Normal to mildly enlarged
Uterine shape	Lobulated	Globular
Lesion	• Well-defined mass • Whorled appearance • Secondary changes, calcifications, etc.	• Heterogenic echotexture • Scattered areas of myometrial cysts • Echogenic nodule and echogenic striations
Uterine cavity	Well-defined except in fibroids in contact with endometrium	Poorly defined borders
Doppler (Feeling vessels around the mass)	Capsular vascularity	Radial/penetrating vascular arrangement

Ovarian Cyst

If a cystic lesion is detected, concern for an ovarian cystic neoplasm is raised when a cyst is large, or if there are complex features, including:
- Thick septations: >3 mm
- Papillary projections in the cyst
- Frank solid components or heterogeneous echogenicity
- Increased vascularity
- Presence of ascites
- Associated regional lymphadenopathy.

Other Imaging Modalities

Computed tomography, magnetic resonance imaging (MRI), and positron emission tomography are not recommended initial evaluation of pelvic masses as they are of high cost and are of limited value in initial investigation.

■ MANAGEMENT

Should be tailored to the symptoms, age, socioeconomic status, pathology, compliance, and preference of the women.

Adenomyosis

Management algorithm of adenomyosis is shown in **Flowchart 1**.

Ovarian Cyst

Management algorithm of ovarian cyst is shown in **Flowchart 2**.

Fibroid Uterus

Management algorithm of fibroid management is shown in **Flowchart 3**.

Pharmacotherapy

Nonsteroidal Anti-inflammatory Drugs[8]

Mefenamic acid is the most common medicine used in menorrhagia and dysmenorrhea. Mefenamic acid will cause reduction of blood loss by 25–50%. Side effects are gastrointestinal and it should be avoided in women with peptic ulcer.

Progesterone

Progesterone is the mainstay of medical treatment in case of symptomatic fibroid.

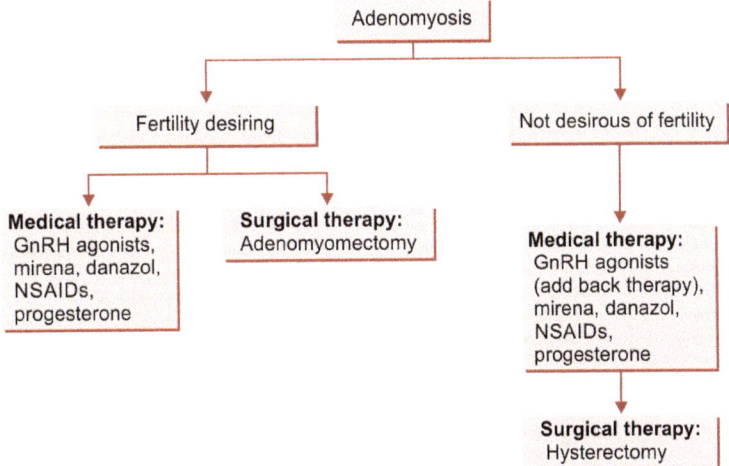

Flowchart 1: Management algorithm of adenomyosis.

(GnRH: gonadotropin-releasing hormone; NSAIDs: nonsteroidal anti-inflammatory drugs)

Flowchart 2: Management algorithm of ovarian cysts.

```
                          Ovarian cyst
                         /            \
                  Asymptomatic      Symptomatic
                       |                 |
          • Normal pap smear, CA-125    • Clinical lesion
          • Simple cyst on USG          • Elevated CA-125
                 /        \              • Complex cyst
          Cyst < 3 cm   Cyst > 3 cm           |
                |           |             • Laparotomy
         Follow-up with  Malignancy       • Oophorectomy
         USG and CA-125  workup           • Surgical staging
                          /      \
                  No malignancy   Evidence of
                                  malignancy
                        |              |
                • Oophorectomy    Surgical staging
                • Peritoneal cytology
```

(CA-125: cancer antigen-125; USG: ultrasonography)

Flowchart 3: Management algorithm of fibroid uterus.

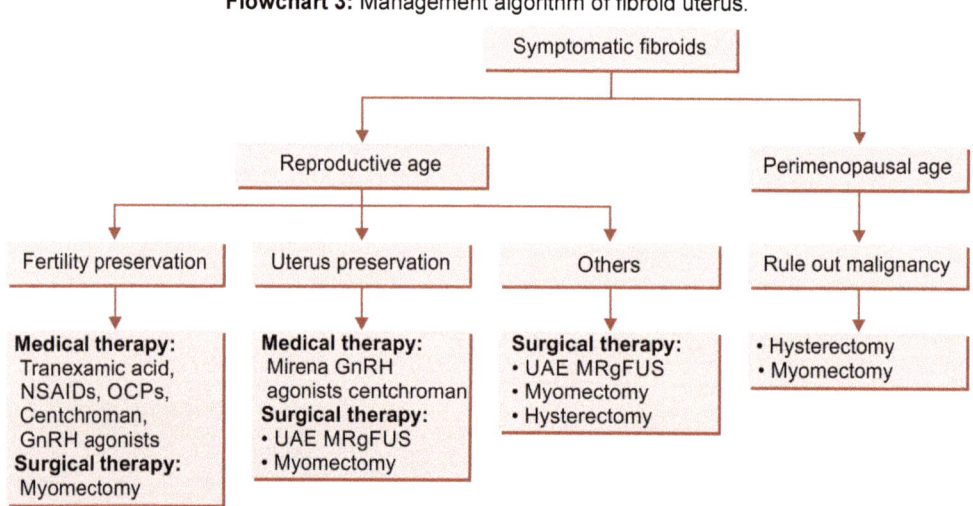

(GnRH: gonadotropin-releasing hormone; MRgFUS: magnetic resonance high-intensity focused ultrasound; NSAIDs: nonsteroidal anti-inflammatory drugs; OCPs: oral contraceptive pills; UAE: uterine artery embolization)

Medroxyprogesterone, norethisterone, and duphaston are the various progesterone. Contraindicated in women with history of vascular thrombosis, current or past history of breast cancer and impaired liver function.

Combined Oral Contraceptives

They are given for adenomyosis. Women with risk of thromboembolism, cerebrovascular disease, ischemic heart disease, migraine, hypertension, severe liver disease, breast cancer, diabetes with vascular complications, and heart disease are some of the contraindications of using oral contraceptive pills.

Danazol

Limited role due to androgenic side effects. It is used in a dose of 200 mg daily. Not to be used in adolescent girls or women trying to conceive.

Gonadotropin-releasing Hormone Agonists

Reduces estrogen and progesterone. To be given as depot injections 3.6 mg monthly, for 4-6 months. It is not useful in acute episodes because of its long onset of action. It causes menopausal symptoms and osteoporosis. Hence, it should not be given for more than 6 months. Osteoporosis should be counteracted with add back therapy by giving norethisterone or tibolone.

Surgical Management

Uterine Artery Embolization

It can be done if the cause of fibroid. It is not to be used in women desiring fertility. Symptoms of heavy menorrhagia, pressure symptoms, and volume of fibroid were found to be reduced. Symptoms were relieved in 70–80% of women. The drawback is that the procedure requires expertise and cannot be performed at all places.

Myomectomy

Submucosal fibroids are to be removed by hysteroscopic removal. Intramural and subserosal fibroids are to be removed if they are causing heavy menstrual bleeding, pressure symptoms or infertility. Care must be taken to avoid hemorrhage which may ultimately lead to hysterectomy. Using gonadotropin-releasing hormone (GnRH) agonists can reduce the size of fibroids but surgical difficulty may be experienced due to thinning of capsule.

Newer techniques like MRI-guided focused ultrasound and laparoscopic myolysis have been introduced to manage fibroids.

Adenomyomectomy

It is a conservative surgery to be offered in women with strong desire to retain the uterus like women trying to conceive.

Hysterectomy

Can be done in laparoscopic, abdominal, and vaginal route. Though hysterectomy is the most effective treatment for AUB, this has to be considered after thorough evaluation of cause, optimum trial of medical treatment, and discussion with the patient because of high risk of adverse effects like hemorrhage, surgical complications, wound-related complications, and thromboembolic events.[9]

Vaginal masses either benign or malignant are rare entity. Most of them are discovered incidentally on examination or during USG for some other indication. Due to close proximity of vagina to other pelvic structures like bladder anteriorly and rectum posteriorly, lesions in these structures might also present as vaginal masses. Most of these lesions are asymptomatic. Larger lesions may present with pressure symptoms, vaginal discomfort, and dyspareunia. Malignant lesions usually present with foul smelling discharge and bleeding per vaginum.

CLASSIFICATION

Vaginal lesions may be divided into benign and malignant. Benign lesions may be either cystic or solid **(Table 2)**. There are few related conditions from adjacent structures also presenting as mass per vaginum.

Malignancies in vagina may present as vaginal masses with AUB. They can be divided into primary and secondary malignancies. Primary malignancies of vagina are rare and can be primary squamous cell carcinoma or adenocarcinoma. Secondary malignancies are metastatic lesions from primary elsewhere.

Benign Cystic Lesions

Gartner Duct Cyst

It arises from remnant of mesonephric duct or Wolffian duct in fetal life. Its incidence of all the vaginal cysts is 12.5%.[9] It usually presents as a mass arising from lateral wall in upper vagina. It is lined by nonsecretory and columnar epithelium. Small cysts are asymptomatic and usually are detected incidentally on pelvic examination. Larger cysts may extend to lateral aspect of cervix and may present with pressure symptoms or dyspareunia. If the cyst is small and asymptomatic, usually no treatment is required. Larger symptomatic cysts need to be excised. In case, where diagnosis is inconclusive or there is history of in utero diethylstilboestrol (DES) exposure, biopsy to rule out adenosis is indicated.

Bartholin Cyst

Bartholin glands are located in lateral part of lower aspect of vagina. Bartholin cyst arises from occlusion to duct opening resulting in collection of secretions inside duct. It usually presents as a cystic fluid-filled swelling in lower aspect of vagina. It can get infected very often and presents as painful tender swelling containing purulent discharge. Infected cyst may also get ruptured spontaneously. Small asymptomatic cysts do not usually require any treatment. Treatment of symptomatic cyst and Bartholin abscess includes antibiotics and marsupialization of the cyst. It has a tendency for recurrence; excision of the gland is required in such cases.

Paramesonephric Duct Cyst

It is of müllerian origin and can be located anywhere in the vagina. These are differentiated from Gartner's duct cyst by being lined with secretory epithelium similar to endocervix or fallopian tube. Large symptomatic cysts require excision. Biopsy of the lesion is required to exclude adenosis.

Inclusion Cyst

Inclusion cyst arises from entrapment of vaginal mucosa in to submucosal area during surgical procedures like repair of

TABLE 2: Differentiating features between cystic and solid lesions.

Cystic	Solid	Related conditions
Gartner duct cyst	Leiomyoma	Urethral caruncle
Bartholin cyst	Fibroepithelial polyp	Fibroid polyp
Inclusion cyst	Foreign body	Hematocolpos
Paramesonephric duct cyst		Inversion uterus
Endometriosis		Cystocele
		Uterine prolapse

episiotomy, colpoperineorrhaphy or perineal trauma during childbirth. These are lined by squamous epithelium and contain keratin and squamous debris. Enlargement of cysts may cause symptoms requiring excision and approximation of normal vaginal mucosa.

Endometriosis

Endometriosis is a condition characterized by presence of ectopic endometrial tissue outside endometrial cavity. Aberrant endometrial tissue can be present in vagina also, accounting for 0.02% of cases,[10] most common site being the posterior fornix. Lesion can be either entirely cystic or may be solid in nature. It undergoes cyclical changes in menstrual cycle. Examination may reveal nodularity in posterior fornix on per vaginal examination or bluish lesions can be seen on speculum examination. Definitive diagnosis can be made by excisional biopsy. In case of larger lesions, preoperative therapy with GnRH analogs might be helpful in shrinking the size of the lesion. Treatment involves excision of the lesion, and as vaginal endometriosis may be coexistent with endometriosis in other locations, laparotomy or laparoscopic surgery might be indicated depending upon extent of disease.

Benign Solid Lesions

Leiomyoma

Vaginal leiomyoma is benign smooth muscle neoplasm usually solitary lesion located in anterior vaginal wall. It may arise from proliferation of vaginal smooth muscles or local vasculature muscle and are usually benign in nature, malignant transformation being rare. It presents as vaginal mass with pressure symptoms like urinary retention, dyspareunia, vaginal discharge, and bleeding. Histologically, it resembles leiomyoma uteri and is estrogen dependent. Differential diagnosis includes other midline vaginal masses like urethral diverticulum, cystocele, fibroepithelial polyp, Gartner's duct cyst, and vaginal malignancy. Treatment involves excision of the mass. Recurrence is rare.

Fibroepithelial Polyp

Fibroepithelial polyps of the vagina are mucosal polypoid lesions. These are uncommon, as only a few cases have been reported in literature. These are usually small and asymptomatic, but can be multiple. Histologically, it is composed of connected tissue core covered by squamous epithelium. It probably arises from granulation tissue reaction after injury to vaginal mucosa. Differential diagnosis includes sarcoma botryoides (infants and young girls), rhabdomyosarcoma, and mixed mesodermal tumor.[11] Diagnosis is confirmed by histological examination. Treatment involves simple excision and recurrence is uncommon.

Foreign Body

Foreign bodies in vagina include forgotten pessaries, tampons in adults, and small objects in children. These may remain asymptomatic for a long time. When present for a long time these may become infected producing foul smelling vaginal discharge, vaginal bleeding or may erode in to vaginal wall. These may be seen as a very echogenic mass with shadowing on USG. Examination with a speculum, visualization, and removal with the help of forceps can be done in outpatient setting in adults. In children, it may require examination and removal under anesthesia.

Related Conditions

Urethral Caruncle

Urethral caruncles are usually seen in postmenopausal women and result due to prolapse of urethral mucosa with secondary inflammation. It presents as localized, red, and friable lesions at the urethral meatus. Urethral malignancy must be ruled out in patients with larger urethral caruncles. Symptoms include pain, dysuria or bleeding. Small asymptomatic lesions may not require any treatment. Larger or symptomatic lesions can be treated by topical application of estrogen after excluding malignancy by small tissue biopsy under local anesthesia. Excision of mass and reapproximation of mucosa is required in large or persistent lesions.

Hematocolpos

It is a condition characterized by collection of menstrual blood in vagina due to outflow tract obstruction due to abnormalities in of development of müllerian system. Most common entity encountered is imperforate hymen. The transverse vaginal septum also presents with similar symptoms and differentiation is usually made by the presence of a hymeneal ring distal to the site of obstruction. Most of the cases are associated with coexistent genitourinary abnormalities. Patients usually present around period of menarche with primary amenorrhea, cyclic pain in lower abdomen, pressure symptoms like urinary retention and constipation. Examination reveals bulging bluish membrane in cases with imperforate hymen. USG can reveal collection in vagina, cervix, and uterus. Treatment involves cruciate incision over imperforated hymen and drainage of secretions. Vaginal septum requires excision followed by reconstruction of segment of vagina.

Fibroid Polyp and Uterine Inversion

Fibroids and polyps are benign neoplasms of uterus. They can be single or multiple and sessile or pedunculated. In rare instances, pedunculated submucosal fibroids or polyps may protrude through the external os and present as vaginal mass. Patients present with heavy menstrual bleeding, foul smelling discharge per vaginum, dysmenorrhea, heaviness, and pain in lower abdomen. On speculum examination, there can be red fleshy mass sometimes with infected surface coming through os. On per vaginum examination, same mass can be felt with pedicle. USG helps in confirming the origin of the mass. Treatment involves polypectomy under hysteroscopic guidance.

Extrusion of large submucosal fundal fibroid can result in to rare phenomena of nonpuerperal uterine inversion. Patient can be asymptomatic or may present with heavy menstrual bleeding, sepsis, and shock. Diagnosis is made by clinical examination and USG reveals heterogeneous mass protruding in vagina with absence of uterus in pelvic cavity. As patients present with heavy menstrual bleeding, malignancy needs to be ruled out by biopsy. In younger patients, conservative operations are done either by abdominal or vaginal or by combined abdominovaginal approach. In parous women or in cases of extensive necrosis of the tissue hysterectomy might be indicated.

Cystocele

It is a condition characterized by prolapse of bladder in to anterior vaginal wall due to weakening of pelvic tissue support. It may go unnoticed if small in size and asymptomatic. Large cystocele presents with heaviness lower abdomen, sensation of incomplete evacuation of bladder, urinary retention, and frequent urinary infection. It can be differentiated from anterior vaginal wall cyst by Valsalva maneuver. Diagnosis can be established by clinical examination and treatment involves repair of anterior vaginal wall defect by colporrhaphy.

Uterovaginal Prolapse

It is a condition in which there is descent of uterus and cervix in vagina due to relaxation of pelvic muscle and fascia. First- and second-degree uterine prolapse might present as mass per vaginum. Diagnosis is made by clinical examination and site of defect can be ascertained followed by site-specific tissue repair.

Malignant Lesions

Primary cancer of the vagina comprises approximately 3% of all malignant neoplasms of the female genital tract.[12] Most of the primary lesions are squamous cell carcinomas, but other histologic types like melanoma and adenocarcinoma also occur. Primary vaginal cancer is a rare entity, most of the lesions in vagina are metastatic from other sites like uterus, cervix, vulva, breast, and rectum. Involvement of vagina by metastatic tumors can occur either by direct extension from adjacent structures or by hematogenous and lymphatic spread. Clinical presentation is by abnormal bleeding per vaginum, pressure symptoms by mass, and discharge per vaginum. Diagnosis is made by clinical examination, aided by Pap smear, colposcopy, USG, and MRI.[13] In extensive disease, cystoscopy and proctoscopy can also help in delineating the extent of disease. Staging of disease is done by International Federation of Gynecology and Obstetrics (FIGO) staging. Treatment is either surgical or by radiotherapy depending on stage of the disease.

SUMMARY

- Pelvic mass may present as abdominal/vaginal mass, among abdominal masses uterine fibroids are the most common benign pelvic tumors among women.
- The causes of abdominal mass could be either gynecological/surgical.
- Women presents with pain abdomen, vomiting, changes in bowel habits, abdominal heaviness, distension, frequent urination, dysuria, polyuria, and mass abdomen , women with fibroid most commonly presents with heavy menstrual bleeding and dysmenorrhea.
- Ultrasonography is the baseline investigation of choice to diagnose the abdominal mass.
- Management includes medical/ surgical depending upon patients age, symptoms, pathology, socioeconomic status, compliance, completion of family.
- Vaginal lesions could be benign/malignant are rare entity, mostly asymptomatic. Larger lesions may present with pressure symptoms, vaginal discomfort, and dyspareunia. Malignant lesions usually present with foul smelling discharge and bleeding per vaginum.
- Malignancies in vagina most commonly present as vaginal masses with AUB and foul smelling discharge. Diagnosis is made by clinical examination, aided by Pap smear, colposcopy, USG, and MRI.

CONCLUSION

Pelvic mass includes both abdominal and vaginal mass, needs to differentiate between benign and malignant lesions, treatment depends on patient age and fertility status.

REFERENCES

1. Castillo G, Alcazar JL, Jurado M. Natural history of sonographically detected simple unilocular adnexal cysts in asymptomatic postmenopausal women. Gynecol Oncol. 2004;92:965-9.
2. Curtin JP. Management of the adnexal mass. Gynecol Oncol. 1994;55:S42-6.
3. Musey VC, Collins DC, Brogan DR. Long term effects of a first pregnancy on the hormonal environment: estrogens and androgens. J Clin Endocrinol Metab. 1987;64:111-8.
4. Musey VC, Collins DC, Musey PI. Long-term effect of a first pregnancy on the secretion of prolactin. N Engl J Med. 1987;316:229-34.
5. Windham GC, Elkin E, Fenster L. Ovarian hormones in premenopausal women: variation by demographic, reproductive and menstrual cycle characteristics. Epidemiol. 2002;13:675-84.
6. Siegel R, Ward E, Brawley O, et al. Cancer statistics, 2011. CA Cancer J Clin. 2011;61: 212-36.
7. Graham L. ACOG releases guidelines on management of adnexal masses. Am Fam Physician. 2008;77(9):1320-3.
8. Cameron IT, Haining R, Lumsden MA, et al. The effects of mefenamic acid and norethisterone on measured menstrual blood loss. Obstet Gynecol. 1990;76(1):85-8.
9. Matteson KA, Abed H, Wheeler TL, et al. Schaffer and Ethan M. Balk. A systematic review comparing hysterectomy to less invasive treatments for abnormal uterine bleeding. J Minim Invasive Gynecol. 2012;19(1):13-28.
10. Kondi-Pafiti A, Grapsa D, Papakonstantinou K, et al. Vaginal cysts: A common pathologic entity revisited. Clin Exp Obstet Gynecol. 2008;35:41-4.
11. Lee HJ, Park YM, Jee BC, et al. Various anatomic locations of surgically proven endometriosis: a single-center experience. Obstet Gynecol Sci. 2015;58:53-8.
12. Siegel RL, Miller KD, Jemal A. Cancer statistics, 2015. CA Cancer J Clin. 2015;65:5-29.
13. Hiniker SM, Roux A, Murphy JD, et al. Primary squamous cell carcinoma of vagina: prognostic factors, treatment patterns, and outcomes. Gynecol Oncol. 2013;131:380-5.

CHAPTER 12

Ovarian Hyperstimulation Syndrome

Nivedita Shetty

■ INTRODUCTION

Ovulation induction and controlled ovarian stimulation for in vitro fertilization (IVF) can cause some extent of hyperstimulation; however, ovarian hyperstimulation syndrome (OHSS) is a life-threatening complication, which may occur due to stimulation of the ovaries in excess.[1-5]

Ovarian stimulation needs to be a balance between collecting appropriate number of oocytes for adequate success, while avoiding the risks of OHSS.

■ DEFINING OVARIAN HYPERSTIMULATION SYNDROME

Ovarian hyperstimulation syndrome is an iatrogenic complication which is characterized by ovarian enlargement and rapid fluid shifts from the intravascular compartment to the third space.[6] It can be a life-threatening condition in its severe form.

■ PATHOPHYSIOLOGY

The causative mechanism is the increase in *vascular permeability*, which results in fluid shifts into the third space. OHSS is triggered by either *exogenous or endogenous human chorionic gonadotropin (hCG)*. Various ovarian factors have been implicated as a cause for the vascular permeability, most important being, *vascular endothelial growth factor (VEGF)*.[7-9]

The fluid shift into the third space can cause hemoconcentration and hypovolemia. The low volume leads to reduced renal and hepatic perfusion causing oliguria and alteration of coagulation. The hemoconcentration and the hyperestrogenic state increases the risk of thromboembolism. The fluid shift also causes electrolyte imbalance resulting in hyponatremia and hypokalemia.[10,11]

CLASSIFICATION OF OVARIAN HYPERSTIMULATION SYNDROME

One classification is according to the time of onset, i.e. early (presenting within 7 days of oocyte retrieval) and late (from 10 days after egg collection).

- Early onset OHSS occurs as a result of exogenous hCG administration as a trigger for egg collection.
- Late onset OHSS occurs as a result of endogenous hCG from an early pregnancy.

Another classification, based on its severity, of OHSS can be classified into mild, moderate, severe, and critical **(Table 1)**.

TABLE 1: Classification of ovarian hyperstimulation syndrome (OHSS) based on disease severity.

Grade based on severity	Symptoms
Mild OHSS	• Abdominal bloating • Mild abdominal pain • Ovarian size usually <8 cm
Moderate OHSS	• Moderate abdominal pain • Nausea vomiting • Ultrasound evidence of ascites • Ovarian size usually 8–12 cm
Severe OHSS	• Clinical (ascites hydrothorax) • Oliguria (<300 mL/day) • Hemoconcentration (hematocrit > 45%) • Hyponatremia (sodium < 135 mmol/L) • Hypoproteinemia (albumin <35 g/dL) • Ovarian size usually >12 cm
Critical OHSS	• Tense ascites • Large hydrothorax • Hematocrit > 55% • White cell count > 25,000/mL • Oliguria/anuria • Thromboembolism • Acute respiratory distress syndrome

PREVENTION

Complete avoidance of OHSS is difficult but identifying the risk factors and individualizing the management to reduce the risk without compromising the success rate.

Primary prevention involves individualizing the treatment by identifying the risk factors. The risk factors can be grouped into:

- *Demographics*: Age, body mass index (BMI), race,[11-14] polycystic ovaries,[15] history of previous hyper response to ovarian stimulation
- *Ovarian reserve markers*: Anti-müllerian hormone (AMH)[16-18] and antral follicle count (AFC)[19,20]
- *Ovarian stimulation parameters*: Number of follicles,[21] oocytes,[22,23] and serum estradiol.[24]

Primary Prevention

- *Metformin*: A Cochrane review has shown that metformin reduces the risk of OHSS by 63%, the live birth rate being similar, with or without metformin.[25-27] 4 months prior to the treatment, up to 2,000 mg can be administered, which can be continued till the first serum β-hCG or until 12 weeks of pregnancy is recommended.
- *Reducing the gonadotropin dose and duration of controlled ovarian stimulation*: Milder stimulation protocols may play a role in achieving this.[28]
- *Gonadotropin-releasing hormone antagonist protocols*: As compared with agonist cycles, antagonist protocols are associated with a reduced risk of OHSS without a significant difference in the live birth rate.[29-33]
- *Avoiding hCG for triggering ovulation*: hCG either urinary or recombinant even at a dose as low as 5,000 IU as ovulatory trigger

can increase the risk of OHSS. Hence, alternatives to hCG like gonadotropin-releasing hormone (GnRH) agonists and recombinant luteinizing hormone (LH) have been explored. GnRH agonists reduce the risk of OHSS,[34,35] however, the standard luteal phase support was found to be inadequate. Hence, when using GnRH agonists as ovulatory trigger the embryos are all frozen and transferred in another cycle after preparing the endometrium. Regarding recombinant LH the costs are higher, as at least 300 IU is needed when used as ovulatory trigger.
- Use of progesterone instead of hCG for luteal phase support: Significantly reduces the risk of OHSS without reducing the pregnancy rate.

Secondary Prevention

- *Freezing all oocytes/embryos*: After egg collection, all the oocytes or embryos are frozen and transferred in a cycle after endometrial preparation, which will prevent the late onset OHSS.[36] However to reduce the early onset OHSS, using GnRH agonists as trigger for ovulation along with freezing of embryos reduces the risk of early and late onset OHSS.
- *Cycle cancellation*: This along with nonadministration of hCG prevents OHSS,[37] but is a waste of finances.
- *Albumin and hydroxyethyl starch (HES)*: The routine use of intravenous albumin is not recommended as a Cochrane review found only limited evidence of benefit.[27] HES is relatively safer alternative to albumin and a statistically significant decrease in the incidence of severe OHSS has been concluded by a Cochrane meta-analyses.

- *Dopamine agonists*: Reduce the incidence of OHSS with no effect on the pregnancy rate.[38] Cabergoline 0.5 mg is taken daily from the day of hCG injection and continued for 8 days.

■ MANAGEMENT

The treatment varies with the severity of the symptoms. Mild and moderate OHSS can be treated on an outpatient basis as most are self-limiting and usually resolve within 1014 days and conservative treatment is adequate.

Outpatient Management

Reassurance and adequate hydration forms the main stay of the treatment. Women are counseled to drink to thirst with a minimum intake of at least 1 L daily. Simple analgesia like paracetamol and codeine can be advised for relief from abdominal discomfort and pain. Nonsteroidal anti-inflammatory drugs (NSAIDs) should be avoided, as they may affect renal function. Nausea and vomiting can be managed with antiemetic medications. Patients should be counseled about avoiding intercourse as ovarian torsion is known to occur. It is also important, to avoid pregnancy, especially when embryos have been cryopreserved to avoid late OHSS. If pregnant, the symptoms may take up to 8 weeks to resolve, due to the endogenous hCG. Mobilization is another important issue as complete bed rest may increase the risk of thromboembolism due to the dehydration.

Inpatient Management

Admission is recommended for increasing abdominal distension, intractable vomiting, oliguria, and hematocrit >45%, respiratory discomfort either due to pleural effusion or due to excessive abdominal distension.

Fluid replacement forms the main stay of management as the patient is dehydrated due to fluid displacement into third spaces. It is important for both organ perfusion and also to prevent thromboembolic phenomenon that may occur. The replaced fluid also enters the third space, due to the leaky capillaries; hence, it is important to monitor fluid intake and urine output. Fluid replacement should be enough to maintain an adequate output of more than 30 mL/hour. If administration of crystalloids is unable to maintain urine output, plasma expanders like HES and albumin can be infused.

Diuretics are to be avoided unless there is no urinary output in spite of adequate hydration. Antiemetics can be administered parenterally, which enables the patient to increase oral fluid intake.

Paracentesis can be considered for abdominal discomfort and breathlessness and if causing oliguria.[39] Thromboprophylaxis is recommended as there is an increased risk of thromboembolism.[40] Adequate hydration, avoiding immobilization and administration of low molecular weight heparin should help reduce the risk of thromboembolism. Multidisciplinary involvement with the IVF clinician in the lead is ideal. In patients resistant to medical treatment termination of pregnancy could be considered.

SUMMARY

- Ovarian hyperstimulation syndrome is an iatrogenic complication which in its severe form can be life-threatening.
- According to the severity it can be classified into mild, moderate and severe OHSS.
- Complete avoidance of OHSS is difficult but identifying the risk factors and individualizing the management to reduce the risk without compromising the success rate is possible.
- Primary prevention can involve metformin, GnRH antagonist protocols and using GnRH agonist instead of hCG as ovulation trigger.
- Secondary prevention can be done by freezing all the oocytes and transferring the embryos in another cycle. This can prevent late OHSS, however, using GnRH agonist as trigger as well as freezing the embryos may prevent both early and late OHSS.
- Mild and moderate OHSS can be treated on an outpatient basis as most are self-limiting and usually resolve within 10–14 days.
- Reassurance and adequate hydration forms the main stay of the treatment.
- Nonsteroidal anti-inflammatory drugs (NSAIDs) should be avoided, as they may affect renal function.
- Mobilization is another important issue as complete bed rest may increase the risk of thromboembolism due to the dehydration.
- Admission is recommended for increasing abdominal distension, intractable vomiting, oliguria, and hematocrit >45%, respiratory discomfort either due to pleural effusion or due to excessive abdominal distension.
- Fluid replacement forms the main stay of management as the patient is dehydrated and should be enough to maintain an adequate output of more than 30 mL/hour.
- Diuretics are to be avoided unless there is no urinary output in spite of adequate hydration.
- Paracentesis can be considered for abdominal discomfort and breathlessness and if causing oliguria. Thromboprophylaxis is recommended as there is an increased risk of thromboembolism. Adequate hydration, avoiding immobilization and

administration of low molecular weight heparin should help reduce the risk of thromboembolism.
- In patients, resistant to medical treatment termination of pregnancy could be considered.

CONCLUSION

- Ovarian hyperstimulation syndrome is an iatrogenic complication but its risk can be reduced by individualizing the management.
- Steps for primary and secondary prevention of OHSS may reduce the risk.
- Adequate hydration forms the main stay of management.
- Mild and moderate OHSS can be managed on an outpatient basis while severe OHSS may sometimes require admission.

REFERENCES

1. Steward RG, Lan L, Shah AA, et al. Oocyte number as a predictor for ovarian hyperstimulation syndrome and live birth: an analysis of 256,381 in vitro fertilization cycles. Fertil Steril. 2014;101:967-73.
2. Luke B, Brown MB, Morbeck DE, et al. Factors associated with ovarian hyperstimulation syndrome (OHSS) and its effect on assisted reproductive technology (ART) treatment and outcome. Fertil Steril. 2010;94:1399-404.
3. Jayaprakasan K, Chan Y, Islam R, et al. Prediction of in vitro fertilization outcome at different antral follicle count thresholds in a prospective cohort of 1,012 women. Fertil Steril. 2012;98:657-63.
4. Kahnberg A, Enskog A, Brännström M, et al. Prediction of ovarian hyperstimulation syndrome in women undergoing in vitro fertilization. Acta Obstet Gynecol Scand. 2009;88:1373-81.
5. Papanikolaou EG, Pozzobon C, Kolibianakis EM, et al. Incidence and prediction of ovarian hyperstimulation syndrome in women undergoing gonadotropin-releasing hormone antagonist in vitro fertilization cycles. Fertil Steril. 2006;85:112-20.
6. Balakumar V, Ramalingam M, Vanessa Kay. Ovarian hyperstimulation syndrome. Obstetrics, Gynaecology & Reproductive Medicine; 2017.
7. Pellicer A, Albert C, Mercader A, et al. The pathogenesis of ovarian hyperstimulation syndrome: In vivo studies investigating the role of interleukin-1beta, interleukin-6, and vascular endothelial growth factor. Fertil Steril. 1999;71:482-9.
8. Whelan JG, 3rd, Vlahos NF. The ovarian hyperstimulation syndrome. Fertil Steril. 2000;73:883-96.
9. Naredi N, Talwar P, Sandeep K. VEGF antagonist for the prevention of ovarian hyperstimulation syndrome: Current status. Med J Armed Forces India. 2014;70:58-63. doi: 10.1016/j.mjafi.2012.03.005.
10. Herr D, Bekes I, Wulff C. Local Renin-Angiotensin system in the reproductive system. Front Endocrinol (Lausanne). 2013;4:58-63. doi: 10.3389/fendo.2013.00150.
11. Mathur R. Prevention and management of ovarian hyperstimulation syndrome. Obstetrics, Gynaecology & Reproductive Medicine; 2008.
12. Ashrafi M, Bahmanabadi A, Akhond MR, et al. Predictive factors of early moderate/severe ovarian hyperstimulation syndrome in non-polycystic ovarian syndrome patients: a statistical model. Arch Gynecol Obstet. 2015;292:1145-52.
13. Johnson MD, Williams SL, Seager CK, et al. Relationship between human chorionic gonadotropin serum levels and the risk of ovarian hyperstimulation syndrome. Gynecol Endocrinol. 2014;30:294-7.
14. Sousa M, Cunha M, Teixeira da Silva J, et al. Ovarian hyperstimulation syndrome: a clinical report on 4894 consecutive ART treatment cycles. Reprod Biol Endocrinol. 2015;13:66.
15. Swanton A, Storey L, McVeigh E, et al. IVF outcome in women with PCOS, PCO and normal ovarian morphology. Eur J Obstet Gynecol Reprod Biol. 2010;149:68-71.
16. Lee TH, Liu CH, Huang CC, et al. Serum anti-müllerian hormone and estradiol levels as predictors of ovarian hyperstimulation

syndrome in assisted reproduction technology cycles. Hum Reprod. 2008;23:160-7.
17. Nakhuda GS, Chu MC, Wang JG, et al. Elevated serum müllerian-inhibiting substance may be a marker for ovarian hyperstimulation syndrome in normal women undergoing in vitro fertilization. Fertil Steril. 2006;85:1541-3.
18. Tal R, Seifer DB, Khanimov M, et al. Characterization of women with elevated anti-müllerian hormone levels (AMH): correlation of AMH with polycystic ovarian syndrome phenotypes and assisted reproductive technology outcomes. Am J Obstet Gynecol. 2014;211:59.e1-8.
19. Ocal P, Sahmay S, Cetin M, et al. Serum anti-müllerian hormone and antral follicle count as predictive markers of OHSS in ART cycles. J Assist Reprod Genet. 2011;28:1197-203.
20. Moos J, Rezabek K, Filova V, et al. Comparison of follicular fluid and serum levels of inhibin A and inhibin B with calculated indices used as predictive markers of Ovarian Hyperstimulation Syndrome in IVF patients. Reprod Biol Endocrinol. 2009;7:86.
21. Jayaprakasan K, Herbert M, Moody E, et al. Estimating the risks of ovarian hyperstimulation syndrome (OHSS): implications for egg donation for research. Hum Fertil (Camb). 2007;10:183-7.
22. D'Angelo A, Davies R, Salah E, et al. Value of the serum estradiol level for preventing ovarian hyperstimulation syndrome: a retrospective case control study. Fertil Steril. 2004;81:332-6.
23. Reljic M, Vlaisavljevic V, Gavric V, et al. Number of oocytes retrieved and resulting pregnancy. Risk factors for ovarian hyperstimulation syndrome. J Reprod Med. 1999;44:713-8.
24. Hendriks DJ, Klinkert ER, Bancsi LF, et al. Use of stimulated serum estradiol measurements for the prediction of hyper-response to ovarian stimulation in in vitro fertilization (IVF). J Assist Reprod Genet. 2004;21:65-72.
25. Palomba S, Falbo A, Carrillo L, et al. METformin in High Responder Italian Group. Metformin reduces risk of ovarian hyperstimulation syndrome in patients with polycystic ovary syndrome during gonadotropin-stimulated in vitro fertilization cycles: a randomized, controlled trial. Fertil Steril. 2011;96:1384-90.e4.
26. Qublan HS, Al-Khaderei S, Abu-Salem AN, et al. Metformin in the treatment of clomiphene citrate-resistant women with polycystic ovary syndrome undergoing in vitro fertilisation treatment: a randomised controlled trial. J Obstet Gynaecol. 2009;29:651-5.
27. Youssef MA, Al-Inany HG, Evers JL, et al. Intra-venous fluids for the prevention of severe ovarian hyperstimulation syndrome. Cochrane Database Syst Rev. 2011:CD001302.
28. Oudshoorn SC, van Tilborg TC, Eijkemans MJC, et al. Individualized versus standard FSH dosing in women starting IVF/ICSI: an RCT. Part 1: The predicted poor responder. Hum Reprod. 2017;32(12):2496-505.
29. Humaidan P, Quartarolo J, Papanikolaou EG. Preventing ovarian hyperstimulation syndrome: guidance for the clinician. Fertil Steril. 2010;94(2):389-400.
30. Pfeifer S, Butts S, Dumesic D, et al. Prevention and treatment of moderate and severe ovarian hyperstimulation syndrome: a guideline. Fertil Steril; 2016.
31. Ludwig M, Katalinic A, Diedrich K. Use of GnRH antagonists in ovarian stimulation for assisted reproductive technologies compared to the long protocol. Meta-analysis. Arch Gynecol Obstet. 2001;265:175-82.
32. Mancini F, Tur R, Martinez F, et al. Gonado-trophin-releasing hormone-antagonists vs long agonist in in-vitro fertilization patients with polycystic ovary syndrome: a meta-analysis. Gynecol Endocrinol. 2011;27:150-5.
33. Xiao J, Chen S, Zhang C, et al. Effectiveness of GnRH antagonist in the treatment of patients with polycystic ovary syndrome undergoing IVF: a systematic review and meta- analysis. Gynecol Endocrinol. 2013;29:187-91.
34. Youssef MA, Van der Veen F, Al-Inany HG, et al. Gonadotropin-releasing hormone agonist versus hCG for oocyte triggering in antagonist-assisted reproductive technology. Cochrane Database Syst Rev. 2014:CD008046.
35. Humaidan P, Polyzos NP, Alsbjerg B, et al. GnRHa trigger and individualized luteal phase hCG support according to ovarian response to stimulation: two prospective randomized controlled multi-centre studies in IVF patients. Hum Reprod. 2013;28:2511-21.

36. Ferraretti AP, Gianaroli L, Magli C, et al. Elective cryopreservation of all pronucleate embryos in women at risk of ovarian hyperstimulation syndrome: efficiency and safety. Hum Reprod. 1999;14:1457-60.
37. Dhont M, Van der Straeten F, De Sutter P. Prevention of severe ovarian hyperstimulation by coasting. Fertil Steril. 1998;70:847-50.
38. Leitao VM, Moroni RM, Seko LM, et al. Cabergoline for the prevention of ovarian hyperstimulation syndrome: systematic review and meta-analysis of randomized controlled trials. Fertil Steril. 2014;101:664-75.
39. Sabahov A, Mitev D, Kirilova I, et al. Ovarian hyperstimulation syndrome (OHSS) and associated complications. Anaesth Intens Care. 2016;45:6-10.
40. Sander T, Borcard A. Ovarian hyperstimulation syndrome (OHSS). Journal for Gynecol Endocrinol. 2011;21:12-4.

CHAPTER 13

Ovarian Torsion

B Ramesh

INTRODUCTION

Torsion of ovary is a gynecological emergency accounting for approximately 2–3% of cases. Most of the cases present with abdominal pain which is sudden, acute, and severe in nature. The diagnosis is often delayed as a variety of other conditions have similar presentation. This may lead to loss of ovary and poor outcomes like infertility. As the clinical features are nonspecific and the ultrasound is the mainstay to make preoperative diagnosis,[1,2] the exact incidence of the condition is unknown and definitive diagnosis is often made intraoperatively.

DEFINITION

Ovarian Torsion

Complete or partial rotation of ligamentous supports which include lymphatics, arteries, and veins due to mechanical obstruction resulting in ischemia and infarction (**Fig. 1**).[3]

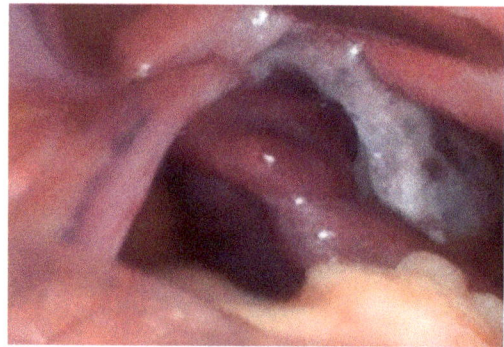

Fig. 1: Torsion of vessels and ovarian ligament.

Adnexal Torsion

It is torsion of the fallopian tubes and ovaries together. It occurs in 67% of cases of adnexal torsion.[4,5]

NORMAL ANATOMY OF OVARIES (FIG. 2)

The infundibulopelvic and utero-ovarian ligaments suspend the movable ovary, and also contain the arterial, venous, and lymphatic

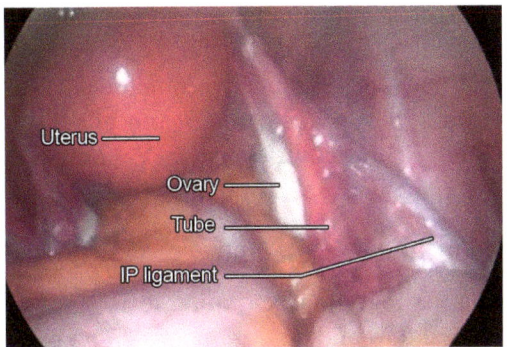

Fig. 2: Normal anatomy of ovaries.

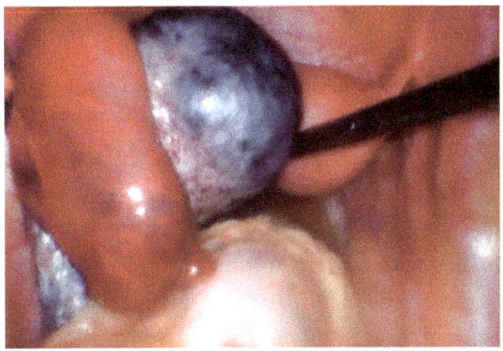

Fig. 3: Pathophysiology of torsion. Torsion of ovarian pedicle leads to twisting of ligaments and vascular pedicles followed by venous occlusion and congestion. In severe and advanced cases, arterial flow is also occluded leading to ischemia and necrosis.

supply to the ovaries.[6] As the ovaries are mobile, they are capable of undergoing twisting by any benign or malignant growth within it.

PATHOPHYSIOLOGY OF TORSION

Ovarian torsion results due to rotation of enlarged ovary on its supports.

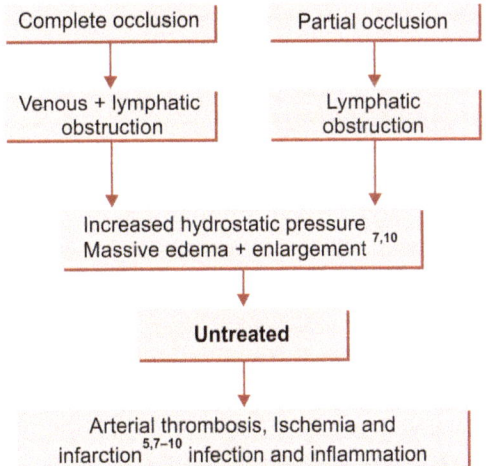

- Torsion of a normal sized ovary is more commonly seen in adolescents. It can occur due to:
  - Marked mobility of fallopian tubes or mesosalpinx
  - Lengthening of pelvic support ligaments
  - Sudden changes in intra-abdominal pressure.[5,16,17]
- Pelvic inflammatory disease, endometriosis, or malignancies are not associated with torsion commonly as adhesions, make the ovaries immobile.[7,8,18]
- Ovarian torsion can be seen after laparoscopic hysterectomy.[19] This is due to less adhesion formation, which is the result of lesser peritoneal trauma and inflammatory response in laparoscopic surgeries.[20,21]
- Torsion involving paratubal or paraovarian cysts have also been found.[22-24]

ETIOLOGY

- The most common cause is cysts in the ovaries[11-13] which includes benign cystic teratoma, cystadenoma,[4,14] hemorrhagic cyst, and cysts caused by ovulation inducing agents.[15]

CLINICAL FEATURES

Most commonly seen in adolescents and young women in childbearing age groups and less common in postmenopausal age groups.[8]

A history of acute pain in a lower abdomen associated with nausea and vomiting should alert the clinician to raise the suspicion of ovarian torsion. On bimanual examination, a palpable mass is felt with adnexal tenderness.[12,25] These classical symptoms and signs are rarely present, leading to delay in diagnosis and treatment. In some cases, due to repeated episodes of torsion and detorsion, acute pain is interspersed with asymptomatic intervals. The following differentials should be considered while evaluating such a patient.

DIFFERENTIAL DIAGNOSIS

- Appendicitis
- Ruptured ovarian cyst
- Urinary tract infection
- Nephrolithiasis
- Pelvic inflammatory disease
- Uterine leiomyoma
- Diverticulitis
- Bowel obstruction
- Ectopic pregnancy.

DIAGNOSIS

Definitive diagnosis of ovarian torsion requires laparoscopy. There is no serum marker for a diagnosis of adnexal torsion. Some studies have found an association between an increased level of serum interleukin-6[26,27] and ovarian torsion, although further research is needed.[28]

IMAGING FEATURES OF OVARIAN TORSION

Grayscale Ultrasonography

As the clinical features are nonspecific, ultrasound is the mainstay to make preoperative diagnosis.[1,2]

The most common ultrasound features include unilateral ovarian enlargement that may be associated with heterogeneous stroma due to hemorrhage and edema. A complex adnexal mass may be found cystic predominately, solid, or both.[4,7,18]

Color Doppler Imaging

The pathognomonic finding is absence of arterial flow and the whirlpool sign on color Doppler. However, it may be associated with normal findings[4,29] because of dual blood supply of ovaries by ovarian and ovarian branches of uterine artery.[9] The abnormal arterial flow is almost always accompanied by either reduced or absent venous flow, which shows that veins are affected earlier in the pathogenesis of torsion.[4] The whirlpool sign is visualization of coiled circular vessels around the enlarged ovaries. It has been associated with necrotic or infarcted ovaries intraoperatively.[10,30]

MANAGEMENT

The gold standard to treat ovary torsion is surgery, and this is also the only way to confirm the torsion. There are two surgical methods, laparoscopy and laparotomy. A laparoscopic approach has become a popular procedure.

The current recommendations suggests surgical detorsion and ovarian conservation[30,31] rather than salpingo-oophorectomy is the best surgical practice **(Figs. 4A and B)**.

If malignancy is suspected, a salpingo-ophorectomy is warranted. According to many observational studies, detorsion is associated with preserved ovarian function.[32-35] The earlier the approach to torsion, the higher is the chance to preserve function. An animal study showed that necrosis might develop after occlusion of ovarian vessels for 36 hours

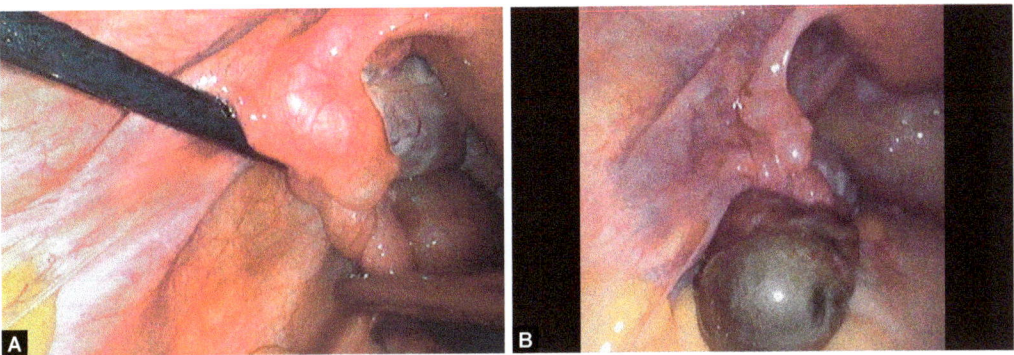

Figs. 4A and B: Laparoscopic image of torsed and detorsed ovaries.

or longer **(Fig. 5)**.[36] After the symptoms have developed, ovarian conservation reportedly decreases with time.[37,38] No evidence suggests that detorsion increases adverse events postoperatively.[39]

Laparoscopic management in pregnancy is controversial. Nezhat et al. (1997) in their study demonstrated operative laparoscopy to be beneficial with subsequent successful pregnancy outcomes.[40] In another study, by Schelling et al. (2000) they advised to avoid laparoscopic management due to difficult access, prolonged operative time, and increase in intra-abdominal pressure leading to decreased uterine blood flow with a theoretical risk of fetal acidosis.[41] Pucci and Seed (1991) reported that pneumoperitoneum with carbon dioxide does not lead to any adverse fetal effects.[42] Taking all these points into consideration, following recommendations need to be followed while operating on pregnant women. These include:
- Monitoring of arterial blood gas and CO_2 level
- Pneumoperitoneum pressure to be kept below 12 mm Hg
- Left lateral position.

Neonates with ovarian torsion often present with irritability and the condition can be treated with laparoscopic surgery.[43-45]

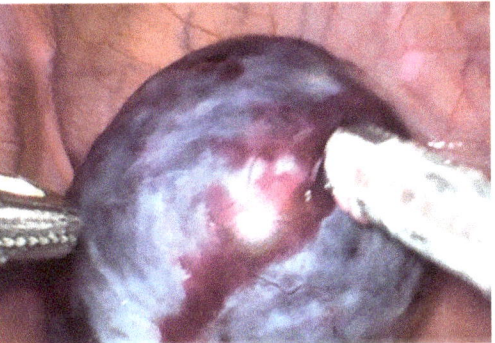

Fig. 5: Laparoscopic image of gangrenous ovary.

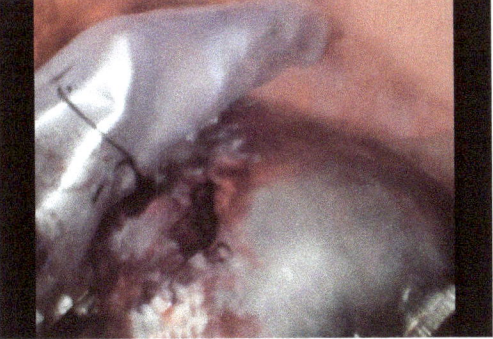

Fig. 6: Laparoscopic oophorectomy in postmenopausal woman and tissue retrieval in endobag.

Bilateral oophorectomy, however is considered treatment of choice in postmenopausal women **(Fig. 6)**.[8]

Oophoropexy is fixation of ovary aiming to decrease further episodes of ovarian torsion for

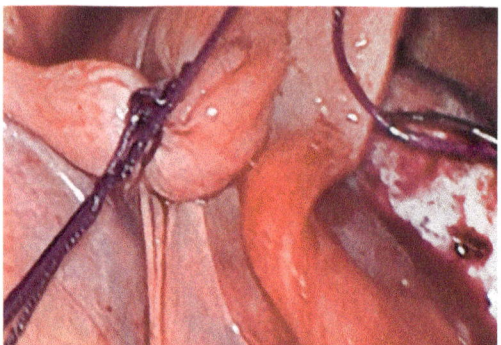

Fig. 7: Laparoscopic oophoropexy.

the purpose of maintaining fertility. However, this management approach has sparked debate recently. At present, there is a lack of substantial evidence relating to the long-term outcome of this conservative approach. Theoretical concerns in regard to oophoropexy include concerns regarding the disruption of tubal blood supply or altered tubo-ovarian communication.[46] There is also controversy over the appropriateness of fixation of the contralateral ovary in children who have lost one ovary due to torsion and necrosis.

Oophoropexy can be done by fixing the ovary to:
- Lateral pelvic wall **(Fig. 7)**
- Posterior abdominal wall
- Utero-ovarian ligament plication—to prevent recurrence.

The plication of utero-ovarian ligament is the preferred technique of oophoropexy. A combined approach of plication of ligament and fixation of ovary to either posterior abdominal wall or lateral pelvic wall may be more efficacious in prevention of recurrence.[47]

KEY NOTES

1. Diagnosis of ovarian torsion is mainly on laparoscopy.
2. An enlarged ovary on ultrasound is most consistent with the diagnosis, in the absence of which the diagnosis is unlikely to be torsion ovary. Also, presence of and comparison with normal contralateral side is very useful in establishing the diagnosis.
3. Conservative approach of management is ideal with majority of cases occurring in young women.
4. The most important factor in preservation of ovarian function is early recognition and treatment. Several studies have reported high salvage rates when treatment is initiated within the first 24 hours of the onset of symptoms.

SUMMARY

- Ovarian torsion is a gynecological emergency and accounts for 2–15% of cases.
- It occurs due to rotation of ovary over its attachment and can result in partial or complete occlusion of the blood supply.
- Clinical symptoms include acute severe abdominal pain, nausea and vomiting. Ultrasonography is the first modality used for diagnostic assessment. Doppler evaluation and MRI can be used as adjunct.
- Surgery is the mainstay of the management and also helps in confirmation of diagnosis. Both laparoscopic and laparotomy are equally effective approaches, though laparoscopy is preferred due to shorter recovery period.

CONCLUSION

The diagnosis of ovarian torsion is difficult due to overlapping of symptoms with other acute abdominal conditions. Careful evaluation of presenting symptoms, physical examination and use of imaging modalities is very critical for early diagnosis and treatment. Conservative treatment with detorsion, cystectomy or oophorectomy can be done based on extent of occlusion and tissue viability.

REFERENCES

1. Bharathan R, Ramsawak L, Kelly A. Ovarian torsion: opportunities to improve clinical management. J Obstet Gynaecol. 2012;32:683-6.
2. Swenson DW, Lourenco AP, Beaudoin FL, et al. Ovarian torsion. Case-control study comparing the sensitivity and specificity of ultrasonography and computed tomography for diagnosis in the emergency department. Eur J Radiol. 2014;84:733-8.
3. Sasaki KJ, Miller CE. Adnexal torsion: review of the literature. J Minim Invasive Gynecol. 2014;21:196-202.
4. Albayram F, Hamper UM. Ovarian and adnexal torsion: spectrum of sonographic findings with pathologic correlation. J Ultrasound Med. 2001;20(10):1083-9.
5. Breech LL, Hillard PJ. Adnexal torsion in pediatric and adolescent girls. Curr Opin Obstet Gynecol. 2005;17(5):483-9.
6. Anne A, Dalley A. Grant's Atlas of Anatomy, 13th edition. Philadelphia: Lippincott Williams & Wilkins; 2012.
7. Warner MA, Fleischer AC, Edell SL. Uterine adnexal torsion: sonographic findings. Radiology. 1985;154(3):773-5.
8. Oelsner G, Shashar D. Adnexal torsion. Clin Obstet Gynecol. 2006;49(3):459-63.
9. Rosado WM, Trambert MA, Gosink BB, et al. Adnexal torsion: diagnosis by using Doppler sonography. AJR Am J Roentgenol. 1992;159(6):1251-3.
10. Lee AR, Kim KH, Lee BH, et al. Massive edema of the ovary: imaging findings. AJR Am J Roentgenol. 1993;161(2):343-4.
11. Varras M, Tsikini A, Polyzos D, et al. Uterine adnexal torsion: Pathologic and gray scale ultrasonographic findings. Clin Exp Obstet Gynecol. 2004;31:34-8.
12. Houry D, Abbott JT. Ovarian torsion: a fifteenyear review. Ann Emerg Med. 2001;38:156-9.
13. White M, Stella J. Ovarian torsion: 10 year perspective. Emerg Med Australas. 2005;17:231-7.
14. Lee EJ, Kwon HC, Joo HJ, et al. Diagnosis of ovarian torsion with color Doppler sonography: depiction of twisted vascular pedicle. J Ultrasound Med. 1998;17(2):83-9.
15. Gorkemli H, Camus M, Clasen K. Adnexal torsion after gonadotrophin ovulation induction for IVF or ICSI and its conservative treatment. Arch Gynecol Obstet. 2002;267:4-6.
16. Littman ED, Rydfors J, Milki AA. Exercise induced ovarian torsion in the cycle following gonadotrophin therapy: case report. Hum Reprod. 2003;18(8):1641-2.
17. Mordehai J, Mares AJ, Barki Y, et al. Torsion of uterine adnexa in neonates and children: a report of 20 cases. J Pediatr Surg. 1991;26(10):1195-9.
18. Graif M, Shalev J, Strauss S, et al. Torsion of the ovary: sonographic features. AJR Am J Roentgenol. 1984;143(6):1331-4.
19. Mashiach R, Canis M, Jardon K, et al. Adnexal torsion after laparoscopic hysterectomy: description of seven cases. J Am Assoc Gynecol Laparosc. 2004;11(3):336-9.
20. Gutt CN, Oniu T, Schemmer P. Fewer adhesions induced by laparoscopic surgery? Surg Endosc. 2004;18(6):898 906.
21. Roberston D, Lefebvre G, Clinical Practice Gynaecology Committee. Adhesion prevention in gynaecological surgery. J Obstet Gynaecol Can. 2010;32:598-608.
22. Muolokwu E, Sanchez J, Bercaw JL, et al. The incidence and surgical management of paratubal cysts in a pediatric and adolescent population. J Pediatr Surg. 2011;46:2161-3.
23. Schrager J, Robles G, Platz T. Isolated fallopian tube torsion: A rare entity in a premenarcheal female. Am Surg. 2012;78:118-9.
24. Said MR, Bamigboye V. Twisted paraovarian cyst in a young girl. J Obstet Gynaecol. 2008;28:549-50.
25. Gillmer MD. Morris PJ, Wood WC. Ovarian accidents. Oxford Textbook of Surgery, 2nd edition. New York, NY: Oxford University Press; 2000.
26. Cohen SB, Wattiez A, Stockheim D, et al. The accuracy of serum interleukin-6 and tumour necrosis factor as markers for ovarian torsion. Hum Reprod. 2001;16:2195-7.
27. Daponte A, Pournaras S, Hadjichristodoulou C, et al. Novel serum inflammatory markers in

patients with adnexal mass who had surgery for ovarian torsion. Fertil Steril. 2006;85:1469-72.
28. Laganà AS, Sofo V, Salmeri FM, et al. Oxidative stress during ovarian torsion in pediatric and adolescent patients: Changing the perspective of the disease. Int J Fertil Steril. 2016;9:416-23.
29. Pena JE, Ufberg D, Cooney N, et al. Usefulness of Doppler sonography in the diagnosis of ovarian torsion. Fertil Steril. 2000;73(5):1047-50.
30. Vijayaraghavan SB. Sonographic whirlpool sign in ovarian torsion. J Ultrasound Med. 2004;23(12):1643-9.
31. Hubner N, Langer JC, Kives S, et al. Evolution in the management of pediatric and adolescent ovarian torsion as a result of quality improvement measures. J Pediatr Adolesc Gynecol. 2017;30:132-7.
32. Harkins G. Ovarian torsion treated with untwisting: Second look 36 hours after untwisting. J Minim Invasive Gynecol. 2007;14:270.
33. Mashiach S, Bider D, Moran O, et al. Adnexal torsion of hyperstimulated ovaries in pregnancies after gonadotropin therapy. Fertil Steril. 1990;53:76-80.
34. Bider D, Mashiach S, Dulitzky M, et al. Clinical, surgical and pathological findings of adnexal torsion in pregnant and non-pregnant women. Surg Gynecol Obstet. 1991;173:363-6.
35. Dolgin SE, Lublin M, Shlasko E. Maximizing ovarian salvage when treating idiopathic adnexal torsion. J Pediatr Surg. 2000;35:624-6.
36. Taskin O, Birincioglu M, Aydin A, et al. The effects of twisted ischaemic adnexa managed by detorsion on ovarian viability and histology: An ischaemia reperfusion rodent model. Hum Reprod. 1998;13:2823-7.
37. Anders JF, Powell EC. Urgency of evaluation and outcome of acute ovarian torsion in pediatric patients. Arch Pediatr Adolesc Med. 2005;159:532-5.
38. Aziz D, Davis V, Allen L, et al. Ovarian torsion in children: Is oophorectomy necessary? J Pediatr Surg. 2004;39:750-3.
39. Zweizig S, Perron J, Grubb D, et al. Conservative management of adnexal torsion. Am J Obstet Gynecol. 1993;168(6):1791-5.
40. Nezhat FR, Tazuke S, Nezhat CH, et al. Laparoscopy during pregnancy: a literature review. JSLS. 1997;1:17-27.
41. Schelling M, Adnextumoren in der Schwangerschaft. In: Schneider H, Husslein P, Schneider KTM (Eds). Heidelberg: Springer-Verlag; 2000.
42. Pucci RO, Seed R. Case report of laparoscopic cholecystectomy in the third trimester of pregnancy. Am J Obstet Gynecol. 1991;165(2):401-2.
43. Crombleholme TM, Craigo SD, Garmel S, et al. Fetal ovarian cyst decompression to prevent torsion. J Pediatr Surg. 1997;32:1447-9.
44. Alrabeeah A, Galliani CA, Giacomantonio M, et al. Neonatal ovarian torsion: Report of three cases and review of the literature. Pediatr Pathol. 1988;8:143-9.
45. Bryant AE, Laufer MR. Fetal ovarian cysts: Incidence, diagnosis and management. J Reprod Med. 2004;49:329-37.
46. Fuchs N, Smorgick N, Tovbin Y. Oophoropexy to prevent adnexal torsion: how, when, and for whom? J Minim Invasive Gynecol. 2010;17(2):205-8.
47. Simsek E, Kilicdag E, Kalayci H, et al. Repeated ovariopexy failure in recurrent adnexal torsion: Combined approach and review of the literature. Eur J Obstet Gynecol Reprod Biol. 2013;170(2):305-6.

CHAPTER 14

Management of Ovarian Mass in Premenopausal Women

Kavita Manchanda, Jahnavi Esanakula

INTRODUCTION

Woman of any age can present with a mass abdomen. It is important to identify a potentially life-threatening disease. 1 in 1,000 premenopausal women have a chance of symptomatic ovarian cyst which is three times higher in women more than 50 years.[1]

Japan and Asian countries have rates of 2–6.5 new ovarian cancer cases per 100,000 women per year. Ovarian carcinoma represents the sixth most common female cancer and the fourth leading cause of death due to cancers in women and is seen predominantly after third decade. Lifetime risk of dying of ovarian cancer is 1 in 95.[2]

An ovarian mass can be managed either conservatively or surgically. Preoperative assessment of ovarian mass whether the mass is of ovarian origin or not and whether the mass is benign or malignant is of at most importance. However, no algorithm was found to be superior to the others in terms of differentiating benign and malignant tumors.

CLASSIFICATION

Ovarian tumors can be classified according to WHO 2014.
- Serous tumors:
    - Benign
        - Cystadenoma, adenofibroma, and surface papilloma
    - Borderline
        - Atypical proliferating tumor and micropapillary type
    - Malignant
        - Serous low grade and high grade carcinoma
- Mucinous tumors:
    - Benign
        - Mucinous cystadenoma
    - Borderline
        - Atypical proliferating mucinous tumor

- Malignant
  - Mucinous carcinoma
- Endometrioid tumor:
  - Benign
    - Cyst, cystadenoma, and adenofibroma
  - Borderline
    - Endometrioid borderline tumor
  - Malignant
    - Endometrioid carcinoma
- Clear cell tumor:
  - Benign
    - Cystadenoma and adenofibroma
  - Borderline
    - Atypical proliferating clear cell tumor
  - Malignant
    - Clear cell carcinoma
- Transitional cell tumor:
  - Benign
    - Brenner tumor
  - Borderline
    - Atypical proliferating transitional cell tumor
  - Malignant
    - Malignant Brenner tumor
- Seromucinous tumors:
  - Benign tumor—cystadenoma and adenofibroma
  - Borderline tumor—atypical proliferating seromucinous tumor
  - Malignant tumor—seromucinous carcinoma
- Mixed epithelial tumors
- Undifferentiated and unclassifiable tumors.

DIFFERENTIAL DIAGNOSIS

Tubal cysts, hydrosalpinx, paraovarian cysts, tubo-ovarian abscess, and peritoneal cysts.

Symptoms

Pain abdomen, vomiting, changes in bowel habits, abdominal heaviness, distension, frequent urination, dysuria, polyuria, and mass abdomen are some of the symptoms a woman can present with in mass abdomen. Rapid growth, loss of weight, and appetite is a sign of malignant ovarian mass. More often than not the woman can be asymptomatic and mass detected on physical examination.

Goff et al. symptomatic index was designed to identify women at risk with ovarian cancer. Pelvic or abdominal pain, urinary urgency or frequency, increased abdominal size or bloating, and difficulty in eating or feeling full when they were present in <1 year and occurred >12 days per month.

Index has a sensitivity of 56.7 for early stage disease and 79.5% for advanced stage disease. Specificity was 90% for women aged >50 years and 86.7% for women aged <50 years.[3]

The difference can be made out with clinical examination and an ultrasonography (USG).

On examination malignant tumors more often bilateral, fixed, solid or semisolid, nodular or lobulated often with ascites containing malignant cells.

Pseudomyxoma Peritonei

It is a condition where mucin accumulates within the peritoneal cavity. It is differentiated from simple mucinous ascites from the fact that mucinous ascites is usually acellular and in pseudomyxoma peritonei has presence of cells either inflammatory of malignant.

Meigs' Syndrome

It accounts for about 1% of ovarian tumors. It is a triad of ovarian fibroma or thecoma or granulosa cell tumor, pleural effusion, and ascites. Around 70% of pleural effusions are right sided, 15% of them are left sided, and the rest of them are bilateral. It is resolved spontaneously after the resection of tumor.

Pseudo-Meigs' Syndrome

Benign cysts of the ovary other than fibroma, thecoma or granulose cell tumor like struma ovarii, mucinous cystadenoma and teratoma, fibroid uterus, and secondary metastatic disease associated with hydrothorax and ascites.

DIAGNOSIS

Ultrasound Examination

It is the most valuable tool for assessment of ovarian tumor. Transvaginal USG is usually used to diagnose the ovarian tumor. In case of tumors extended into the abdomen or suspicion of metastasis transabdominal ultrasound has to be added.

Functional Cyst

It is usually less than 5 cm unilateral, thin walled clear, unilocular, and no solid components. Functional cyst is one of the most common cysts in premenopausal women **(Figs. 1A and B)**.

Endometriotic Cyst

Endometriotic cysts can have variable appearance on USG. The classical presentation includes single cyst with acoustic enhancing echoes giving ground-glass appearance due to hemorrhagic debris **(Figs. 2A and B)**.

Malignant cyst features **(Fig. 3)**:
- Bilateralism
- Solid component
- Thick septations: >2–3 mm
- Presence of ascites
- Metastatic deposits
- Peritoneal masses
- Enlarged lymph nodes.

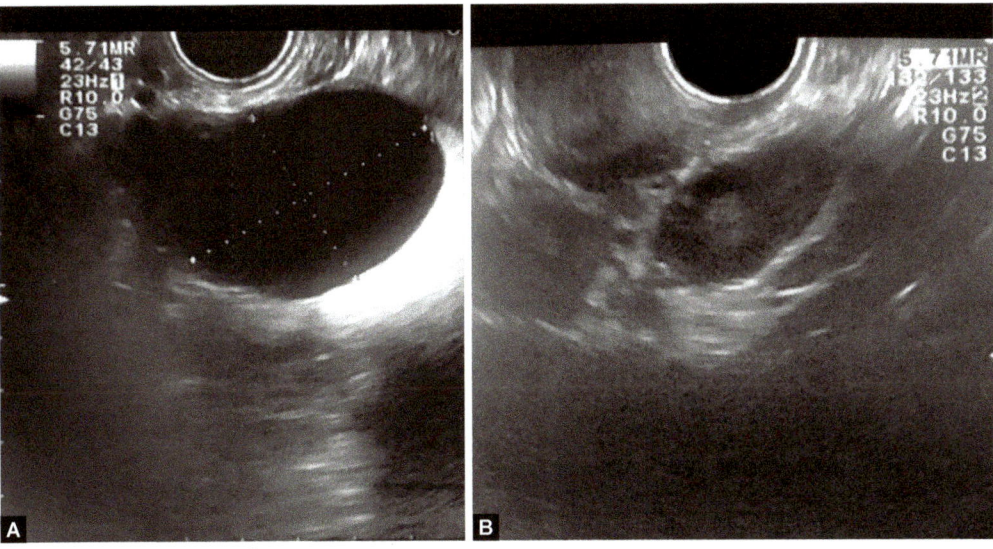

Figs. 1A and B: (A) Simple cyst of ovary; (B) Normal ovary.

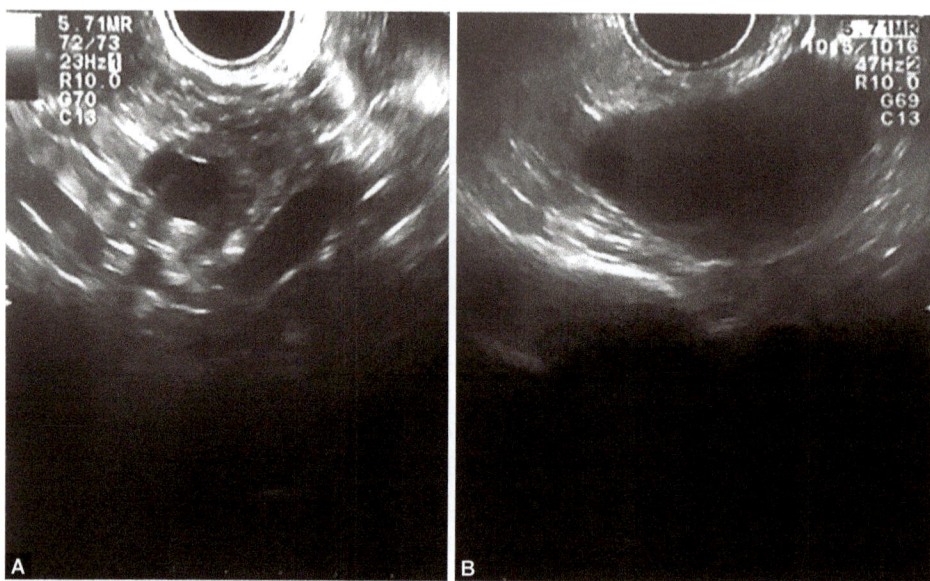

Figs. 2A and B: (A) Normal ovary; (B) Endometriotic cyst of ovary with ground-glass appearance.

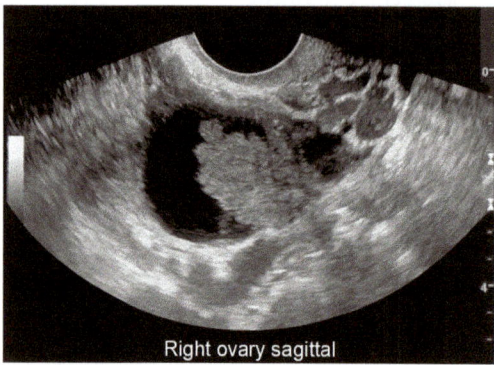

Fig. 3: Malignant lesion of ovary with solid areas and papillary projections.

Magnetic Resonance Imaging/ Computed Tomography/Positron Emission Tomography-Computed Tomography

These are the modalities used when ultrasound is inconclusive or when the origin of a pelvic mass cannot be determined.

Tumor Markers

These are not entirely diagnostic, but they help to characterize the tumor.

Cancer antigen-125 (CA-125): Elevated in ovarian carcinoma. It is also increased in other conditions like endometriosis, pelvic infections, tuberculosis, fibroids, inflammatory bowel disease, hepatic dysfunction, etc. CA-125 is not needed in all premenopausal women, especially when an USG of simple ovarian cyst is made.[4]

- *Alpha-fetoprotein (AFP):* Yolk sac tumor
- *Lactate dehydrogenase (LDH):* Dysgerminoma
- *Inhibin:* Granulosa cell tumor
- *Human chorionic gonadotropin (hCG):* Choriocarcinoma.

AFP, LDH, hCG, and inhibin are to be done in women with <40 years of age with symptoms and signs of germ cell tumors.[1]

Chapter 14: Management of Ovarian Mass in Premenopausal Women

Primary elsewhere:
- *Carcinoembryonic antigen (CEA):* Suspected colorectal
- *Carbohydrate antigen 19-9 (CA 19-9):* Suspected pancreatic or colorectal

INDICATIONS FOR OVARIAN CANCER GENETIC RISK ASSESSMENT AND GENETIC COUNSELING

- Known mutation of gene susceptibility gene
- Ovarian cancer history
- Breast cancer <45 years or 46–50 years with more than two primary breast cancers or 51–60 years with triple negative breast cancer
- Family history of ovarian cancer
- Family history of breast cancer in young or more than two relatives
- Male blood relative with breast cancer
- High-risk population like Ashkenazi Jewish population.

RISK ASSESSMENT

Risk Factors

- *Genetic syndromes:* Hereditary breast and ovarian cancers (BRCA1 and BRCA2), Lynch syndrome, MUTYH associated polyposis, Peutz–Jeghers syndrome, and PTEN hamartoma tumor syndrome
- Postmenopausal hormone replacement therapy
- Obesity
- Weight gain
- Early menarche and late menopause
- Talc exposure
- Usage of oral contraceptive pill (OCP), salpingectomy, tubal ligation, and breast-feeding are protective against ovarian carcinoma.

Risk of Malignancy Index

A risk of malignancy index (RMI) score of more than 200 has sensitivity of 78% and specificity of 87%[5] of predicting of ovarian carcinoma.

CA-125 (value) × Menopausal status (M) × Ultrasound score (U)

- Numerical value of CA-125 in IU/mL
- *Menopausal status:* 1 = premenopausal and 3 = postmenopausal (postmenopausal women is defined as women with no period for one year or more)
- *Ultrasound score:* 0 if none of the following features is noted, 1 if one of the following features is noted, and 3 if two or more of the following features are noted.
  - Multilocular cysts
  - Solid areas
  - Metastasis
  - Ascites
  - Bilateral lesions.

Risk of Malignancy Algorithm (ROMA)

It is based on serum levels of human epididymis protein 4 (HE-4) and CA-125.

OVA1 Test

This uses beta-2 microglobulin, transferrin, transthyretin, and apolipoprotein.

Risk of Ovarian Cancer Algorithm (ROCA)

Uses age of the women and CA-125 profile to triage women into various risk categories.

Proteomics

Matrix-assisted laser desorption and ionization-time of flight (MALDI-TOF) and surface-enhanced laser desorption and ionization-time of flight (SELDI-TOF) are the techniques that allow for the entire protein compliment of a patient to be evaluated.

International Ovarian Tumor Analysis Rules

International Ovarian Tumor Analysis (IOTA) group derived simple ultrasound rules to differentiate benign and malignant lesions.[6] Women with any of the features in M-rules should be referred to a gynecological oncologist.

- *B-rules*:
    - Unilocular cysts
    - Solid components largest <7 mm
    - Acoustic shadowing
    - Smooth multilocular tumor largest <100 mm
    - No blood flow.
- *M-rules*:
    - Irregular solid tumor
    - Ascites
    - Minimum of four papillary structures
    - Irregular multilocular solid tumor largest >100 mm
    - High blood flow.

MANAGEMENT OF OVARIAN MASSES

Management of ovarian mass in premenopausal women can be challenging considering the reproductive choices of the women. Most of the ovarian masses in premenopausal women are benign with overall incidence of approximately 1:1,000 for asymptomatic cysts being malignant. Management decisions are to be guided by nature of the cyst either benign or malignant.

Benign Ovarian Mass

Majority of cysts encountered in premenopausal age group women are found to be functional cysts in luteal phase with diameter 30–50 mm.

Functional cysts ranging in size from 30–50 mm can be managed expectantly with observation if there are no signs of malignancy on USG and RMI is <200. These physiological cysts in most of the cases resolve in three menstrual cycles. According to consensus statement by The Society of Radiologists in Ultrasound, routine follow-up is not required in asymptomatic simple cysts 30–50 mm in diameter. Follow-up with repeat USG at 6 months is done in cysts 50–70 mm. Cysts more than 70 mm in diameter should be further evaluated by either further imaging with MRI or surgical intervention,[7] as there are concerns regarding accurate assessment of cysts as the size increases. Further evaluation is also required in cases of persistent cysts with increase in complexity of the lesion.

Hormonal suppression with OCPs for 3–6 months can be offered for functional cysts less than 50 mm in diameter. However, according to a recent Cochrane review administration of OCPs does not hasten the resolution of the cyst.

Cyst aspiration can be done as a temporary measure, usually in patients undergoing ovulation induction for fertility. However, it is not advised routinely as there are high chances of reaccumulation of fluid and moreover it does not offer any advantage over routine observation.

Surgical management is done in case of persisting cysts, size > 7 cm, increase in size and complexity of the cyst and when there is suspicion of cyst being malignant or borderline malignant. Surgical management can be done either laparoscopically or by laparotomy. Simple ovarian cysts in premenopausal women are usually managed by laparoscopic approach, which offers the advantage of being minimally invasive with less adhesion formation and less postoperative morbidity.

Surgical options include laparoscopic ovarian cystectomy or aspiration of cystic fluid followed by removal of cyst wall. Informed consent should be taken prior to the procedure explaining the risks of laparoscopic surgery,[8] impact of surgery on ovarian reserve, chances of recurrence, and procedure being converted to laparotomy in case need arises. Oophorectomy might be needed in some unexpected scenarios, chances of which should be explained to the women preoperatively.

Patients can present with acute complications like torsion, rupture or hemorrhage in the cyst. Torsion is common in dermoid cyst usually in second trimester of pregnancy. Complete occlusion (arterial and venous) compromises the blood supply of the ovary resulting in necrosis of ovarian tissue. If on clinical examination, patient is stable and there is low risk of a surgical emergency, analgesics and outpatient management is appropriate. For outpatient management, patient is instructed to report immediately in case symptoms worsen. For a patient who appears toxic or is in shock, an immediate surgical exploration is warranted.

Cystectomy involves intact removal of the cyst without rupture and is preferred in cases of dermoid cyst. Intraperitoneal spillage of contents of dermoid cyst can result in chemical peritonitis. Hence, cyst should be removed carefully in endobag to avoid spilling of the contents. Chemical peritonitis due to spillage of dermoid cyst contents has been reported in different series to occur in less than 0.2% of cases.[9] Cystectomy is also preferred in young women with malignancy in whom ovarian preservation is desired for fertility to avoid spill of malignant cells.

Endometriotic cysts can be managed medically or surgically depending upon the symptoms, extent of the disease, and fertility preferences.

Medical management with nonsteroidal anti-inflammatory drugs (NSAIDs) can be offered initially for pain relief explaining risk of recurrence of symptoms after discontinuation. Hormonal treatment with OCPs, progestins, danazol, and gonadotropin-releasing hormone (GnRH) analogs is advised in patients with confirmed or recurrent endometriosis. These agents usually induce either pregnancy-like state or menopause, resulting in suppression of the lesion and hence relief of symptoms. But, there are high chances of recurrence of symptoms after discontinuation of medications.

Surgical management options should be discussed with women, explaining the risks of surgery, its impact on the ovarian reserve, and chances of recurrences. Surgical approach includes adhesiolysis, cystotomy with drainage of contents of the cyst followed by ablation or stripping of cyst wall. Chances of recurrence are more in cases of ablation of cyst wall as compared to stripping, but there is less damage to primordial follicles. Stripping of follicular wall also carries more risk of bleeding and adhesion formation. Chances of spontaneous conception are increased after surgery, but degree of improvement is unclear. Hormonal treatment with GnRH analogs can be offered postsurgically to improve benefits of surgery and associated symptoms. In women, in whom fertility is not an issue definitive management includes hysterectomy with bilateral salpingo-oophorectomy and removal of all visible lesions.

Management of Premenopausal Ovarian Cysts

Management of simple ovarian cyst **(Flowchart 1)** and management of complex ovarian cyst **(Flowchart 2)**.

Flowchart 1: Management of simple ovarian cyst.

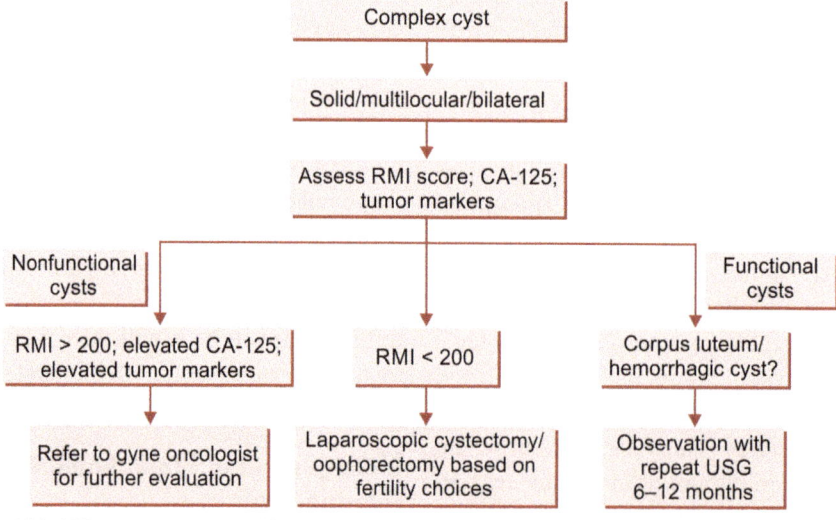

(CA-125: cancer antigen-125).

Flowchart 2: Management of complex ovarian cyst.

(CA-125: cancer antigen-125; RMI: risk of malignancy index; USG: ultrasonography)

Management of Malignant Ovarian Masses

The lifetime risk of developing ovarian cancer is approximately 1 in 70. The risk is even low in premenopausal women, but malignancy should be ruled out in every women presenting with an adnexal mass. The incidence of ovarian cancer increases with age (1.8 to 2.2 per 100,000 women for ages 20–29 years; 3.1 to 5.1 for ages 30–39 years; and 9.0 to 15.2 for ages 40–49 years).[10]

Management of borderline and frankly malignant lesions can be challenging considering the need for future fertility. Management decision should preferably be taken by multidisciplinary team involving gynecologist, radiologist, oncologist, and fertility specialist. Referral to oncologist is required in cases with:

- Elevated CA-125 levels >200 IU
- Presence of ascites
- Presence of metastatic disease
- Family history of breast or ovarian cancer with complex ovarian mass.

Early suspicion, prompt diagnosis, and referral to oncologist can make difference in outcome and survival.

Surgery is the mainstay of therapy in case of malignant ovarian masses. Patient should be well informed about the procedure, the risks associated with surgery, its impact on future fertility, need for postoperative chemotherapy/radiotherapy, chances of recurrence, and survival rate.

Borderline ovarian tumors in young women pose a real clinical dilemma. Most of these tumors are diagnosed in early stage (stage I) and have good 5-year survival rates. However, presence of invasive implants carries high risk of recurrence.

Patients who are keen on fertility preservation should be explained about need for regular surveillance, risk of recurrence of tumor, decrease in ovarian reserve associated with surgery, and the need for second surgery. Unilateral oophorectomy or cystectomy with surgical staging can be done laparoscopically or by laparotomy in early stage disease with noninvasive implants. Spillage of contents should be minimized by removing the tissue in tissue recovery bag as it can upstage the disease. There are high chances of recurrence in cases where cystectomy is performed because of intraoperative rupture of the cyst and presence of multifocal disease. Regular follow-up with USG and CA-125 measurement (if elevated at initial presentation) should be done at 6 monthly intervals for 2 years and annually after that.

Ovarian tissue biopsy from contralateral ovary is not recommended until there is suspicion of malignant lesion on examination. In case of large cysts, aspiration of cyst fluid followed by removal of tissue can be done avoiding intraperitoneal spill. Adjuvant therapy has not been proven to be of much value in cases of borderline malignant tumors.

Patients who have completed child bearing and ones with advanced stage of disease treatment strategy involves exploration of pelvis, abdominal viscera, and peritoneum for metastatic implants, peritoneal fluid cytology, and assessment of lymph node status followed by hysterectomy with bilateral salpingo-oophorectomy. All visible implants should be excised and multiple peritoneal biopsies to be taken in cases with no visible lesions.

Malignant Tumors

Surgical therapy is mainstay of management of malignant ovarian tumors. Proper staging and risk assessment should be done preoperatively. Malignant tumors usually present in advanced stages, with massive ascites and metastasis to distant organs. Abdominal fluid tapping can be done in patients presenting with massive ascites and respiratory discomfort, to provide symptomatic relief. Patient should be referred to gynecology oncology specialist.

Definitive management includes surgical exploration for staging debulking of the tumor mass. Adjuvant chemotherapy depends on the stage of the disease and of residual disease.

INTERNATIONAL FEDERATION OF GYNECOLOGY AND OBSTETRICS (FIGO) STAGING OF OVARIAN TUMORS

- *Stage I:* Tumor confined to ovaries
  - *IA:* Tumor limited to one ovary, intact capsule, no tumor on surface and negative washings
  - *IB:* Tumor involved in both ovaries
  - *IC:* Tumor limited to one or both ovaries
    - *IC1:* Surgical spill
    - *IC2:* Capsule rupture before surgery or tumor on ovarian surface
    - *IC3:* Malignant cells in ascites or peritoneal washings
- *Stage II:* Tumor involves one or both the ovaries with pelvic extension or primary peritoneal cancer
  - *IIA:* Extension and/or implant on uterus and/or Fallopian tubes
  - *IIB:* Extension to other pelvic intraperitoneal tissues.
- *Stage III:* Tumor involves 1 or both ovaries with cytologically or histologically confirmed spread to the peritoneum outside the pelvis and/or metastasis to the retroperitoneal lymph nodes
  - *IIIA:*
    - *A1:* Positive retroperitoneal lymph nodes only
    - *A2:* Microscopic extrapelvic peritoneal involvement
  - *IIIB:* Macroscopic, extrapelvic peritoneal metastasis <2 cm includes extension to capsule of liver and spleen.
  - *IIIC:* Macroscopic, extrapelvic peritoneal metastasis <2 cm includes extension to capsule of liver and spleen.
- *Stage IV:* Distant metastasis excluding peritoneal metastasis
  - *IVA:* Pleural effusion with positive cytology
  - *IVB:* Hepatic and/or splenic parenchymal metastasis, metastasis to extra-abdominal organs

Unilateral oophorectomy may be optimal in patients who desire to preserve fertility, disease confined to the one ovary, stage I disease with no evidence of metastasis, and tumors with low grade malignant potential.

Neoadjuvant chemotherapy followed by debulking surgery has been shown to offer better long-term survival and improved quality of life in patients with advanced stage disease.

Postadjuvant chemotherapy is recommended in advanced stage disease, but is not indicated in patients with disease confined to one ovary.[11]

Post-treatment surveillance should be provided by oncologist with 3 monthly follow-up for 2 years followed by 6 monthly for 3 years, as in most of the cases recurrence occurs in first 5 years. Surveillance should be done by complete physical examination, pelvic examination, imaging modalities like USG and positron emission tomography (PET) scan, and tumor markers like CA-125 and inhibin B if they were found to be raised at initial presentation.

SUMMARY

- Women of any age can present with mass abdomen, 1 in 1000 premenopausal women have a chance of symptomatic ovarian cyst.

- Most of the women present with vague abdominal symptoms like heaviness in abdomen, nausea, pain lower abdomen, urinary symptoms, distension and mass in abdomen.
- Functional cysts are most common in premenopausal age group.
- Ultrasound is the most valuable tool for diagnosis of ovarian masses. Various features on ultrasound can help in differentiation of benign lesions from malignant lesions.
- Treatment can be done by laparoscopy or laparotomy based upon nature of lesion, stage of disease in cases with malignancy and fertility wishes of woman.

CONCLUSION

Ovarian cysts are common in women of reproductive age group. These can be distressing to the patient for the anxiety about malignancy and concern for future fertility. Treatment should be individualized based on the results of lab investigations, radiological assessment and patient's fertility choices. Multidisciplinary approach involving gynecologist, reproductive medicine specialist and gynecological oncologist should be sought in cases with malignancy.

REFERENCES

1. RCOG/BSGE. (2011). Management of Suspected Ovarian Masses in Premenopausal Women. RCOG Green-top Guidelines No.62. [online] Available from https://www.rcog.org.uk/globalassets/documents/guidelines/gtg_62.pdf [Last accessed August, 2019].
2. Siegel R, Ward E, Brawley O, et al. Cancer statistics, 2011. CA Cancer J Clin. 2011;61:212-36.
3. Goff BA, Mandel LS, Drescher CW, et al. Development of an ovarian cancer symptom index. Cancer. 2007;109:221-7.
4. Kahraman K, Ozguven I, Gungor M, et al. Extremely elevated serum CA-125 level as a result of unruptured unilateral endometrioma: the highest value reported. Fertil Steril. 2007;88:968.e15-7.
5. Morgante G, la Marca A, Ditto A, et al. Comparison of two malignancy risk indices based on serum CA125, ultrasound score and menopausal status in the diagnosis of ovarian masses. Br J Obstet Gynaecol. 1999;106:524-7.
6. Timmerman D, Testa AC, Bourne T, et al. Logistic regression model to distinguish between the benign and malignant adnexal mass before surgery: a multicenter study by the International Ovarian Tumor Analysis Group. J Clin Oncol. 2005;23:8794-801.
7. Levine D, Brown DL, Andreotti RF, et al. Management of asymptomatic ovarian and other adnexal cysts imaged at US: Society of Radiologists in Ultrasound Consensus Conference Statement. Radiology. 2010;256:943-54.
8. Clements RV. Major vessel injury. Clinical Risk. 1995;1:112-5.
9. Nezhat CR, Kalyoncu S, Nezhat CH, et al. Laparoscopic management of ovarian dermoid cysts: ten years' experience. JSLS. 1999;3:179-84.
10. American College of Obstetricians and Gynecologists. ACOG Practice Bulletin. Management of adnexal masses. Obstet Gynecol. 2007;110:201-14.
11. Winter-Roach BA, Kitchener HC, Lawrie TA. Adjuvant (post-surgery) chemotherapy for early stage epithelial ovarian cancer. Cochrane Database Syst Rev. 2012;(3):CD004706.

CHAPTER 15

Emergencies and Complications Related to Contraception

Shashikala KT

INTRODUCTION

Contraception is one of the vital interventions in gynecological practice. Thorough understanding of the emergencies and complications related to various contraceptive methods is highly essential, to facilitate informed clinical decision making.

CONTRACEPTION: A BRIEF HISTORY AND EVOLUTION

Contraception or birth control has been one of the ancient and most debated practices among almost every society of the world. Since ancient times to modern day newer contraceptives predominantly target two processes in the process of childbirth, i.e. preventing the ovulation and preventing the fertilization the ovum. Once it was predominantly natural methods, based on understanding of the menstrual cycle. With the advances in medical sciences and enhanced understanding of the process of ovulation, fertilization, and development of fetus, it has evolved into one of the major medical intervention over centuries.

Barrier method of contraception by the use of condoms was one of earliest method. The concept of intrauterine devices (IUDs), which came into existence in 1920s, has evolved as one of the important methods following invention of new generation copper-based IUDs in 1960s. The contraceptive landscape has taken its major turn with the invention of hormonal contraceptives in 1960s. Various technical innovations of permanent methods of contraception including tubectomy and vasectomy also came into existence in later part of 20th century. The advancement has been even more rapid over last four to five decades, with exponential increase in the number and type of contraceptive agents or devices coming into regular clinical practice. With this rapid and unprecedented expansion of the basket of contraceptive agents, also has resulted in corresponding raise in the concerns regarding their safety.

Chapter 15: Emergencies and Complications Related to Contraception

Once considered as an individual prerogative, contraception has evolved into a public health intervention of unprecedented scale in the 20th century. Many countries across the globe, including the most popular countries like India and China have undertaken birth control as nationwide public health measure to contain the uncontrolled growth of their populations. Many of these programs have been criticized for their paternalistic and target-based approach. With the time, these programs also have witnessed a major change in the approach, more towards counseling and informed decision making. Healthcare providers of modern times are required to council the couple thoroughly regarding the advantages, disadvantages, cost, and other aspects of each of contraceptives and to facilitate an informed decision.

EFFECTIVENESS AND SAFETY OF CONTRACEPTIVES: PRACTICE IMPLICATIONS

Both effectiveness and safety of contraceptive methods is of extreme practical importance not only for the couple and their family, but also for the healthcare provider and the sanctity of the community level birth control programs. Failed contraception can end up in unwanted pregnancy and can lead to a cascade of subsequent events, which puts the couple in tremendous amount of mental agony and also the women at risk of major complications due to abortion or child birth.

Major complications occurring due to any contraceptive method, apart from resulting in physical ill health to the women, may have medicolegal consequences to the healthcare providers and may damage the credibility of the birth controls programs at community level. Hence, it is of paramount importance for a healthcare provider to have a thorough understanding of the complications of commonly used contraceptive methods, in order to avoid these adverse consequences.

EMERGENCIES AND MAJOR COMPLICATIONS DUE TO VARIOUS CONTRACEPTIVE METHODS

Female Sterilization (Tubectomy)

Sterilization is the purposeful exclusion of fecundity without sexual and endocrine function compromise.[1,2] Nowadays, the female sterilizations are performed laparoscopically. There are many complications and emergencies related to the female sterilization.

Immediate Complications

- *Bleeding*: Complications of bleeding resulting from laparoscopic sterilization usually occur only if there has been resection or transection of the segment of the tube as part of ligation.[3]
- *Infections*: Wound infection or infection of the pelvic organ might occur in less than 1% of female sterilization. They are more common with the laparoscopy than minilaparotomy approach.[4]
- *Hemorrhage*: One of the rare complications of female sterilization is hemorrhage. It is reported to occur in 30–90 cases per 100,000 female sterilization cases. It follows usually after major vessel (aorta, inferior vena cava or iliac) injury during laparoscopic entry and infrequently subsequent to mesosalpingeal vessel injury during the occlusion procedure. Mesosalpingeal bleeding occurs more commonly with rings and clips and in the course of tube resection during bipolar or unipolar occlusion (level III).[4,5]

- *Pelvic organ injuries:* Pelvic organ injury usually occurs as a result of sharp trauma (i.e. trocar, a Veress needle, and scalpel), blunt trauma (e.g. dissecting adhesions), or electrical-thermal trauma. Organ injuries may infrequently occur during careless application of the occlusion device to the inappropriate structure.[4,6]
- *Death*: The major cause of mortality in female sterilization is attributable to anesthesia and infection. Anesthesia and infection are major causes of death owing to sterilization. Other reasons are due to hypoventilation, hemorrhage, and myocardial infarction.[4]
- *Other complications:* Mule VD et al. evaluated the complication of the female sterilization over a decade at district tertiary care hospital in Maharashtra, India. The most common medical complications were gastritis, fever, convulsions, chest pain, puerperal psychosis, septicemia, skin rash, hypertension, pelvic inflammatory disease (PID), endometritis, encephalitis, hypoglycemia, carpopedal spasm, abdominal tuberculosis, pulmonary embolism, transverse sinus thrombosis, jaundice, and gastroenteritis. The most common surgical complications were bowel injury, bladder injury, wound infection, bleeding in muscle, uterine perforation (lap TL), peritonitis, paralytic ileus, mesosalpingeal tear, adhesions (could not perform tubectomy), urinary retention, burst abdomen, pyosalpinx, omental prolapse, and tubal stump bleeding.[7]

Long-term Complications

- *Regret*: A smaller proportion of women regrets for being sterilized at some point of time after the procedure. Measuring regret is always a challenge since factors indicating regret are unknown. The most common reasons associated with regret are sterilization at an early age and events that are unpredictable such as child death or new marriage.[4]
- *Failure*: Recanalization can occur in females even 20 years after sterilization. Female sterilization performed at primary health center and minilap procedures attributes to the highest failure cases. Undetected luteal pregnancy, partial or inadequate occlusion, occlusion of the inappropriate structure (round ligament mostly), mechanical device slippage, tuboperitoneal fistula development, and spontaneous reanastomosis or recanalization of the cut ends are the most common reasons.[8]
- *Ectopic pregnancy*: One of the major causes of maternal mortality is ectopic pregnancy. Out of 36 patients with ectopic pregnancy, 8 (22.2%) had history of PID, 1 (2.7%) had previous tubal surgery in one of the Indian study.[9]
- *Menstrual changes*: Some of the earlier studies have reported that menstrual variations do occur after sterilization. However, these studies are confounded by factors such as earlier use of contraceptive and irregular menstruation that can affect menstrual cycles.[4]
- *Hernia*: When the puncture site is 8 mm or greater, the bowel can rarely herniate through the site of an umbilical or lower abdominal puncture.[4]
- *Breast cancer, endometrial cancer, and bone density*: Few studies have reported that female sterilization increases the incidence of breast and endometrial cancer while some other studies reported it decreases bone density.[4]

Hormonal Contraceptives

Worldwide the most commonly used hormonal contraceptive is oral contraceptives (OCs). They are generally considered safe and highly effective. OC provides a range of noncontraceptive benefit.[10] However, they do have complications.

- *Cardiovascular effect*: The relative risk for developing venous thromboembolism (VTE) and arterial embolism increases by fourfold and twofold respectively with the use of combined oral contraceptives (COCs). Several studies have reported increased risk of myocardial infarction with OC. However, the OC duration does not seem to correlate with increased risk and becomes nil after discontinuation of treatment. Careful screening of high-risk females reduces the risk further.
- *Venous thromboembolism*: It is a severe adverse complication of hormonal contraception. The VTE incidence among nonusers of OC in fertile age and in oral contraceptive users are respectively, 4–5/10,000 women per year and 9–10/10,000 women per year. The type of progestin and the dose of the estrogen constituent determines the risk of VTE.[11]
- *Metabolic effects*: The use of high-dose, progestogen-dominant OCs raises the atherogenic lipoprotein profile [high low-density lipoprotein (LDL):high-density lipoprotein (HDL) ratio].
- *Liver disorders*: Oral contraceptive may lead to hepatocellular adenoma and gallbladder disease. Rarely, occurrence of cholestatic jaundice was also reported.[12]
- *Subsequent fertility*: In general, oral contraceptive use seems to be followed by a slight delay in conception. The proportion of women becoming pregnant within 2 months of discontinuing the pill may range from 15% to 35%.
- *Ectopic pregnancies*: Ectopic pregnancies mostly occur in women taking progestogen-only pills than in those taking combined pills.[13] Literature have reported an increased risk with intrauterine contraceptive device (IUCD) even after discontinuation of its use.[14]
- *Breast tenderness*: Studies have reported incidence of breast fullness, tenderness, and discomfort among women taking oral pills. Breast engorgement and fullness dependents on the level progestogen; whereas pain and tenderness are estrogen dependent.
- *Migraine*: The use of COC is always contraindicated in case of migraine with aura. Also ones it develops, continuation of therapy is terminated.[15]
- *Bleeding*: Highest number of bleeding/spotting days are reported by OC users.[16]

Complications associated with injectable hormonal contraceptives like depot medroxyprogesterone acetate (DMPA) and norethisterone enanthate (NET-EN) includes cancer of the breast, all genital cancers, undiagnosed abnormal uterine bleeding, and a suspected malignancy.

Intrauterine Devices

Intrauterine devices are birth control devices placed in the uterine cavity to prevent pregnancy in a long-term basis.[17] IUDs are used by around 14.5% of women in reproductive age in the developing countries. Its use constitutes 7.6% in developed countries.[18,19] The copper containing IUDs are the best known and levonorgestrel (LNG) is the next.[20]

There are several complications associated with IUDs which are either immediate or delayed.

Immediate Complications

Perforation of the uterus, vasovagal reaction, bleeding, and pain constitutes the immediate complication. Stenosis of the cervical canal predominantly in emotive and/or nulliparous women occurs with vagal reaction. Any trauma caused by the IUD to the mucus of the endocervix and/or endometrium results in bleeding. Pain appears at the moment of insertion, more frequently in young nullipara than multipara, and disappears spontaneously after 5–10 minutes and it is more constant.

Perforation of intrauterine walls: One of the most serious complications of IUD insertion is uterine perforation. For currently available IUDs, risk is estimated to be less than 1/1,000 for insertions. Perforation risk increases at 4–8 weeks postpartum and mostly occurs at the time of insertion. An IUD device can perforate anywhere in uterine wall.

Intrauterine devices of appropriate size to the endometrial cavity should be chosen always. Displacement of IUDs into the peritoneal cavity is extremely rare. Often it occurs when an inexperienced physician inserts an IUD soon after delivery. The ante- or retroverted uterus further increases the risk. In those cases, removal of IUDs is recommended. Once the IUD becomes embedded in the intestinal wall, laparotomy is usually recommended. An IUD displaced into the peritoneum, might adhere to the peritoneal wall. Therefore, immediate withdrawal of device is advised.[21]

Bleeding: One of the major reasons for IUD removal is uterine bleeding. However, the exact reason is not known. Greater amount of blood loss is reported to be from large inert devices and less with small copper-containing devices. The least is reported to be from progesterone-containing IUD. IUD users are advised for periodic detection of hemoglobin level.

Delayed Complications

Menometrorrhagia, often accompanied by dysmenorrhea, lost IUD, total or partial expulsion, ectopic pregnancy, and pelvic inflammatory disease (PID) constitutes the delayed complications.

Menometrorrhagia: Menometrorrhagia usually occurs due to an increase of fibrinolytic activity of the endometrium in contact with the IUD.

Intrauterine device failure: The rate of IUD failures leading to pregnancy varies between 1.6 and 5.3/100 women per year. The rate of ectopic pregnancy is extremely low among IUD users. However, pregnancy in an IUD user is considered as ectopic until proven otherwise. The protective effects of IUDs are the highest during the 1st and 2nd year. Fallopian tubes are also protected with its contraceptive effect. If pregnant, spontaneous abortion occurs among half of the women with removal of IUD. Nevertheless, spontaneous expulsion occurs in 20–30%, if an IUD is left in situ.[22] Even though rare, intrauterine pregnancies once develop, often end up in miscarriage among IUD users. Within 5 years, in about 5–10% of cases the IUD is expelled. Among 30% of these women expulsion recurs.[23]

According to Howard B et al.,[24] the major complications with IUDs are amenorrhea (7.36–11.59%), heavy menstrual bleeding (HMB) (4.85–15.69%), and pelvic pain (11.12–14.27%).

Pelvic inflammatory disease: The risk for PID ranges from 1.6% to 10.5% among IUD users and are the highest compared with other modes of contraception. The risk is highest in the initial months following insertion and persists higher than normal as long as the IUD is used. PID risk is reduced with hormonal contraceptives. Among IUD users, 6 out of 1,000 women are susceptible to PID in a year. However, routine antibiotic prophylaxis is not recommended. For mild infection, tetracycline 500 mg orally four times daily is advised. In more severe cases a regimen consisting of an aminoglycoside plus penicillin is required.

Emergency Contraception

Emergency contraception pill (ECP) is often referred as the morning-after pill. It is an effective way to prevent pregnancy after unprotected intercourse. It is also advised after a condom breaks, or if another contraceptive has been used inconsistently.[25] ECP is effective only in the first few days following intercourse before the ovum is released from the ovary and before the sperm fertilizes the ovum. Currently the widely used ECPs are single use of a combination of estrogen and gestagen (ethinylestradiol together with LNG); the single use of a progestin (LNG); the use of the mifepristone (mifegyne and mifeprex) and the insertion of a copper IUD.[26]

Complications

The complications or side effects associated with ECPs are very rare and when present are mild and normally resolve without further medications. Some of the most common side effects with emergency contraceptives are:

Nausea and vomiting: When estrogen-containing ECPs are given without antiemetics, nausea and vomiting frequently occurs. Nausea and vomiting are reported in 23% and 6% of women using LNG ECPs and in about 12% of women using the ulipristal regimen.[27] The side effects associated with these newer regimen is far less compared to the earlier combined estrogen-progestin regimen; which causes nausea in about 50% of users, and vomiting in 20%. If vomiting occurs within 2 hours after taking a dose repetition of the dose is recommended.

Abdominal pain: Levonorgestrel ECPs are associated with abdominal pain in 18% of cases.[27]

Short or delayed menstrual cycle: Subsequent to the use of ECPs, temporary disruption of the menstrual cycle is always common. It varies depending on when in the menstrual cycle the pills are taken. ECPs taken after ovulation might extend the duration of luteal phase, thereby delaying menstruation by few days. Whereas higher dose of progesterone might lead to progesterone withdrawal bleeding few days after, if ECPs are taken before ovulation. ECPs cause the disruption of cycle in which it is taken. Following cycle length are not affected generally.[28]

Fatigue or headache: Levonorgestrel ECPs are associated with fatigue in 17% of cases.[27]

Pregnancy: The results are inconclusive on live birth following consumption of combined ECPs by pregnant ladies. Even though lower dose of mifepristone (10 mg) has no effect on endometrium, at higher dose it affects endometrial receptivity. Moreover, if administered during follicular phase of ovarian cycle it inhibits ovulation and in the early luteal phase it prevents implantation.

Emergency contraception pills are beneficial for women with failed contraception or who had unprotected sex. Nevertheless, it cannot be considered as a substitute for regular contraception. Follow-up is always important in ECPs since contraception is not 100% effective.

RECOMMENDATIONS AND FUTURE DIRECTION

All the practitioners at different levels of healthcare system need to have thorough understanding of the complications associated with contraceptive methods. This will facilitate appropriate risk communication to the couple seeking contraceptive advice and aid in informed decision making. Patients often may not report the contraceptive use, hence having a high index of suspicion regarding the contraception-related adverse effects, is vital for timely diagnosis of these events. Establishing database at facility level and periodic audit of the contraceptive associated complications may aid us in understanding the changing trends and help in providing safe and effective contraception.

SUMMARY

The chapter highlighted the spectrum of complications associated with various contraceptive methods. Clinicians at various levels involved in providing contraceptive advise to couples must be completely aware of these complications.

CONCLUSION

All the contraceptive methods are associated with wide range of complications. The spectrum of these complications varies widely from a mild discomfort to often life-threatening complications.

REFERENCES

1. Park K. Female sterilization. Park's Textbook of Preventive and Social Medicine, 24th edition. New Delhi: M/s Banarasidas Bhanot Publications; 2018.
2. Gizzo S, Bertocco A, Saccardi C, et al. Female sterilization: update on clinical efficacy, side effects and contraindications. Minim Invasive Ther Allied Technol. 2014;23(5):261-70.
3. Huggins GR, Sondheimer SJ. Complications of female sterilization: Immediate and delayed. Fertil Steril. 1984;41(3):337-55.
4. Pati S, Cullins V. Female sterilization. Evidence. Obstet Gynecol Clin North Am. 2000;27(4):859-99.
5. Miesfeld RR, Giarratano RC, Moyers TG. Vaginal tubal ligation—is infection a significant risk? Am J Obstet Gynecol. 1980;137(2):183-8.
6. Ansari AH, Sealey RM, Gay JW, et al. Silicone rubber band for laparoscopic tubal sterilization. Fertil Steril. 1977;28(12):1306-9.
7. Mule VD, Date SV, Gadekar MS. Complications of female sterilization procedure: Review over a decade at district tertiary care hospital. Int J Reprod Contracept Obstet Gynecol. 2017;6(10):4309-13.
8. Date SV, Rokade J, Mule V, et al. Female sterilization failure: Review over a decade and its clinicopathological correlation. Int J Appl Basic Med Res. 2014;4(2):81-5.
9. Madan A, Nitin KH, Kaur A, et al. Ectopic Pregnancy: A life threatening emergency. Int J Curr Res Med Sci. 2017;3(7):144-51.
10. Khan S, Smulders YM, de Vries JIP, et al. Life-threatening complications of hormonal contraceptives: A case history. Case Rep Obstet Gynecol. 2013;2013:1-3.
11. Reid R, Leyland N, Wolfman W, et al. Oral contraceptives and the risk of venous thromboembolism: An update. 2011;112(3):252-6.
12. Adlercreutz H. Oral contraceptives and liver damage. Br Med J. 1964;2(5417):1133.
13. Stoll BA, Andrews JT, Motteram R, et al. Oral contraceptives and liver damage. Br Med J. 1965;1(5436):723.
14. Mol BWJ, Ankum WM, Bossuyt PMM, et al. Contraception and the risk of ectopic pregnancy: A meta-analysis. Contraception. 1995;52(6):337-41.
15. Allais G, Gabellari IC, De Lorenzo C, et al. Oral contraceptives in migraine. Expert Rev Neurother. 2009;9(3):381-93.
16. Bachmann G, Korner P. Bleeding patterns associated with oral contraceptive use: A

Chapter 15: Emergencies and Complications Related to Contraception

review of the literature. Contraception. 2007;76(3):182-9.
17. Intrauterine devices: an effective alternative to oral hormonal contraception. Prescrire Int. 2009;18(101):125-30.
18. d'Arcangues C. Worldwide use of intrauterine devices for contraception. Contraception. 2007;75(6 Suppl):S2-7.
19. Aoun J, Dines VA, Stovall DW, et al. Effects of age, parity, and device type on complications and discontinuation of intrauterine devices. Obstet Gynecol. 2014;123(3):585-92.
20. ESHRE Capri Workshop Group. Intrauterine devices and intrauterine systems. Human Reprod Update. 2008;14(3):197-208.
21. Kiilholma P, Mäkinen J, Mäenpää J. Perforation of the uterus following IUD insertion in the puerperium. Adv Contracept. 1990;6(1):57-61.
22. Nagel TC. Intrauterine contraceptive devices. Complications associated with their use. Postgrad Med. 1983;73(3):155-64.
23. Rowlands S, Oloto E, Horwell DH. Intrauterine devices and risk of uterine perforation: current perspectives. Open Access J Contracept. 2016;7:19-32.
24. Howard B, Grubb E, Lage MJ, et al. Trends in use of and complications from intrauterine contraceptive devices and tubal ligation or occlusion. Reprod Health. 2017;14(1):70.
25. World Health Organization. (2018). Emergency Contraception. [online] Available from: http://www.who.int/news-room/fact-sheets/detail/emergency-contraception [Last accessed September, 2019].
26. Lee JK, Schwarz EB. The safety of available and emerging options for emergency contraception. Expert Opin Drug Saf. 2017;16(10):1163-71.
27. Emergency contraception. Paediatr Child Health. 2003;8(3):181-92.
28. Mittal S. Emergency contraception—potential for women's health. Indian J Med Res. 2014;140 (Suppl):S45-52.

SECTION 3

Postmenopausal Age Group

- Pyometra
  Arveen Vohra
- Postmenopausal Bleeding
  Arveen Vohra
- Management of Ovarian Mass in Postmenopausal Women
  Sonal Agarwal
- Gynecological Emergencies in Postmenopausal Women with Mass per Vaginum
  Anu Joseph

CHAPTER 16

Pyometra

Arveen Vohra

INTRODUCTION

The word "pyometra" is derived from Latin "pyo" meaning pus and "metra" meaning uterus. Pyometra is a rare condition characterized by the accumulation of pus within the uterine cavity, with an incidence of 0.01–0.5% of female patients. The incidence of pyometra becomes much higher with age and decline in activity, most frequently seen in postmenopausal women but can affect younger women also.[1,2]

The first case was described in 1812 by John and Clarke of London.

DEFINITION

Accumulation of pus in uterine cavity, caused by interference with natural drainage of uterus is pyometra.

ETIOLOGY

It is primarily caused by impairment of natural drainage of the cervix due to malignant diseases of genital tract and consequences of their treatment with radiotherapy. The common causes of pyometra are given in **Table 1**.[2]

TABLE 1: Common causes of pyometra.

Endometrial carcinoma	Genital tuberculosis[3]
Cervical carcinoma	Cervical occlusion after surgery (prolapse surgery, endometrial ablation)[4,5]
Obstetrical puerperal sepsis	Radiation effect for uterine carcinoma
Senile endometritis	Congenital cervix anomalies[6]
Senile cervicitis	Secondary to intrauterine infection
Submucous fibroid polyp	Forgotten intrauterine device **(Fig. 1)**
Leiomyoma	Actinomycotic pyometra—complication of forgotten intrauterine device **(Fig. 1)**
Uterovaginal prolapse	After ovum retrieval for in vitro fertilization (IVF)[7,8]

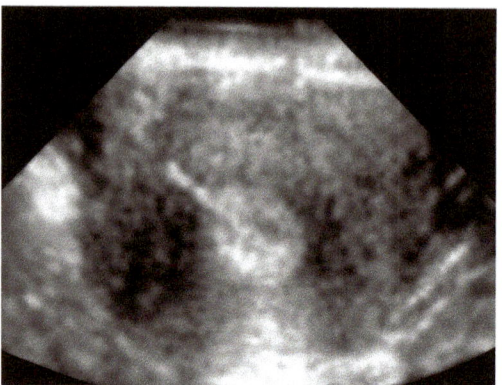

Fig. 1: Forgotten intrauterine contraceptive device (IUCD) with pyometra.

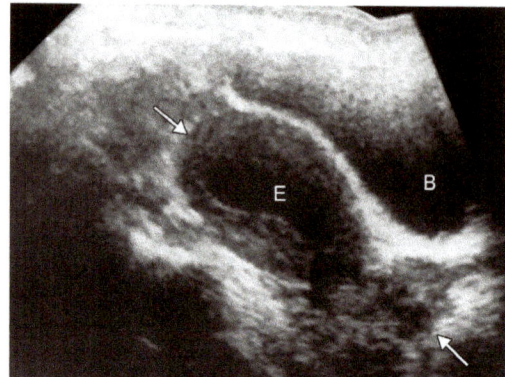

Fig. 2: Endometrial fluid collection. (E: endometrial fluid; B: bladder).

PATHOGENESIS

- Association with squamous metaplasia of endometrium reported with varying frequency. It may precede squamous carcinoma of endometrium.
- Pyometra chiefly appears to be a result of malignancy as cervical canal is blocked by big tumor growth or presence of big necrotic growth in endometrium.
- After menopause, when endometrium loses its resistance; not being shed repeatedly, infection that enters uterus persists as senile endometritis.
- The pus, which tends to collect in uterus forms pyometra, as cervix is narrowed by senile change and atrophied myometrium is unable to expel it.

SIGNS AND SYMPTOMS

Pyometra often does not cause any symptom and can be found during an ultrasonography of pelvis. Signs and symptoms include:[6,9,10]

- Purulent vaginal discharge with traces of blood
- Postmenopausal bleeding
- Lower abdominal pain
- Symmetrical enlargement of the uterus
- Nausea and vomiting
- Diarrhea
- Pyrexia (rarely).

DIFFERENTIAL DIAGNOSIS

Rule out other causes of uterine enlargement including:
- Uterine causes—fibroids and adenomyosis
- Endometrial causes—polyps, hematometra, endometrial tumor, and gestational trophoblastic neoplasia
- Congenital abnormalities.

Causes of blood-stained vaginal discharge that need to be excluded are: vaginosis, vulvar vestibulitis, and different infections of genital tract.

Perforated pyometra should be considered as a differential diagnosis in women with pneumoperitoneum and fever. Hypoalbuminemia is a predisposing factor for pyometra perforation.[10,11]

DIAGNOSIS

The diagnosis of pyometra is usually difficult because it is often asymptomatic. Transvaginal ultrasound scanning is the mainstay of diagnosis but sometimes CT and MRI can be used **(Fig. 2)**.[12]

INVESTIGATIONS

- The mainstay of investigation is imaging. Ultrasound scanning has been employed for over 20 years, and transvaginal ultrasound (TVUS) remains the chosen modality in most cases.[7]
- When pyometra complicates endometrial carcinoma, Doppler scanning may be used to detect blood flow changes.[13]
- CT scanning seems as a sensitive tool as compared to ultrasound, but the latter is often easier to access and cheap.
- Vaginal swabs may be negative in up to 50% of cases, since the principle organisms are anaerobes and these are difficult to culture.
- If tuberculosis is suspected, tuberculin testing, culture, histology, and nucleic acid amplification testing may be indicated.
- X-ray is used to confirm spontaneous perforation of the uterus (free gas under diaphragm).[14]

MANAGEMENT (FLOWCHART 1)

Primary Treatment

- Pyometra can be potentially lethal hence considered as an abscess and treated promptly by dilation of the cervix, evacuation and continued drainage of the uterine cavity.[1,2,9]
- Gentle curettage of the cavity and the endocervical canal after dilatation is essential to rule out associated malignant disease as well as to debride the necrotic tissue.
- Antibiotics effective against aerobic and anaerobic bacteria should be given to all patients with evidence of invasive infection, in the form of generalized malaise, pyrexia, or altered laboratory parameters. It should cover *Bacteroides* species, anaerobic *Staphylococcus* and *Streptococcus* species, and aerobic coliform bacterial infection.[9]
- Current research is focused on a group of drugs called carbapenems, which have an exceptionally wide spectrum of activity.
- Tubercular pyometra should be treated with appropriate antitubercular chemotherapy.[3]
- Once the infection is controlled, the underlying problem can be treated with regular monitoring to detect recurrent or persistent disease.

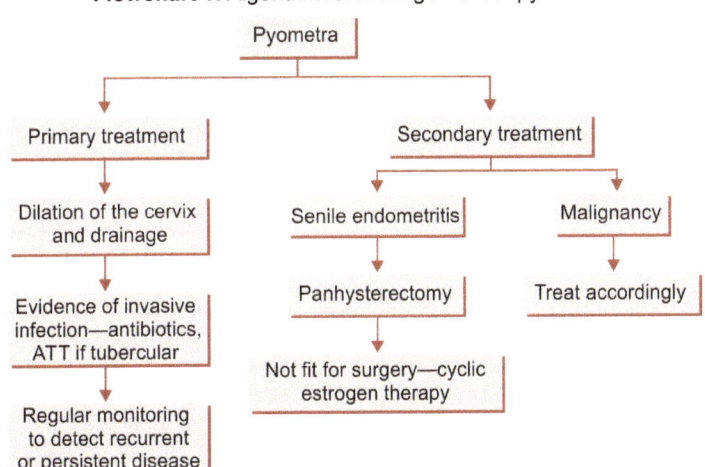

Flowchart 1: Algorithm for management of pyometra.

(ATT: antitubercular therapy)

Secondary Treatment

- When cause of pyometra is malignant or other specific disease, management is as per case. Radiotherapy is contraindicated in active disease.
- Hysterectomy is recommended in pyometra due to senile endometritis. Those not fit for surgery may benefit from prolonged cyclic estrogen therapy (premarin 0.625 mg daily) as it helps in healing of senile endometritis.[1,8-10]

Prognosis

Recurrences can occur.
The prognosis in pyometra will depend on:
- Underlying cause (e.g. malignancy)
- Possibility of spontaneous perforation

Spontaneously perforated pyometra has better prognosis if it not associated with malignancy. Prompt recognition and treatment of the condition improves the prognosis considerably.[14,15]

CONCLUSION

Gynecological malignancy and the sequelae of radiotherapy are the common causes of pyometra and can mislead clinicians. Pyometra occurs predominantly in elderly postmenopausal women. Most patients with spontaneously perforated pyometra will require surgery. Meanwhile, meticulous clinical judgment is required in discerning which patients may benefit from conservative management.

REFERENCES

1. Muram D, Drouin P, Thompson FE, et al. Pyometra. Can Med Assoc J. 1981;125(6):589-92.
2. Lien WC, Ong AW, Sun JT, et al. Pyometra: a potentially lethal differential diagnosis in older women. Am J Emerg Med. 2010;28(1):103-5.
3. Hasselgren PO, Bolin T. Postmenopausal tuberculous pyometra. Acta Obstet Gynecol Scand. 1977;56(1):23-5.
4. Toglia MR, Fagan MJ. Pyometra complicating a LeFort colpocleisis. Int Urogynecol J Pelvic Floor Dysfunct. 2009;20(3):361-2.
5. Schlumbrecht M, Balgobin S, Word L. Pyometra after thermal endometrial ablation. Obstet Gynecol. 2007;110(2 Pt 2):538-40.
6. Yildizhan B, Uyar E, Sişmanoğlu A, et al. Spontaneous perforation of pyometra. Infect Dis Obstet Gynecol. 2006;2006:26786.
7. Hofmann GE, Warikoo P, Jacobs W. Ultrasound detection of pyometra at the time of embryo transfer after ovum retrieval for in vitro fertilization. Fertil Steril. 2003;80(3):637-8.
8. Zohreh NA, Neekianand K, Muhammad FA, et al. Pyometra after ovum retrieval for in vitro fertilization resulting in hysterectomy. Fertil Steril. 2010;93(1):268.e1-2.
9. Chan LY, Lau TK, Wong SF, et al. Pyometra. What is its clinical significance? J Reprod Med. 2001;46(11):952-6.
10. Ou YC, Lan KC, Lin H, et al. Clinical characteristics of perforated pyometra and impending perforation: specific issues in gynecological emergency. J Obstet Gynaecol Res. 2010;36(3):661-6.
11. Kim TH, Lee HH, Chung SH. Presenting features of pyometra including an increase in iatrogenic causes. J Low Genit Tract Dis. 2011;15(4):316-7.
12. Kim J, Cho DH, Kim YK, et al. Sealed-off spontaneous perforation of a pyometra diagnosed preoperatively by magnetic resonance imaging: a case report. J Magn Reson Imaging. 2010;32(3):697-9.
13. Emoto M, Tamura R, Shirota K, et al. Clinical usefulness of color Doppler ultrasound in patients with endometrial hyperplasia and carcinoma. Cancer. 2002;94(3):700-6.
14. Sahoo SP, Dora AK, Harika M, et al. Spontaneous uterine perforation due to pyometra presenting as acute abdomen. Indian J Surg. 2011;73(5):370-1.
15. Shapey IM, Nasser T, Dickens P, et al. Spontaneously perforated pyometra: an unusual cause of acute abdomen and pneumoperitoneum. Ann R Coll Surg Engl. 2012;94(8):e246-e248.

Postmenopausal Bleeding

Arveen Vohra

INTRODUCTION

Postmenopausal bleeding (PMB) is a common clinical problem and one of the most frequent complaints with which women present in the outpatient gynecology clinic. Patients with PMB have 10-15% chance of having endometrial carcinoma and therefore, the diagnostic workup is aimed at excluding malignancy. Contributory factors are perhaps increasing longevity, obesity, hormone therapy, and increasing numbers of women seeking help or reassurance for this problem due to increased awareness. Bleeding occurs in >3% of postmenopausal women, and the use of hormones increases the likelihood of bleeding by >5-fold.[1]

DEFINITION

The menopause is defined by the World Health Organization (WHO) as the permanent cessation of menstruation resulting from the loss of ovarian follicular activity.[2]

The definition of PMB and what is clinically significant is however varied. By definition, PMB is bleeding that occurs 12 months after the last normal period.[2] However, it is recommended that any vaginal bleeding that occurs 6 months after the last period (presumed menopause) should be investigated.

SIGNIFICANCE OF POSTMENOPAUSAL BLEEDING

In postmenopausal women, the endometrial thickness is considerably less than premenopausal women. Endometrial thickness is directly related to endometrial pathology. The risk of endometrial cancer at the age of 50 in a woman with PMB is approximately 1% and rises to 25% at the age of 80.[3] More than 90% of women diagnosed with endometrial carcinoma present with irregular perimenopausal bleeding or PMB. The incidence of significant pathology in women with PMB is only 20%.[4]

CAUSES OF POSTMENOPAUSAL BLEEDING

Clinical risk factors for endometrial cancer, including but not limited to age, obesity, specific medical comorbidities like polycystic ovary syndrome, type 2 diabetes mellitus, and atypical glandular cells on screening cervical cytology; use of unopposed estrogen, and family history of gynecologic malignancy should be considered when evaluating PMB.

The common causes of PMB include atrophic vaginitis, vaginal, cervical and endometrial polyps, endometritis, trauma and genital tract malignancy. Pruritus vulva due to vulval dystrophies, exogenous sources of estrogen like hormone therapy and especially plant sources of estrogen have to be kept in mind. Bleeding disorders, although rare, should be considered. Hypertension, obesity, and diabetes have been associated with an increased risk of malignancy **(Table 1)**.

Causes of abnormal bleeding in women using HRT include the following:[5]
- Poor compliance
- Poor gastrointestinal absorption for oral medications
- Drug interactions
- Liver disease
- Coagulation defects

TABLE 1: Etiology of postmenopausal bleeding (PMB).

Common factors for PMB	Approximate %
Exogenous estrogens	30
Atrophic endometritis/vaginitis	30
Endometrial cancer	15
Endometrial or cervical polyps	10
Endometrial hyperplasia	05
Miscellaneous (e.g. cervical cancer, uterine sarcoma, urethral caruncle, trauma)	10

- Gynecologic disorders, including but not limited to endometrial cancer, endometrial polyps, and cervical or vaginal lesions
- Nonreproductive tract origins like urinary tract, gastrointestinal tract.

EVALUATION OF POSTMENOPAUSAL BLEEDING

As with all clinical presentations, a thorough history, clinical examination and set of investigations are indicated. These should be conducted with urgency to exclude malignancy. Goldstein, in 2010, recommended postmenopausal asymptomatic endometrial thickening be evaluated on a case-by-case basis as opposed to American College of Obstetricians and Gynecologists (ACOG) guidelines.[6]

Women with spontaneous PMB should be primarily evaluated with either endometrial biopsy (EB), or transvaginal sonography (TVS) to measure the thickness of the endometrial echo complex (EEC) (Grade A).

Postmenopausal bleeding can be a presenting symptom of cancer in the cervical canal. Consequently, if there is no endometrial explanation for PMB, appropriate steps to evaluate patients for cervical cancer should be undertaken considering Pap smear, colposcopy, and curettage of the endocervical canal (Grade C).

History

The nature of current bleeding—first episode, persistent or recurrent, along with history of perimenopausal dysfunctional bleeding and/or endometrial hyperplasia should be elicited. A detailed history of duration, frequency, length, and quantity of bleeding and association with pain should be elicited. The presence of other comorbid factors such as diabetes, hypertension,[7] nulliparity, and use of unopposed estrogen therapy should be recorded. History of treatment with tamoxifen,[8] tibolone, and cyclical/continuous combined hormonal therapy (HT) should be noted. Postmenopausal women receiving tamoxifen therapy for more than five years are at increased risk of endometrial cancer.[9] Early menarche and late menopause are also associated with increased likelihood of endometrial hyperplasia/carcinoma. A history of thyroid, kidney, easy bruising or liver conditions may be reported.

Examination

A thorough general and local examination is mandatory. Examination of the vulva, vagina, and uterus both by visual and palpation examination may reveal signs of atrophy, and areas of bleeding, ulcers, or tumors. A uterus that is larger than normal may be indicative of the presence of fibroids or polyps or cancer. Hematuria and bleeding per rectum (Hemorrhoids) should be kept in mind. The conventional Pap smear or liquid-based cytology can detect abnormal endometrial cells in up to 30% of the cases.[10]

Investigations

The principal aim of investigation of PMB is to identify or exclude endometrial pathology, most notably endometrial carcinoma. The best diagnostic strategy for diagnosing endometrial carcinoma in patients with PMB still remains controversial. ACOG recommends transvaginal ultrasonography as a reasonable alternative to endometrial sampling as a first approach in evaluating a postmenopausal woman with an initial episode of bleeding. If blind sampling does not reveal endometrial hyperplasia or malignancy, further testing, such as hysteroscopy with dilation and curettage, is then warranted in the evaluation of women with persistent or recurrent bleeding.[6]

Women with spontaneous PMB should be primarily evaluated with TVS to measure the thickness of the EEC.

When the thickness is more than 4 mm, an outpatient endometrial sampling is performed.[11]

Further evaluation by saline infusion sonography (SIS) and/or 3D ultrasound is recommended when the tissue yield is inadequate. Endometrial, cervical, and ovarian malignancies must be ruled out in the presence of PMB. A Pap test is essential when PMB is noted, although the Pap test is an insensitive diagnostic test for detecting endometrial cancer **(Flowchart 1)**.

Transvaginal Sonography

The initial assessment in all cases of PMB should be using the ultrasonography (USG) especially TVS. It is not an appropriate screening tool for endometrial cancer in postmenopausal women without bleeding.[6]

Endometrial thickness is measured as the maximum anterior-posterior thickness of the endometrial echo on a long-axis transvaginal view of the uterus **(Fig. 1)**.

USG also provides an opportunity to evaluate the pelvis for any related or incidental pathology especially the ovaries. As opposed to diffuse thickening of the endometrium focal pathology like submucous fibroids and endometrial polyps can be diagnosed using SIS and/or 3D USG. The addition of color Doppler imaging does not add benefit to the diagnosis or influence further management.[12]

About 96% of women with endometrial carcinoma and 92% of women with benign endometrial pathology can be identified when a 4 mm cut off is used for endometrial

Flowchart 1: Possible diagnostic pathways for postmenopausal bleeding.

```
Patient with postmenopausal bleeding
         │
         ├──────────────────────────┐
         ▼                          ▼
                          Patient characteristics
                          prediction model
                                    │
                                    ▼
                          Based on predicted
                          probability bleeding
                                    │
    ┌───────────────────────────────┼──────────────────────┐
    ▼                                                      ▼
Transvaginal                                          Expectant
sonography                                            management
    │                                                      │
    ├──────────────┐                                       ▼
    ▼              ▼                                   Recurrent
Endometrial    Endometrial         Endometrial ◄──── bleeding
thickness ≤ 4 mm   thickness ≥ 4 mm   sampling
    │              │                     │
    ▼              ▼                     │
Expectant      Recurrent                 │
management ◄── bleeding                  │
                                         │
            ┌────────────────┬───────────┴──────────┐
            ▼                ▼                      ▼
        (Pre-) malignancy  Insufficient        (Pre-) malignancy
        rule out           endometrial sample
            │                │
            ▼                ▼
        Expectant        Hysteroscopy
        management           │
            │                │
            ▼                │
        Recurrent ───────────┘
        bleeding
```

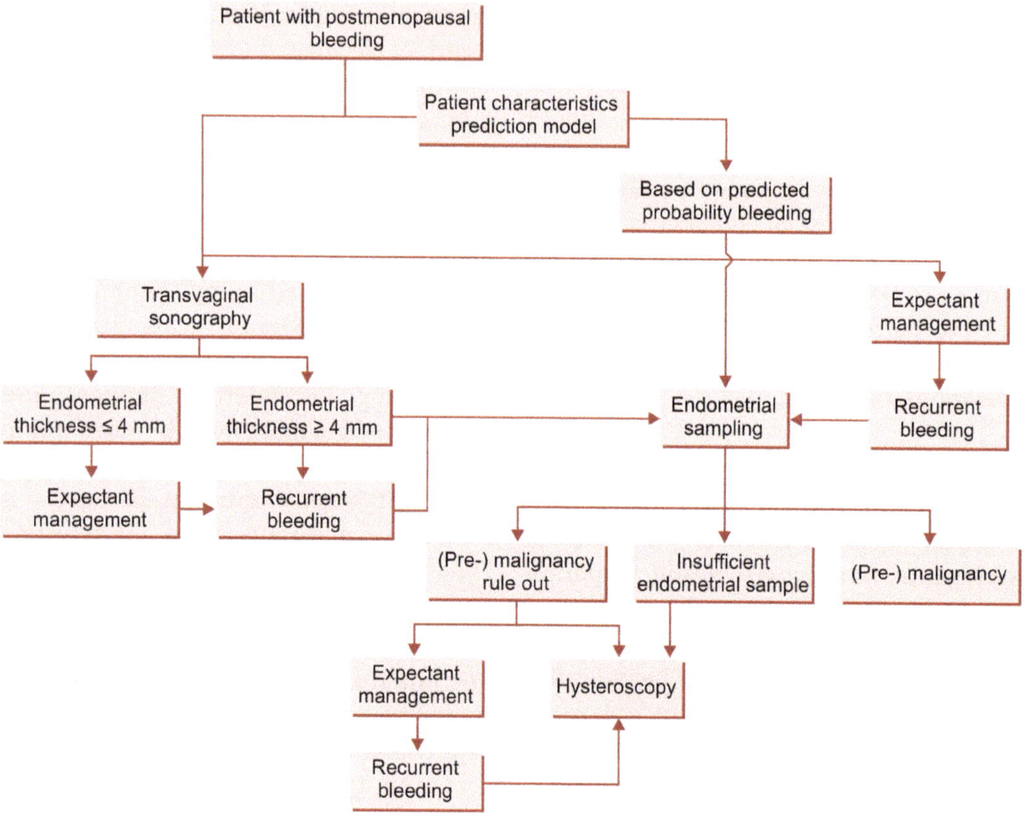

thickness using TVS.[12] The pretest probability of endometrial cancer of 10% in a woman with spontaneous PMB will be reduced to 1% following a normal TVS.[13]

Endometrial thickness of >4 mm warrants histological evaluation either as outpatient endometrial sampling or hysteroscopy-directed EB. For the patients on conservative management (endometrial thickness <4 mm), repeat TVS is indicated if bleeding persists or recurs.[14] TVS has a high sensitivity but a relatively poor specificity. In women on HT, the cut off of 4 mm results in a high false-positive rate. Interpretation of endometrial thickness should be related to the phase of HT, i.e ideally 5–10 days from the end of the progesterone

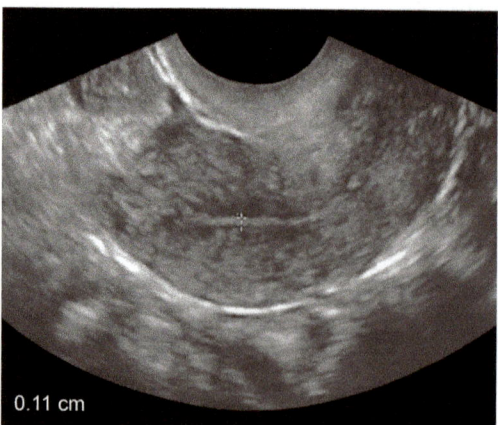

Fig. 1: Measurement of endometrial thickness. The endometrial thickness measured at its thickest portion as the distance between the echogenic borders (calipers) perpendicular to the midline longitudinal plane of the uterus.

phase and any time during continuous combined treatment.

In women on cyclical HT, withdrawal bleeding outside the time of progestin therapy should be evaluated.[15]

However, a routine ultrasound for endometrial thickening should not be performed in asymptomatic women on tamoxifen.[16,17]

However, women having uterine bleeding while receiving tamoxifen (usually used as an adjuvant therapy for breast cancer) should be assessed primarily with endometrial sampling because, in such patients, TVS is neither sensitive nor specific for neoplasia.[5]

Endometrial Biopsy

Outpatient sampling of the endometrium is comparable to hysteroscopy for diagnosing endometrial hyperplasia.[18] The Pipelle endometrial curette samples only 4.2% of the endometrial surface.[19,20] The endometrial aspirator samples about 41.6% of the endometrial surface but is less well tolerated.[21] The 10% failure rate of outpatient sampling procedure is due to cervical stenosis in postmenopausal women.

Fractional Curettage

Fractional curettage was traditionally the method of choice for investigating patients with PMB. However, in approximately 60% of the fractional curettage procedures less than half of the uterine cavity is curetted. Fractional curettage is now considered to be outdated practice and is replaced by less invasive outpatient evaluation using EB devices and outpatient hysteroscopy-guided biopsies. Lesions can be missed in up to 10% of the cases.[22] It has been suggested that an endometrial thickness of less than 6-10 mm measured by TVS is unlikely to indicate endometrial cancer. A meta-analysis of studies comparing endometrial pathology with ultrasonography findings suggested that an endometrial thickness of less than 6 mm essentially excludes malignancy. Patients with an increased endometrial thickness should undergo more invasive testing, like office endometrial sampling, hysteroscopy or fractional curettage, to exclude endometrial pathology.

In women with PMB, the sensitivity of endometrial sampling to detect endometrial cancer and especially atypical hyperplasia and endometrial disease, including endometrial polyps, is lower than previously thought. Endometrial sampling fails in 42% of cases (either technical failure or insufficient material) and (pre)malignancy is found in 7% of these cases. Hence, further diagnostic work-up for focal pathology is warranted, even after a benign result of endometrial sampling.[23]

Endometrial sampling in a postmenopausal woman without bleeding should not be routinely performed. Indications for tissue sampling of the endometrium in bleeding postmenopausal women with an endometrial thickness of greater than 4-5 mm should not be extrapolated to asymptomatic women.[17]

Hysteroscopy

It is the gold standard investigation for postmenopausal bleeding. Hysteroscopy may be performed as an outpatient procedure. Hysteroscopy may reveal the presence of uterine polyps, atrophy, endometrial hyperplasia, or cancer. It is especially useful in evaluating focal thickening and helps in diagnosis and management of uterine polyps and abnormal pathology detected **(Flowchart 1)**.[18]

Magnetic Resonance Imaging

Magnetic resonance imaging (MRI) is of value only in endometrial carcinoma for delineating the size of the primary tumor and myometrial invasion. The presence of enlarged lymph nodes and cervical involvement can be made out.

MANAGEMENT OF BENIGN DISORDERS

The management of bleeding caused by atrophic vaginitis includes topical or systemic use of estrogens after other causes of abnormal bleeding have been excluded. Cervical polyps can easily be removed in the office.

Endometrial polyps are best removed during the hysteroscopic evaluation and sent for histopathological examination (HPE).

The endometrium should also be sampled and sent for HPE as the likelihood of endometrial hyperplasia is high (3% of polyps).

Women with PMB and endometrium <4 mm can be followed up with a repeat USG 3 months later unless the patient has further episodes of bleeding.

If the endometrial thickness is > 4mm, a biopsy is performed either as outpatient or hysteroscopy directed. Endometrial hyperplasia without atypia responds well to hormonal therapy. The use of Levonorgestrel intrauterine system is preferred to systemic therapy.

Hyperplasia with atypia, simple or complex, warrants definitive surgical management.[24]

For patients receiving tamoxifen therapy, having persistent episodes of PMB, but no evidence of focal lesions, and for whom both the cervical canal and endometrial cavity have been adequately evaluated with imaging and adequate endometrial sampling showing benign tissue, annual repeated sampling is indicated.[5]

Endometrial Hyperplasia

Benign endometrial patterns include anovulatory, proliferative, cystic glandular hyperplasia, simple cystic hyperplasia, simple hyperplasia, and adenomatous hyperplasia without atypia. In most cases, benign endometrial hyperplasia is resolved with fractional curettage or progestin therapy but it requires continuous surveillance. Architectural complexity and crowding poses a greater risk for progression than the presence of cytologic atypia alone. Hysterectomy is recommended for treatment of atypical endometrial hyperplasia in postmenopausal women. Patients who do not respond are at a significantly increased risk of progressing to invasive cancer and should be advised to have a hysterectomy.

COMPLICATIONS

Profuse bleeding can cause anemia. Prolonged use of estrogen replacement therapy (ERT) that is not combined with progestin increases the risk of endometrial hyperplasia and endometrial cancer in women who have not had a hysterectomy. Endometrial and cervical cancers can spread to other areas of the body.

CONCLUSION

Postmenopausal bleeding (PMB) is often the first sign of endometrial cancer. Hence, the principal aim of the investigation of postmenopausal bleeding is to identify or exclude endometrial pathology, most notably endometrial carcinoma. It is also important to ensure that women are sufficiently reassured following normal tests, that symptomatic benign disease is identified.

Fractional curettage is no longer used as the first-line method of investigating PMB in most cases. Hysteroscopy and biopsy (curettage) is the preferred diagnostic technique to detect polyps and other benign lesions.

Timely diagnosis and management can avoid fatalities due to cancer.

REFERENCES

1. Collins J, Crosignani PG; ESHRE Capri Workshop Group. Endometrial Bleeding. Hum Reprod Update. 2007;13(5):421-31.
2. Research on the menopause in the 1990s. Report of a WHO Scientific Group. World Health Organ Tech Rep Ser. 1996;866:1-107.
3. Gredmark T, Kvint S, Havel G, et al. Histopathological findings in women with postmenopausal bleeding. Br J Obstet Gynaecol. 1995;102(2):133-6.
4. Oehler MK, MacKenzie I, Kehoe S, et al. Assessment of abnormal bleeding in menopausal bleeding: an update. J Br Menopause Soc. 2003;9(3):117-21.
5. Munro MG; The Southern California Permanente Medical Group's Abnormal Uterine Bleeding Working Group. Investigation of Women with Postmenopausal Uterine Bleeding: Clinical Practice Recommendations. Perm J. 2014;18(1):55-70.
6. American College of Obstetricians and Gynecologists. The Role of Transvaginal Ultrasonography in Evaluating the Endometrium of Women With Postmenopausal Bleeding. ACOG Committee Opinion May 2018. [online] Available from https://www.acog.org/Clinical-Guidance-and-Publications/Committee-Opinions/Committee-on-Gynecologic-Practice/The-Role-of-Transvaginal-Ultrasonography-in-Evaluating-the-Endometrium-of-Women-With-Postmenopausal?IsMobileSet=false. [Last accessed September, 2019].
7. Feldman S, Cook EF, Harlow BL, et al. Predicting endometrial cancer among older women who present with abnormal vaginal bleeding. Gynecol Oncol. 1995;56(3):376-81.
8. Kedar RP, Bourne TH, Powles TJ, et al. Effects of Tamoxifen on uterus and ovaries of postmenopausal women in a randomized breast cancer prevention trial. Lancet. 1994;343(8909):1318-21.
9. Scottish Intercollegiate Guidelines Network. The investigation of postmenopausal bleeding: a national guideline: SIGN 61. Edinburgh: SIGN; 2002.
10. Demirkiran F, Arvas M, Erkun E, et al. The prognostic significance of cervico vaginal cytology in endometrial cancer. Eur J Gynecol Oncol. 1995;16(5):403-9.
11. Moodley M, Roberts C. Clinical Pathway for the evaluation of PMB with an emphasis on endometrial cancer detection. J Obstet Gynaecol. 2004;24(7):736-41.
12. Wilialak S, Jirapinyo M, Theppisai U, et al. Transvaginal Doppler Sonography: is there a role for this modality in the evaluation of women with PMB? Maturitas. 2005;50(2):111-6.
13. Smith-Bindman R, Kerlikowske K, Feldstein VA, et al. Endovaginal ultrasound to exclude endometrial cancer and other endometrial abnormalities. JAMA. 1998;280:1510-7.
14. Garuti G, Sambruni I, Cellani F, et al. Hysteroscopy and transvaginal Ultrasonography in postmenopausal women with uterine bleeding. Int J Gynaecol Obstet. 1999;65(1):25-33.
15. Amann M, Anguino II, Bauman RA, et al. Postmenopausal uterine bleeding. Pasadena (CA): Kaiser Permanente Southern California; 2006.
16. Berlière M, Galant C, Gillerot S, et al. Endometrial evaluation prior to Tamoxifen: preliminary results of a prospective study. Bull Cancer. 1998;85(8):721-4.
17. Wolfman W. Asymptomatic Endometrial Thickening. J Obstet Gynaecol Can. 2018;40(5):e367-e377.
18. Etherington IJ, Harrison KR, Read MD. A comparison of outpatient endometrial sampling with hysteroscopy, curettage and cystoscopy in the evaluation of PMB. J Obstet Gynaecol. 1995;15(4):259-62.
19. Rodriguez GC, Yaqub N, King ME. A comparison of the Pipelle device and the Vabra aspirator as measured by endometrial denudation in hysterectomy specimens: the Pipelle device samples significantly less of the endometrial surface than the Vabra aspirator. Am J Obstet Gynecol. 1993;168(1 Pt 1):55-9.
20. Kaunitz AM, Masciello A, Ostrowski M, et al. Comparison of endometrial biopsy with

Pipelle and Vabra aspirator. J Reprod Med. 1988;33(5):427-31.
21. Stovall TG, Ling FW, Morgan PL. A prospective, randomized comparison of the Pipelle endometrial sampling device with the Novak curette. Am J Obstet Gynecol. 1991;165(5 Pt 1):1287-90.
22. Stock RJ, Kanbour A. Prehysterectomy curettage. Obstet Gynecol. 1975;45(5):537-41.
23. van Hanegem N, Prins MM, Bongers MY, et al. The accuracy of endometrial sampling in women with postmenopausal bleeding: a systematic review and meta-analysis. Eur J Obstet Gynecol Reprod Biol. 2016;197:147-55.
24. Indian Menopause Society. Evaluation and Management of Post-menopausal Bleeding. Guideline Number 4; 2010.

CHAPTER 18

Management of Ovarian Mass in Postmenopausal Women

Sonal Agarwal

INTRODUCTION

Ovarian mass in postmenopausal women represents benign and malignant tumors of epithelial, sex cord-stromal, and primary peritoneal origin. In postmenopausal women,[1] 90% of ovarian cancer is epithelial in origin. Germ cell and sex cord-stromal tumors have a more favorable prognosis but are not found generally in postmenopausal women. Ovarian malignancies pose the greatest clinical challenge due to high morbidity and mortality rates. Ovarian cancer is the fifth most common cause of death from malignancy in women. Classification of malignant ovarian cancer given by World Health Organization is enlisted in **Table 1**.

EPITHELIAL OVARIAN CANCER

Epidemiology

Epithelial ovarian cancer is one of the leading causes of mortality amongst gynecological cancers. Median age for sporadic disease is around 60 years and for genetic disease, it is fifth decade. Lifetime risk of sporadic incidence is approximately 1.7% while familial predisposition has a higher risk of 10–40%. 30% epithelial neoplasms of ovary are malignant in postmenopausal women whereas only around 7% are malignant in premenopausal women. For borderline tumors, average age is 46 years.

Classification

Histological subtypes of epithelial ovarian cancer are given in **Table 2**. Serous histology constitutes more than 70%, endometrioid 10%, mucinous and clear cell 5%, transitional and undifferentiated carcinomas 1% each of all epithelial cancers.

Serous tumors have psammoma bodies with concentric rings of calcification. Papillary excrescences may be present. Mucinous tumors have loculi lined with mucin-like glands representing endocervix, gastric

TABLE 1: WHO classification of malignant ovarian cancer.

Common epithelial tumors

Malignant serous tumor
- Adenocarcinoma, papillary adenocarcinoma, papillary cystadenocarcinoma
- Surface papillary carcinoma
- Malignant adenofibroma, cystadenofibroma

Malignant mucinous tumor
- Adenocarcinoma, cystadenocarcinoma
- Malignant adenofibroma, cystadenofibroma

Malignant endometrioid tumor
- Carcinoma
- Adenocarcinoma
- Adenoacanthoma
- Malignant adenofibroma, cystadenofibroma
- Endometrioid stromal sarcoma
- Mesodermal (müllerian) mixed tumor: homologous and heterologous

Other
- Clear cell (mesonephroid) tumor, malignant
- Carcinoma and adenocarcinoma
- Brenner tumor, malignant
- Mixed epithelial tumor, malignant
- Undifferentiated carcinoma
- Unclassified

Sex cord-stromal tumors

Granulosa-stromal cell tumor
- Granulosa cell tumor
- Tumor in the thecoma-fibroma group
- Fibroma
- Unclassified

Androblastoma: Sertoli-Leydig cell tumor
- Well differentiated
- Tubular androblastoma, Sertoli cell tumor (tubular adenoma of Pick)
- Tubular androblastoma with lipid storage, Sertoli cell tumor with lipid storage
- Sertoli-Leydig cell tumor (tubular adenoma with Leydig cells)
- Leydig cell tumor, hilus cell tumor
- Of intermediate differentiation
- Poorly differentiated (sarcomatoid)
- With heterologous elements
- Gynandroblastoma
- Lipid (lipoid) cell tumors
- Unclassified

Contd...

Contd...

Germ cell tumor
- Dysgerminoma
- Endodermal sinus tumor
- Embryonal carcinoma
- Polyembryoma
- Choriocarcinoma
- Immature teratoma
- Mature dermoid cyst with malignant transformation
- Monodermal and highly specialized
- Struma ovarii
- Carcinoid
- Struma ovarii and carcinoid
- Others
- Mixed forms

Gonadoblastoma
- Pure
- Mixed with dysgerminoma or other form of germ cell tumor

Source: Young RH. A brief history of the pathology of the gonads. Mod Pathol. 2005;18(Suppl 2):S3-S17.

pylorus or intestine. They reach a size filling entire abdominal cavity. Endometrioid tumors have a complex glandular pattern with variations of epithelia found in uterus. Clear cell carcinomas are made up of clear hobnail cells projecting nuclei into apical cytoplasm. Transitional (Brenner) tumors resemble low-grade papillary urothelial carcinoma of the urinary bladder.

Risk Factors

- Early menarche and late menopause causing prolonged estrogen exposure
- *Polycystic ovary syndrome* (PCOS)
- Nulliparous (having one child reduces risk to 0.3–0.4)
- Obesity
- Smoking
- Family history of ovarian and breast cancer
- Personal history of breast cancer

Chapter 18: Management of Ovarian Mass in Postmenopausal Women

TABLE 2: Common histologic types of epithelial ovarian cancer.

Histology	Features
Papillary serous	The most common type of epithelial ovarian cancer. May contain psammoma bodies and is often associated with CA125 elevation. Identical histology is observed for primary peritoneal serous cancer.
Endometrioid	Sometimes associated with endometriosis or an independent uterine cancer of similar histology. May occur with early-stage disease in younger patients, although advanced disease is also possible.
Mucinous	May rarely be associated with pseudomyxoma peritonei. CA125 levels may not be markedly elevated. Relatively chemoresistant. Differential diagnosis of a mucinous ovarian tumor includes metastatic disease from an appendiceal primary.
Clear cell	The most chemoresistant type of ovarian cancer. Often contains "hobnail" cells with cleared out cytoplasm due to glycogen. Sometimes associated with endometriosis or humorally mediated hypercalcemia.

- Genetic mutations (BRCA 1, BRCA 2, and Lynch syndrome)
- No use of oral contraceptive pill (OCP) (Use for 5 years reduces risk up to 50%)[2]
- Hormone replacement therapy
- Fertility treatment
- Undergone tubal ligation.

Symptoms

Generally asymptomatic. There is very low predictive value for malignancy. For each symptom, it is less than 1% with abdominal distension having a value of 2.5%. Most common symptoms which may be associated with ovarian cancer are:

- Pain abdomen
- Postmenopausal bleeding
- Decreased hunger
- Abdominal distension
- Urinary frequency
- Rectal bleeding
- Abdominal bloating.

Majority of women have nonspecific and vague symptoms. Till advanced stage, there may be no symptoms so it is considered as a silent killer. Acute symptoms, such as pain secondary to rupture or torsion may occur. In advanced stage, patients may have ascites, omental metastases, and bowel metastases.

Signs

Solid, irregular, and fixed pelvic mass on physical examination is suggestive of ovarian malignancy. Upper abdominal mass and ascites are part of diagnostic criteria for ovarian cancer.

Routes of Metastasis, Pathogenesis, and Spread Pattern

Epithelial ovarian cancers arise from surface epithelium of ovary which is contiguous to peritoneal mesothelium by transcoelomic migration, lymphatic route or blood vessels. Malignant transformation occurs and that epithelium gets trapped inside the inclusion cysts of ovary during process of ovulation leading to different types of müllerian type histologies. A small subset of epithelial ovarian cancers may also originate in fimbria of fallopian tube and then spread to peritoneal cavity and ovary.

Transcoelomic

Metastasis is seen in posterior cul-de-sac, hemidiaphragm, paracolic gutters, liver, and intestinal peritoneal surface and omentum.

Lymphatic

Lymphatic dissemination to pelvic and para-aortic lymph nodes is common in advanced-stage disease.

Hematogenous

It is uncommon. About 2–3% women may have spread to lungs and liver.

Diagnosis

- Serum CA125 levels can differentiate between malignant and benign mass. For postmenopausal patient with adnexal mass and serum CA125 level (>200 U/mL), 96% positive predictive value present for malignancy. Other tumor markers such as CA 19-9, which is elevated in mucinous ovarian carcinomas and carcinoembryonic antigen (CEA), are less frequently useful
- Transvaginal ultrasonography has better resolution than transabdominal ultrasonography for adnexal neoplasms. Doppler color flow imaging enhances specificity of ultrasonography[3]
- Confirm diagnosis can be done only on exploratory laparotomy
- Limited value of abdominal and pelvic computed tomography and MRI
- PET scan is still being evaluated for diagnosis.

Risk of Malignancy Index

Helps in decision making whether management has to be dealt by general gynecologist or gynecological oncologist at a tertiary cancer care center.[4] Staging laparotomy is performed by the oncosurgeon to prognosticate the woman.

 Risk of malignancy index (RMI) = $U \times M \times CA125$

- Every ultrasound feature has been given one point each: multilocular cyst, bilateral lesions, evidence of solid areas, evidence of metastases, and presence of ascites.
- $U = 0$ (for ultrasound score of 0); $U = 1$ (for ultrasound score of 1); $U = 3$ (for ultrasound score of 2–5).
- $M = 1$ for premenopausal women and 3 for postmenopausal women
- CA125 is serum CA125 measurement in U/mL

Management According to Risk Stratification[5]

- *Low risk*: Simple cyst < 5 cm in diameter with normal CA125 serum levels can be managed conservatively. Ultrasound and CA125 level surveillance at 3 months, then 6 monthly to be done for 3 years. If above criteria is not met or the patient wants surgery, then laparoscopic oophorectomy is acceptable. It can be taken care of by a general gynecologist.
- *Moderate risk*: Laparoscopic salpingo-oophorectomy is done in selected cases. If malignancy is found, staging laparotomy has to be done.
- *High risk*: To be managed in an oncology center by a gynecological oncologist.

Staging

It is according to FIGO system based on surgical exploration. Preoperative evaluation should exclude extraperitoneal metastases. Categories depend on clinical examination or surgical exploration or both. Histological staging depends on cytologic testing. Suspicious area biopsy is taken. It is important to know whether rupture of capsule was spontaneous or iatrogenic and source of malignant cells whether peritoneal washings or ascites.

Technique of Staging

- Midline or paramedian abdominal incision is made for complete access
- Cytology for pouch of Douglas fluid
- If no free fluid is present, peritoneal washings should be performed by instilling and recovering 50–100 mL of saline from pelvic cul-de-sac, paracolic gutter, and hemidiaphragm
- Systematic exploration of all intra-abdominal surfaces and viscera is performed in a clockwise fashion from cecum cephalad to rectosigmoid colon. Small intestine and its mesentery from the Treitz ligament to the cecum should be inspected. Any suspicious area/adhesion on peritoneal surface should be biopsied
- Pelvic and para-aortic area should be explored and sent for frozen section, if needed.
- Hysterectomy with bilateral salpingo-oophorectomy (BSO), infracolic omentectomy followed by bilateral selective pelvic, and para-aortic lymphadenectomy. In mucinous type, appendicectomy is also done.

FIGO Staging for Primary Carcinoma of the Ovary[6]

- *Stage I: Growth limited to the ovaries*
  IA: Growth limited to one ovary; no ascites containing malignant cells. No tumor on the external surface; capsule intact.
  IB: Growth limited to both ovaries; no ascites containing malignant cells. No tumor on the external surfaces; capsules intact.
  IC: Tumor either stage IA or IB but with tumor on the surface of one or both ovaries; or with capsule ruptured; or with ascites present containing malignant cells or with positive peritoneal washings.
- *Stage II: Growth involving one or both ovaries with pelvic extension.*
  IIA: Extension and/or metastases to the uterus and/or fallopian tubes.
  IIB: Extension to other pelvic tissues.
  IIC: Tumor either stage IIA or IIB but with tumor on the surface of one or both ovaries; or with capsule(s) ruptured; or with ascites present containing malignant cells or with positive peritoneal washings.
- *Stage III:* Tumor involving one or both ovaries with peritoneal implants outside the pelvis and/or positive retroperitoneal or inguinal nodes. Superficial liver metastasis equals stage III. Tumor is limited to the true pelvis, but with histologically proven malignant extension to small bowel or omentum.
  IIIA: Tumor grossly limited to the true pelvis with negative nodes but with histologically confirmed microscopic seeding of abdominal peritoneal surfaces.
  IIIB: Tumor of one or both ovaries with histologically confirmed implants of abdominal peritoneal surfaces, none exceeding 2 cm in diameter. Nodes are negative.
  IIIC: Abdominal implants > 2 cm in diameter or positive retroperitoneal or inguinal nodes or both.
- *Stage IV:* Growth involving one or both ovaries with distant metastasis. If pleural effusion is present, there must be positive cytologic test results to allot a case to stage IV. Parenchymal liver metastasis equals stage IV.

Management of Early Stage Disease

Total abdominal hysterectomy, bilateral salpingo-oophorectomy, and surgical staging are the standard treatments for stage I disease. Based on former findings, patients with stage I ovarian cancer can be divided into low-risk and high-risk categories as depicted in **Table 3**.

Stage I low risk: No postoperative adjuvant therapy needed.

Stage I high risk: Postoperative adjuvant therapy needed.

Postoperative chemotherapy: It can be given to patients with stage I, grade 3, stage IC or any stage II disease. Administration of six cycles of adjuvant carboplatin and paclitaxel chemotherapy should be given to high-risk, early stage patients.

Postoperative radiation therapy: Pelvic irradiation has same efficacy as prolonged courses of melphalan or chlorambucil.

TABLE 3: Prognostic variables in early-stage epithelial ovarian cancer.

Low risk	High risk
Low grade	High grade
Intact capsule	Tumor growth through capsule
No surface excrescences	Surface excrescences
No ascites	Ascites
Negative peritoneal cytologic findings	Malignant cells in fluid
Unruptured or intraoperative rupture	Preoperative rupture
Unruptured or intraoperative rupture	Dense adherence
Diploid tumor	Aneuploid tumor

Management of Advanced-stage Disease

Debulking Surgery

It has been thought that tumor debulking leads to enhanced sensitivity to postoperative chemotherapy. Primary cytoreduction is still the preferred option initially for women having stage IIIC and IV disease and good performance status, <5 cm upper abdominal disease.[7]

Interval Debulking Surgery

Cytoreductive procedure can be performed after several cycles of chemotherapy in patients who are not appropriate for primary debulking surgery due to poor performance status or bulky intra-abdominal disease that is not having very promising results. Patients who underwent primary debulking surgery but were suboptimally cytoreduced can undergo interval debulking surgery.

Secondary Cytoreductive Surgery

Secondary cytoreduction is defined as an attempt at cytoreductive surgery after completing first line chemotherapy. Patients with progressive disease already on chemotherapy are not suitable patients for secondary cytoreduction. Tumor resection should be restricted to patients who have disease-free interval of at least 12 months. Complete resection is possible when there are only one or two isolated recurrences with no diffuse carcinomatosis.

Intraperitoneal Chemotherapy

Epithelial ovarian cancers due to their association with peritoneum have been considered as an indication for intraperitoneal chemotherapy recently in past 3 decades. Drugs such as cisplatin and paclitaxel have ability to deliver drugs with effective cytoreduction of disease and lesser tolerable systemic side effects.

Patients with previous history of bowel resection usually tend to have postoperative complications which prevent use of intraperitoneal chemotherapy.[8] At present, intraperitoneal (IP) therapy is equivalent to IV treatment in patients with stage IV disease, suboptimally debulked residual disease, or relapsed disease. Contraindications are renal insufficiency, significant neuropathy, or extensive intra-abdominal adhesions.

Catheter insertion for IP therapy has following steps:
- A separate 5–6 cm transverse incision is made 2–3 inches above left inferior costal margin in the mid-clavicular line and is carried down to the fascia
- Subcutaneous pocket is made for implantable port
- Port is sutured to fascia at four corners using nylon suture
- Proximal end of catheter is grasped with clamp and brought through peritoneal cavity up to the subcutaneous tunnel
- Catheter is flushed with heparinized saline to check patency
- Transverse skin incision is closed.

Premedications for cisplatin and paclitaxel and aggressive IV hydration are given to prevent nephropathy. Potassium and magnesium levels monitoring is required.

Intraperitoneal instillation of cisplatin or paclitaxel is done by mixing drug in volume of 1 L prewarmed solution to avoid discomfort during infusion.

Postoperative Chemotherapy

Early stage, low risk: No adjuvant chemotherapy needed.

Early stage, high risk: Adjuvant chemotherapy given depends on health status and related medical comorbidities.

Systemic multi-agent chemotherapy is the standard treatment for metastatic disease.[9]

Neoadjuvant Chemotherapy

Helpful in selected patients with suboptimal stage III-IV disease, ascites, and pleural effusion.[10]

Radiotherapy after First-line Chemotherapy

Several trials have been done to assess need of radiotherapy after chemotherapy but results are still conflicting. After six cycles of carboplatin, epirubicin, and prednimustine, radiotherapy of 30 Gy in 1.5-Gy fractions, using 12–18 MeV photons, followed by pelvic, para-aortic, and partial diaphragm boosts is given.[11] Only selective cases of ovarian cancer might benefit from this therapy.

Maintenance Therapy

Value of maintenance or consolidation methods after achievement of a clinical complete remission in patients with advanced epithelial ovarian cancer has been tested again and again in many trials. Based on data, single-agent paclitaxel cannot be recommended for people who achieve complete clinical remission after chemotherapy.[12]

Surveillance

Around 50% of patients with advanced-stage epithelial ovarian cancer achieve clinical complete remission after platinum and taxane induction chemotherapy. Complete clinical remission is no evidence of disease on physical examination, normal CA125 level, and normal CT findings. Use of CA125 for surveillance should be individualized. Routine performance of CT without symptoms or any findings on physical examination with normal CA125 level is not needed.

CT is reserved for further evaluation of any symptom, sign or evidence of relapse.[13] There is no benefit of PET scan in settings of post-treatment.

Management of Recurrent Disease

Hormonal Therapy

Recurrence is common in patients with advanced ovarian cancer after first line chemotherapy. Recurrence can be marked by presence of rising titers of CA125 or CT findings. Survival rate after recurrence is very low. Women with only CA125 level raised can be given aromatase inhibitor like tamoxifen with less side effects though response rate is very slow and it can take up to 2–3 months for titer to gradually start falling.

Chemotherapy

Recurrence in the form of tumor-related symptoms, objective disease on examination or CT, or failure of hormonal therapy is an indication for platinum-based chemotherapy. Benefit of therapy depends on previous platinum free interval (PFI). PFI of less than 6 months are less likely to respond to chemotherapy and alternative agents like liposomal doxorubicin, paclitaxel, gemcitabine, docetaxel, topotecan, or oral etoposide. Usually liposomal doxorubicin is well tolerated in dose of 40 mg/m^2 every 4 weeks but development of *palmar-plantar* erythrodysesthesia (hand-foot syndrome) or mucositis may require dose reduction, leading to delay in treatment. Patients with a PFI of >6 months are platinum sensitive and can be treated with either single-agent platinum or a combination of platinum with paclitaxel, gemcitabine, or liposomal doxorubicin. Several investigational agents like bevacizumab which is a humanized antibody and neutralizes VEGF have been studied.[14,15]

Surgery

Criteria for secondary cytoreduction is no gross residual disease >1 cm in diameter. Large bowel obstruction can be relieved by performing colostomy, which can provide significant prolongation of survival and improved quality of life. Palliative surgery can benefit women with recurrent ovarian cancer. Metoclopramide improves motility of upper gastrointestinal tract without stimulating gastric, biliary, or pancreatic secretions.

Radiation Therapy

It is not curative though, it can help in palliative therapy. Pelvic radiotherapy can provide relief in symptoms such as pain, bleeding, and rectal narrowing. It can prevent or delay colostomy need. Doses of 8–10 Gy in a single fraction, 20 Gy in five fractions, 30 Gy in ten fractions, or higher total doses given in smaller fractions have produced acceptable short-term results. Cerebral or bone metastases can be treated with radiotherapy. Whole abdominal radiation is given for persistent and recurrent disease which is associated with very high morbidity due to development of acute and chronic intestinal obstruction needing exploratory surgery.

Hereditary Ovarian Carcinoma

Germline mutation is found in 5–10% of epithelial ovarian carcinomas which potentially increase the risk of developing the disease.[16] Breast-ovarian cancer syndrome accounts for approximately 90% of hereditary ovarian cancers. Patients at high risk of having a hereditary cancer should undergo genetic counseling, and multidisciplinary services should be provided to the patient.

BRCA1 gene is located on chromosome band 17q12-21 and *BRCA2* gene is located on chromosome band 13q12-13 are identified to be associated.[17] The majority of *BRCA1*-associated cancers are serous adenocarcinomas, endometrioid, and clear cell tumors.[18]

Germline mutation in DNA mismatch repair is responsible for the hereditary nonpolyposis colorectal cancer syndrome (HNPCC) phenotype: *hMSH2, hMLH1, hPMS1, hPMS2,* and *hMSH6*. The estimated cumulative risk for ovarian carcinoma by around 70 years of age is 24% for those with germline mutations in *MLH1* and *MSH2*. HNPCC is characterized by right colon cancer, endometrial, ovarian, upper gastrointestinal, genitourinary, and hepatobiliary cancers.[19]

Management of inherited ovarian cancers is complex and confusing due to variable penetrance of germline mutations. Women with high risk of ovarian or breast cancer should be offered genetic testing. Prophylactic, risk reduction bilateral salpingo-oophorectomy (RRSO) is recommended. In women who have a strong family history of breast or ovarian cancer, annual breast screening should begin at age of 30 years with MRI, mammogram and ultrasound.[20] In HNPCC syndrome along with above remedies, periodic colonoscopy, endometrial biopsy, and prophylactic hysterectomy should also be done.

■ BORDERLINE TUMORS

Ovarian borderline tumors are epithelial neoplasms which are histologically distinguished from ovarian carcinomas in the form of stromal invasion. Cells from primary tumor mass can be shed in the peritoneal cavity forming serous implants involving bowel, abdomen, and omentum. It is rare in postmenopausal women as median age is 40 years which is 20 years younger than median age for epithelial carcinoma. They may exhibit either serous or mucinous features. Serous is more common and is bilateral in 10–20% cases. On the other hand, mucinous tumors are larger and usually bilateral and may be associated with pseudomyxoma peritonei. Mortality can occur as result of intestinal obstruction. Borderline serous tumors may harbor foci of stromal microinvasion. They are distinguished from benign cystadenomas by presence of epithelial budding, multi-layered epithelium, increased mitotic activity, and nuclear atypia.

Management

Principal treatment is resection of primary tumor. If retroperitoneal nodes are involved, debulking should be done. Appendectomy is also recommended.

Follow-up of Borderline Tumors

No follow-up needed for stage I and 5-year survival is excellent (99%). From stage II-IV, it should be individualized. If contralateral ovary or both remain (following cystectomy) for stage I: Recurrence risk is approximately 40%.

Sex Cord-Stromal Tumors

Ovarian sex cord-stromal tumors are 5% of all ovarian cancers.[21] Sex cord-stromal tumors arise from ovarian stroma which consists of fibroblasts, granulosa cells, and theca cells or mesenchyme. Granulosa cell tumor presents with cystic/solid mass with cholesterol crystals embedded in it along with a longitudinal cleft resembling coffee bean shape with fluid filled spherical call-exner bodies. These tumors secrete estradiol, inhibin, and müllerian inhibitory substance which are used for surveillance. Every age group has different presentation depending on the characteristics. Postmenopausal women may present with postmenopausal bleeding due to presence of endometrial hyperplasia. Presentation is at stage I generally with an excellent prognosis.

Relapse can happen later in life so long-term follow-up is needed. Low-grade endometrial cancer occurs in association with granulosa cell tumors and endometrial hyperplasia.[22]

Sertoli-Leydig cell tumors present with virilization. Rarely, Sertoli-Leydig tumors can manifest as signs of estrogenization presenting as isosexual precocity, irregular or postmenopausal bleeding.

There is no specific presentation or symptom associated with it and may be diagnosed on presentation as ovarian torsion also.

Management

Surgical staging is same as epithelial ovarian cancer. Surgical management consists of bilateral salpingo-oophorectomy and total abdominal hysterectomy, along with standard surgical staging. Recurrence of lymph nodes is uncommon.

Granulosa cell tumors are potentially hormonally responsive, with about 30% of granulosa tumors expressing estrogen receptors and almost 100% expressing progesterone receptors. Hormonal agents such as progestins or luteinizing hormone releasing hormone agonists can also be used in these elderly women.

Stage II-IV need additional adjuvant therapy after initial therapy. Approximately 30–50% of patients will respond to platinum-based chemotherapy. The most commonly studied platinum combinations are cyclophosphamide, doxorubicin, and cisplatin or bleomycin, etoposide and cisplatin. Bleomycin can cause lung damage, etoposide can cause leukemia, renal dysfunction, hypertension, and Raynaud phenomenon. In those who cannot tolerate this regimen, paclitaxel and carboplatin can be used. Recurrence may be in abdomen-pelvis or reach up to liver, lung or bone through hematogenous route which can be treated with surgical resection followed by chemo or radiotherapy.

Prognosis

DNA ploidy status is related to survival. Patients with residual negative DNA diploid tumors tend to have atleast 10-year progression-free survival of more than 90%.

Krukenberg Tumor

This accounts for 30–40% of metastatic cancers arising in the ovarian stroma. The primary tumor is located in the stomach and less commonly in the colon, appendix, breast or biliary tract. Cervix and bladder are the rare primary sites. They are usually bilateral. Only at advanced stage, lesions are diagnosed and thus patients die of their illness within 1 year.

Metastatic Tumors

About 5–6% of ovarian tumors are metastatic; there may be direct extension, hematogenous or lymphatic spread or transcoelomic extension of tumor cells.

Primary Peritoneal Serous Carcinoma

It is identical to serous carcinoma in respect to its origin. It presents as diffuse peritoneal implants in the absence of dominant ovarian mass.[23] It represents malignant transformation of peritoneal surface epithelium like ovarian surface epithelium which is derived from coelomic mesoderm. It has higher risk of development with germline mutations in BRCA1 and BRCA2. Abdominal examination may reveal ascites and omental mass. Exploratory laparotomy needs to be done to make a histologic diagnosis and to do tumor cytoreduction. All patients present with stage III or IV disease due to diffuse nature of it.

Principles of treatment are same as that of epithelial ovarian carcinomas. Surgery should be followed by combination chemotherapy.

GUIDELINES ON MANAGEMENT OF OVARIAN MASS (NHS 2016)

- Transvaginal ultrasonography is used for initial evaluation of an adnexal mass.
- Functional ovarian cysts are unilocular and thin walled with <5 cm diameter.
- Typical sonographic features associated with ovarian malignancy are: solid component, nodular or papillary, thick septations >2–3 mm, peritoneal masses, enlarged lymph nodes, and ascites.
- MRI tends to determine origin of pelvic mass, i.e. uterine, ovarian or bowel.
- Tumor markers are not diagnostic but can characterize an ovarian mass and help in follow-up of disease. CA125 (normal <35 kU/L) is elevated in 80% women. It is nonspecific as it is also increased in conditions such as endometriosis, pelvic infection, fibroids, diverticulitis, inflammatory bowel disease, and hepatic dysfunction.
- Using an RMI cut-off of 200, a sensitivity of 70% and specificity of 90% can be achieved.
- Surgery should be considered if cyst >5 cm as risk of malignancy is calculated to be in a range of 2–9%.
- Laparoscopic approach should be done with low malignancy cases.
- Spillage of cyst contents should be avoided. Extensive peritoneal lavage is to be done.
- Laparoscopic specimen retrieval should be through umbilical port which is associated with lesser postoperative pain, faster recovery time, improved cosmesis, and decreased chances of incisional hernias.
- Value of prophylactic salpingo-oophorectomy in patients with hereditary ovarian carcinomas is documented and most effective way of reducing risk of occurrence.
- Patients with advanced-stage disease are chosen for debulking or cytoreductive surgery if patient is medically fit for major surgical procedure.
- Combination chemotherapy with carboplatin/cisplatin and paclitaxel is recommended for patients with high-risk, low-stage disease.
- In advanced stage, treatment should be individualized.
- Women should be counseled properly before laparoscopic bilateral salpingo-oophorectomy that if features of malignancy are suspected during the procedure, then it will be abandoned and laparotomy will be done along with assistance from oncology team afterwards.

SUMMARY

- Postmenopausal women with ovarian cyst should be investigated thoroughly by transvaginal ultrasound and CA125 level.
- RMI should be calculated to decide line of management.
- Unilateral simple ovarian cysts with diameter <5 cm can be managed conservatively with CA125 level monitoring and ultrasound surveillance.
- Aspiration is not to be done for postmenopausal ovarian cysts.
- Women who do not fit into criteria for conservative management but have low risk of malignancy can undergo laparoscopic oophorectomy.
- Consider salpingectomy or bilateral salpingo-oophorectomy for women undergoing laparoscopic management of postmenopausal ovarian cysts.

- Women with moderate risk of malignancy index should undergo laparoscopic bilateral salpingo-oophorectomy.

CONCLUSION

As the advancements are day-by-day increasing in the field of imaging, recognition of ovarian cancers is becoming more easier even with subtle symptoms. It is utmost important to distinguish ovarian cysts that can be monitored with repeat sonography from masses that need to be surgically evaluated due to their elevated risk of early ovarian cancer.

REFERENCES

1. American College of Obstetricians and Gynecologists. ACOG Practice Bulletin. Management of adnexal masses. Obstet Gynecol. 2007;110(1):201-14.
2. Holt VL, Cushing-Haugen KL, Daling JR. Oral contraceptives, tubal sterilization, and functional ovarian cyst risk. Obstet Gynecol. 2003;102(2):252-8.
3. Van Calster B, Van Hoorde K, Valentin L, et al. Evaluating the risk of ovarian cancer before surgery using the ADNEX model to differentiate between benign, borderline, early and advanced stage invasive, and secondary metastatic tumours: prospective multicentre diagnostic study. BMJ. 2014;349:g5920.
4. Giede KC, Kieser K, Dodge J, et al. Who should operate on patients with ovarian cancer? An evidence-based review. Gynecol Oncol. 2005;99(2):447-61.
5. Earle CC, Schrag D, Neville BA, et al. Effect of surgeon specialty on processes of care and outcomes for ovarian cancer patients. J Natl Cancer Inst. 2006;98(3):172-80.
6. Prat J; FIGO Committee on Gynecologic Oncology. Staging classification for cancer of the ovary, fallopian tube, and peritoneum. Int J Gynaecol Obstet. 2014;124(1):1-5.
7. Chang SJ, Bristow RE. Evolution of surgical treatment paradigms for advanced-stage ovarian cancer: redefining "optimal" residual disease. Gynecol Oncol. 2012;125(2):483-92.
8. Armstrong DK, Bundy B, Wenzel L, et al. Intraperitoneal cisplatin and paclitaxel in ovarian cancer. N Engl J Med. 2006;354:34-43.
9. Pujade-Lauraine E, Wagner U, Aavall-Lundqvist E, et al. Pegylated liposomal doxorubicin and carboplatin compared with paclitaxel and carboplatin for patients with platinum-sensitive ovarian cancer in late relapse. J Clin Oncol. 2010;28(20):3323-9.
10. Vergote I, du Bois A. Neoadjuvant chemotherapy in advanced ovarian cancer: on what do we agree and disagree? Gynecol Oncol. 2013;128(1):6-11.
11. Albuquerque KV, Singla R, Potkul RK, et al. Impact of tumor volume-directed involved field radiation therapy integrated in the management of recurrent ovarian cancer. Gynecol Oncol. 2005;96(3):701-4.
12. Cannistra SA. Is there a "best" choice of second-line agent in the treatment of recurrent, potentially platinum-sensitive ovarian cancer? J Clin Oncol. 2002;20(5):1158-60.
13. Trimble CL, Kosary C, Trimble EL. Long-term survival and patterns of care in women with ovarian tumors of low malignant potential. Gynecol Oncol. 2002;86(1):34-7.
14. Aghajanian C, Blank SV, Goff BA, et al. OCEANS: a randomized, double-blind, placebo-controlled phase III trial of chemotherapy with or without bevacizumab in patients with platinum-sensitive recurrent epithelial ovarian, primary peritoneal, or fallopian tube cancer. J Clin Oncol. 2012;30(17):2039-45.
15. Pujade-Lauraine E, Hilpert F, Weber B, et al. AURELIA: A randomized phase III trial evaluating bevacizumab (BEV) plus chemotherapy (CT) for platinum (PT)-resistant recurrent ovarian cancer (OC). J Clin Oncol. 2012;30.
16. Levine DA, Argenta PA, Yee CJ, et al. Fallopian tube and primary peritoneal carcinomas associated with BRCA mutations. J Clin Oncol. 2003;21(22):4222-7.
17. Walsh T, Casadei S, Coats KH, et al. Spectrum of mutations in BRCA1, BRCA2, CHEK2, and TP53 in families at high risk of breast cancer. JAMA. 2006;295(12):1379-88.

18. Domchek SM, Friebel TM, Singer CF, et al. Association of risk-reducing surgery in brca1 or brca2 mutation carriers with cancer risk and mortality. JAMA. 2010;304(9):967-75.
19. Watson P, Butzow R, Lynch HT, et al. The clinical features of ovarian cancer in hereditary nonpolyposis colorectal cancer. Gynecol Oncol. 2001;82(2):223-8.
20. Bonadona V, Bonaiti B, Olschwang S, et al. Cancer risks associated with germline mutations in mlh1, msh2, and msh6 genes in lynch syndrome. JAMA. 2011;305(22):2304-10.
21. Brown J, Sood AK, Deavers MT, et al. Patterns of metastasis in sex cord-stromal tumors of the ovary: can routine staging lymphadenectomy be omitted? Gynecol Oncol. 2009;113(1):86-90.
22. Homesley HD, Bundy BN, Hurteau JA, et al. Bleomycin, etoposide, and cisplatin combination therapy of ovarian granulosa cell tumors and other stromal malignancies: a Gynecologic Oncology Group study. Gynecol Oncol. 1999;72(2):131-7.
23. Piver MS, Jishi MF, Tsukada Y, et al. Primary peritoneal carcinoma after prophylactic oophorectomy in women with a family history of ovarian cancer. A report of the Gilda Radner Familial Ovarian Cancer Registry. Cancer. 1993;71(9):2751-5.

CHAPTER 19

Gynecological Emergencies in Postmenopausal Women with Mass per Vaginum

Anu Joseph

INTRODUCTION

Postmenopausal age is one wherein women go through a lot of social, psychological, emotional, hormonal, and physiological changes. This is an age group that can be associated with a variety of gynecological conditions, most importantly malignancy. Among the other pandora of emergency visits to hospital by women of postmenopausal age group, are some not very common gynecological conditions.

In this chapter, we intend to discuss a few of the gynecological emergencies associated with complaints of mass per vaginum. As we all know, the most common emergencies which bring in one's attention are pain and bleeding. But to see things in a better perspective, the conditions which may present to us are being further classified based on the pathology that may present as mass per vaginum and its associated acute complications.

Conditions which can present as mass per vaginum:
- Pelvic organ prolapse
- Uterine inversion
- Submucous myoma or polyp
- Malignancy
- Miscellaneous.

We shall see these conditions in a bit further detail with respect to the emergencies with which each of them may present.

PELVIC ORGAN PROLAPSE

Uterine prolapse means the uterus has descended from its normal position (at the level of ischial spines) in the pelvis farther down into the vagina. Studies have estimated that 50% of parous women have some degree of urogenital prolapse and, of these; 10–20% are symptomatic. The degree of uterine prolapse tends to increase in menopause due to the weakening of the pelvic supports.

Chapter 19: Gynecological Emergencies in Postmenopausal Women with Mass per Vaginum

Emergencies associated with pelvic organ prolapse are as follows:
- Irreducibility
- Pain
- Bleeding
- Acute urinary retention
- Constipation.

The diagnosis and treatment of emergencies related to pelvic organ prolapse is summarized in **Table 1**.

TABLE 1: Emergencies associated with pelvic organ prolapse.

Symptom	Cause	Clinical diagnosis	Investigation	Treatment
Irreducibility	Edema	Signs of prolapse: Not reducible manually with Trendelenburg position	Clinical diagnosis: Ultrasound to rule out associated pathology	Treat infection and edema; Spontaneously reduces vaginal hysterectomy and site specific repair
	Bladder calculi[1] Multiple[2] Large[3]	Presence of hard mass in the cystocele associated	X-ray Ultrasound	Vaginal cystolithotomy
Pain				
• Chronic	Stretching of ligaments/ nerves	Rule out other causes	Clinical diagnosis	Pessary repair
• Acute	Urinary infection	Fever with chills, dysuria, foul smelling urine	Urine microscopy and culture	Antibiotic Correct stasis
	Urinary retention	Cystocele with large amount of residual urine on catheterization	USG: postvoid residual volume	Catheterize Surgical correction Pessary
• Abdominal/flank pain	Ureteric involvement[4]	Colicky flank pain Rule out coexistent malignancy	USG/KUB X-ray showing hydroureteronephrosis[5]	Surgical correction
	Bowel involvement and obstruction	Enterocele Rectocele	X-ray	Correction of prolapse
Bleeding	Decubitus ulcer	Pale sometimes infected ulcer at the dependent area	Rule out malignancy by biopsy	Antibiotics Pessary Hygiene
	Malignancies of cervix/vagina[6]	Eroded margins	Biopsy	Depending on stage and spread
	Atrophic vagina	Pale vagina	Always rule out malignancy	Topical estrogen
Urinary retention	Discussed above			
Constipation				

There has been case reports of urinary obstruction leading to renal failure in patients with prolapsed uterus.[7,8] Hydroureteronephrosis may remain asymptomatic for a prolonged duration and present as fever with pyuria when there is associated urinary tract infection or pyelonephritis.

UTERINE INVERSION

Uterine inversion in a nonpregnant woman is a rare occurrence, with only 150 cases reported from 1887 to 2006, and the large majority occurring in women over 45 years old.[9] Nonpuerperal inversion usually results from a tumor implanted on fundus of the uterus.

Causes

- Unnoticed prolonged puerperal inversion
- Uterine polyp[10] (fundal)
- Fibroid (fundal)[11]
- Malignancies of uterus.[12] Sarcomatous change of a fundal fibroid may soften the uterine wall and cause inversion
- Following previous high amputation of cervix, due to lax cervical tone.

Diagnosis of Uterine Inversion

- Globular mass protruding through the introitus
- No cervical is noticed
- Covering is shaggy (Pelvic organ prolapse has a smooth covering)
- Cervical rim felt high in the vagina on per vaginal examination
- Dimpling at the uterine fundus on bimanual examination; sometimes, better appreciated on a rectoabdominal examination
- Sound test shows absence of uterine cavity. This test is used to clinically differentiate inversion from a prolapsed polyp or a pelvic organ prolapse.

Main Clinical Symptoms

- Abnormal vaginal bleeding[13]
- Lower abdominal pain
- Vaginal pressure
- Rarely acute urinary retention by urethral compression which may be the reason for acute emergency visit to the hospital. Pelvic ultrasonography, CT, and MRI can be beneficial in diagnosis.[14] Treatment depends on the associated pathology and the stage of the inversion. Total hysterectomy by combined laparoscopic and vaginal route is a valid and feasible approach in postmenopausal women. Surgeons should be aware that intra-abdominal morcellation should be avoided, due to a risk that the protruded mass may be a malignant uterine tumor.[15]

SUBMUCOUS POLYP/MYOMA

In today's age, with increasing use of hormone replacement therapy, it is not uncommon to see postmenopausal women presenting with fibroid uterus or polyp. But very rarely presents as a mass at the introitus. When a submucous polyp/fibroid presents as a mass PV, it should be differentiated from pelvic organ prolapse and inversion as described above.

It may also be associated with:

- Foul-smelling discharge
- Irregular vaginal bleeding
- *Pain*: Very rare.

Further diagnosis is made by imaging and biopsy. It is prudent that any mass PV in the postmenopausal age group be viewed with suspicion and histopathological diagnosis made to rule out malignancy.

A benign fibroid polyp is managed with polypectomy and endometrial curettage. Patient should be followed up with serial ultrasound and progesterone therapy for regression of endometrial thickness.

MALIGNANCY

Carcinoma of the cervix and the vagina may sometimes present as mass per vaginum, especially with the polypoidal growth pattern. Malignancies, especially in the latter stages, may present with various emergencies. Some may be diagnosed with carcinoma when they first visit an emergency department with symptoms of vaginal bleeding, pain, or intestinal obstruction.

Vaginal Bleeding

- Any postmenopausal woman with vaginal bleeding should be considered as having reproductive tract malignancy unless proved otherwise.
- A gentle speculum examination should be made after the initial general and systemic examination. An obvious mass should be ruled out, and the exact site of origin of bleed should be established. Further diagnostic and therapeutic management will depend upon the initial evaluation and differential diagnosis.
- Though, carcinoma of cervix and vagina are more common in mass per vaginum presenting as bleeding PV, other malignancies like endometrial carcinoma, gestational trophoblastic disease, vulvar carcinoma, etc. should also be looked for.

Patients may also present with medical emergencies like altered mental or neurological status, electrolyte imbalance, jaundice, pedal edema, etc. or surgical emergencies like urinary obstruction, urinary incontinence, mass abdomen, or intestinal obstruction. It is prudent on the part of the attending doctor to evaluate the reproductive history and do a pelvic examination including a Pap smear or biopsy as the case may demand.

MISCELLANEOUS

Though rare, literature has shown a variety of other lesions which may present as an emergency, which may be associated with a mass PV. For instance, a case report from Malaysia discusses the presentation of a vascular malformation of the vagina in a postmenopausal woman. She was treated with a vascular embolization.[16]

Occasionally, the symptom with which the patient presents may not be associated with the mass. For instance, a lady may present with vaginal bleeding, and have a coexistent benign vaginal cyst. It is prudent to investigate beyond the vaginal mass to find out the actual etiology of the symptom.

CONCLUSION

Vaginal masses may present with a variety of associated emergency symptoms. A thorough history taking and clinical examination would point towards the diagnosis majority of the times. Bleeding and mass per vaginum, whether troubling the patient or not, should be thoroughly examined and investigated to rule out malignancy.

REFERENCES

1. Chuang FR, Lee CH, Chen CS, et al. Bilateral moderate hydroureteronephrosis due to uterine prolapse: two case reports and review of the literature. Ren Fail. 2003;25(5):879-84.
2. Dahiya P, Gupta A, Sangwan K. Multiple bladder calculi: A rare cause of irreducible uterine prolapsed. Arch Gynecol Obstet. 2007;275(5):411-2.

3. Lupovitch A, England ER, Chen R. Non-puerperal uterine inversion in association with uterine sarcoma: case report in a 26-year-old and review of the literature. Gynecol Oncol. 2005;97(3):938-41.
4. MacKenzie TM, Chan LW, Yuen PM, et al. Uterine prolapse and acute renal failure in a Chinese patient. Aust NZJ Obstet Gynecol. 1995;35(4):461-2.
5. Auber M, Darwish B, Lefebure A, et al. Management of non-puerperal uterine inversion using a combined laparoscopic and vaginal approach. Am J Obstet Gyne. 2011;204(6):e7-9.
6. Melser M, Miles BJ, Kastan D, et al. Chronic renal failure secondary to post-hysterectomy vaginal prolapse. Urology. 1991;38(4):361-3.
7. Molinelli EA, Porges RF. Incarcerated uterine prolapse associated with a cul-de-sac abscess. Obstet Gynecol. 1993;82(4 Pt 2 Suppl):664-6.
8. Pandit U. Prolapsed uterine sarcoma causing non-puerperal uterine inversion in a postmenopausal woman. JNMA J Nepal Med Assoc. 2006;45(164):373-4.
9. Darji P, Banker H, Gandhi V, et al. Postmenopausal woman with vaginal mass: do not forget to see for uterine inversion. BMJ Case Reports. 2012;2012. pii: bcr0220125841.
10. Préfontaine M. Complete uterine inversion in a patient with endometrial cancer. J Obstet Gynecol Can. 2012;34(7):609.
11. Pue LB, Lo TS, Wu PY. Vaginal vascular malformation mimicking pelvic organ prolapse requiring serial embolizations. Int Urogynecol J. 2013;24(11):1985-7.
12. Rao K, Kumar NP, Geetha AS. Primary carcinoma of vagina with uterine prolapsed. J Indian Med Assoc. 1989;87(1):10-2.
13. Rocconi R, Huh WK, Chiang S. Postmenopausal uterine inversion associated with endometrial polyps. Obstet Gynecol. 2003;102(3):521-3.
14. Skinner GN, Louden KA. Nonpuerperal uterine inversion associated with an atypical leiomyoma. Aust NZJ Obstet Gynecol. 2001;41(1):100-1.
15. Thompson JD. Pelvic organ prolapse. Basic concepts. In: Rock JA, Thompson JD (Eds). TeLinde's operative gynecology, Lippencott-Raven: Philadelphia/New York; 1996. pp. 951-8.
16. Wai CY, Margulis V, Baugh BR, et al. Multiple vesical calculi and complete vaginal vault prolapsed. Am J Obstet Gynecol. 2003;189(3):884-5.

SECTION 4

Emergencies in Gynecological Surgeries

- Complications in Open Gynecological Surgery
  Jahnavi Esanakula, Varsha Rengaraj
- Complications in Laparoscopy
  Kavita Manchanda, Varsha Rengaraj
- Gynecological Oncology Emergencies
  Ipsita Batra
- Imaging in Gynecological Emergencies
  Aradhana Kalra Dawar, Jahnavi Esanakula

CHAPTER 20

Complications in Open Gynecological Surgery

Jahnavi Esanakula, Varsha Rengaraj

INTRODUCTION

Complications in any surgical procedure are not uncommon. More complex the procedure more likely is the chance of a major operative injury. Thorough understanding of the anatomy of the operating area and optimal surgical technique can reduce the complications. However, the most important part is the timely recognition and management of these events. The most common complications are:
- Injury to urinary tract
- Bowel injury
- Vascular injuries
- Uterine and cervical injuries
- Hematomas
- Wound sepsis and wound dehiscence.

INJURY TO THE URINARY TRACT

Bladder Injury

Bladder injury is one of the most common complications in pelvic surgery. Close anatomic relation between bladder and genital organs predispose the urinary tract to injury during pelvic surgery.

Bladder injury can occur in 1-2% of abdominal hysterectomies and in 4% in vaginal hysterectomies.[1]

If a bladder injury is suspected, bladder should be filled with a dye (methylene blue), leak will identify the site of injury.

Preventive measures to avoid urinary tract injuries and postoperative fistula formation are:
- A detailed anatomical knowledge of operating part and common mode and area of injury.
- High-risk patients should be identified. Alterations in anatomy predisposes to injury. There is possibility of alteration in anatomy in:
  - Fibrosis
  - Chronic pelvic inflammatory disease
  - Endometriosis
  - Fibroids—large or broad ligament

- Malignancy and previous irradiation
- Congenital abnormalities of the urogenital system.
- High-risk patients have to be identified and thorough preoperative evaluation has to be done. It may require renal function tests, intravenous pyelography, cystoscopy, and ureteric catheterization.
- Emptying the bladder before surgery and catheterization in case of prolonged surgery is simple procedure which prevents bladder injury. Urinary output should be monitored during the procedure in case bladder is catheterized.

Surgeon should be conscious about the ureteric position and course of ureter during the surgery. In high risk cases, bladder and ureters should be properly exposed and directly visualized following proper and systematic surgical technique.

Types of Bladder Injuries

Full thickness injuries: In case of full thickness injuries to bladder, it has to be repaired in two layers—first layer involving mucosa and second layer involving muscle and serosa (burying the first layer). Vicryl 3-0 round body is the suture material of choice.

Precautions during repair are:
- Identification of ureters during the bladder repair. If in doubt, ureteric stents should be placed under direct vision.
- Bladder catheterization has to be done for 7–10 days.
- Larger defects will need intra-abdominal drain and suprapubic catheterization. To check voiding function, the catheter has to be clamped intermittently.

Partial thickness defect: In partial defect of bladder, a single layer closure with 2-0 absorbable sutures will suffice.

Small extraperitoneal defect: Need only observation. Indwelling catheter for 7–10 days will usually result in healing. Cystoscopic inspection of bladder is necessary if there is a doubt of bladder injury. Bladder injuries if missed during surgery, present as postoperative urinary incontinence or rarely menouria. These injuries can be diagnosed by a simple speculum examination and three swab test, or may need cystoscopy and intravenous urography.[2]

Ureteric Injury

Incidence of ureteric injury is around 0.1-2%.[3]

Ureteric injury is more commonly seen in complicated surgical procedures such as hysterectomy, lymphadenectomy, and extensive endometriosis especially involving the uterosacral ligaments and rectovaginal septum.

Injury to the ureter can be ligation, crushing, partial or complete transaction, injury due to electrocautery and stripping of ureteric serosa.

During complicated pelvic surgeries, ureter should be identified. If need be, ureteric stenting can be done before surgery.

Ureter can be identified by:
- Peristalsis
- When it crosses over the iliac artery
- Palpation and snap technique.

Special precautions have to be taken at the common sites of ureteric injuries which are:
- Cardinal ligament where ureter crosses the uterine artery
- Under the insertion of the infundibulopelvic ligament
- Tunnel of Wertheim
- Vesicoureteric junction
- Lateral pelvic sidewall above uterosacral ligament.

Diagnosis of Ureteric Injury

Intraoperative:
- Dilatation of proximal portion of ureter
- Presence of urine in the field of surgery
- Absence of ureteric peristalsis
- Dilatation of proximal ureter and urine leakage after giving intravenous diuretics
- Leakage of dye after intravenous 5–10 mL indigo carmine dye
- Cystoscopy showing lack of ureteral jet indicates a coagulated or ligated ureter.

In case of suspicion of ureteric injury during surgery, any obstruction or defect in the wall can be identified by ureteric catheterization and injection of contrast or cystoscopy and retrograde ureteropyelography.

Management:
- In the case of misplaced sutures or clamps, these should be immediately removed.
- If the ureter is not transected, stenting with 6 F double J silicone catheters can be done and conservatively managed.
- In case of a small perforation, repair and stent placement has to be done.
- In partial injury, repair and place stent.
- In complete ureteric transaction, do end-to-end anastomosis and stent.
- *Postoperative*: In bulk (70%) of cases, ureteric injury is detected postoperatively.[4]

Symptoms and signs:
- Postoperative anuria in bilateral ureteric ligation
- Unexplained hematuria
- Flank pain/costovertebral angle tenderness
- Leakage of urine per vaginum
- Lump in the abdomen or ileus
- In case of infection and pyelonephritis loin pain, fever and rigors are the common symptoms
- Signs and symptoms of urinary ascites

Postoperative imaging:
- Renal ultrasound—ascites, retroperitoneal fluid collection, hydronephrosis, hydroureter or pelvic mass
- X-ray erect abdomen shows a ground glass appearance
- CT scan to image kidneys, ureters, and bladder
- Retrograde ureteropyelography with flexible cystoscope or intravenous urography (IVU) to determine the level at which urinary leak is present.

Management:
- *Immediate recognition*: Suturing and end-to-end repair, ureteral reconstruction.
- *Delayed recognition*: End-to-end repair or ureteroneocystostomy.
- Double J-shaped catheter or a ureteric stent insertion is done with cystoscopy and removed after 6–12 weeks.
- Patients with bilateral ureteric damage will present with anuria and develop uremia rapidly. They may require percutaneous nephrostomy as an emergency.

The results of ureteric repair are related to the surgery that caused the lesion.[5]

■ BOWEL INJURY

Bowel injury complicates 0.13% of hysterectomies.[6]

Bowel injury can be avoided by following the guidelines:
- Identifying high-risk cases like previous abdominal surgeries, complicated appendicitis, diverticulitis, endometriosis, pelvic malignancies, ovarian malignancy, and pelvic tuberculosis
- Preoperative preparation of bowel
- Start liquid diet for 1 day prior to surgery
- 24 hours nil by mouth
- Give laxatives to clear the bowel

- Start preoperative antibiotics 24 hours prior to surgery
- Drugs with gram-negative coverage and metronidazole are preferred
- Follow traction and counter traction rule for lysing adhesions
- Vascular adhesions have to be ligated
- In very dense adhesions, the pararectal space should be developed
- Ureter, major blood vessels, and walls of the bowel should be identified before lysing the adhesions
- In benign cases, a sharp uterine serosal incision is often necessary.

Bowel injury is best diagnosed at the time of surgery itself, but injuries caused by diathermy and crush injuries are sometimes missed intraoperatively and present days after a surgery. Surgical repair is needed in such patients. Laparotomy has to be performed and bowel contents have to be washed out.[7]

Injured bowel is identified and isolated. If not done carefully, the bowel contents leak into the peritoneal cavity and cause peritonitis.

A two layer closure with No.1 non-absorbable suture with round body needle is recommended.

Bowel wall is repaired with interrupted sutures with 3-0 absorbable suture material. The sutures are tied to create an air proof seal. If tied too tight it causes ischemia of the bowel wall and leads to dehiscence.[8]

If the injury is longitudinal horizontal closure prevents stricture formation. Fistula formation is one of the complications of a bowel surgery. Mucosa has to be inverted to prevent fistula formation. Suturing 1 mm of either submucosa or mucosa and including 5 mm of serosa and muscularis will invert the mucosa.

For superficial damage, only muscularis and serosa has to be sutured. This buries the defect.

Occasionally, primary anastomosis is required.
Bowel anastomosis can be:
- End to end
- End to side
- Side to side.

Recently, anastomosis with staplers is gaining popularity. GIA and TA stapler can be used for this purpose.[9]

After bowel repair, care has to be taken to check for hemostasis, to check for air leaks, and to check for circulation to the anastomosed bowel region. To prevent development of peritonitis, an abdominal wash with warm normal saline and metronidazole is advocated after completion of the anastomosis before closure of abdomen.

Appropriate intraoperative and postoperative antibiotic coverage is required.

Postoperative Ileus

The duration of postoperative ileus depends on:
- Location of surgery
- Degree of surgical manipulation
- Inflammatory responses.

Symptoms include nausea, vomiting, abdominal pain, distension, and absent bowel movements.

Laboratory investigations include complete blood count (CBC) and serum electrolytes.

X-ray abdomen shows dilated bowel loops.

Treatment involves bowel rest, intravenous fluids, and electrolyte management.[9]

UTERINE AND CERVICAL INJURIES

Cervical injury and uterine perforation are very common in forceful dilatation or with soft uterus. Following are the high risk factors:
- Nulliparity
- Previous cervical surgery
- Postmenopausal women
- During pregnancy

Chapter 20: Complications in Open Gynecological Surgery

- Markedly retroverted uterus
- Prior cone biopsy
- GnRH agonist use
- Uterine malformations.

Management of Uterine Perforation and Cervical Injury

In case of small perforations which are not bleeding—observation and prophylactic course of antibiotics is all that is needed for the perforation to heal.

If the perforation was with a sharp instrument, visceral and vascular injury should be ruled out.

Examination of injury with laparoscopy is indicated if patient is stable, and examination of bowel, adnexa, and pelvic side walls is possible or if the injury has been identified during a laparoscopic surgery.

Laparotomy has to be done in unstable patient and if laparoscopic comprehensive assessment of the extent of the injury is not possible.

Retroperitoneal structure injury is often missed as they are concealed. A broad ligament hematoma or change in the patient vital signs may be the only signs pointing towards a retroperitoneal hemorrhage. Most of the lateral perforations through cervix and broad ligament hematomas can be managed conservatively.[10]

However, if there is any increase in size of hematoma or if the patient becomes unstable exploration has to be done immediately and hemostasis secured. Cervical injury can be managed by tamponade or suturing.

VASCULAR INJURIES

Primary Hemorrhage

Primary hemorrhage is defined as bleeding at the time of surgery.

The main causes are:
- Acute vascular injury
- Ineffective local hemostasis
- Complications of blood transfusion
- Coagulopathy
- Sepsis.

Hemorrhage can be anticipated in the following:
- Fibroids—large sized, cervical or broad ligament fibroid
- Endometriosis altering the pelvic anatomy
- Chronic pelvic inflammatory disease (PID)
- Genital tuberculosis
- Vaginal hysterectomy with extensive pelvic floor repair
- Cases of malignancy
- Previous history of radiotherapy

Management: When primary hemorrhage is anticipated, adequate packing, saline adrenaline infiltration in vaginal surgery, dissection in correct planes, and achieving proper hemostasis at every step is essential. No dead space should be left behind. Use of regional anesthesia and prophylactic antibiotics is recommended.

Reactionary Hemorrhage

It is defined as hemorrhage that occurs within 24 hours of surgery. Patient usually present with cold clammy extremities, become restless, have a rising pulse and low urine output in postoperative period. A strong degree of suspicion is necessary as vital signs may remain normal for 12-14 hours.

Resuscitation is started immediately by making arrangements to shift patient to operation theater. Blood for crossmatching should be taken and reserved. Ultrasonography should be made available. In case of vaginal hemorrhage, examination under anesthesia and ligation of the bleeding vessel is done immediately. Tight packing is done in generalized oozing. If hemorrhage continues or intraperitoneal hemorrhage is detected, relaparotomy is required.[10,11]

Secondary Hemorrhage

Hemorrhage that occurs up to 6 weeks postoperatively is called secondary hemorrhage. It is usually due to infection. Risk can be reduced by good hemostasis, keeping drainage, antibiotics, and use of povidone-iodine to clean the vault.

PELVIC HEMATOMA

A hematoma in the pelvic region causes serious morbidity. It can cause pain and get infected. The incidence of postoperative hematoma varies from 3% to 8%.[11]

Hematomas can develop in the following regions:
- Vaginal vault
- Pelvic side wall
- Paravesical space
- Abdominal wall
- Ischiorectal fossa
- Vulva.

Postoperative pelvic hematomas give a varying clinical picture. Most commonly, these patients may be asymptomatic. Postoperative discomfort, abdominal distension, paralytic ileus, fever, tenesmus, nausea, vomiting, diarrhea, and vaginal discharge are some of the symptoms a postoperative pelvic hematoma may present with. If neglected, grossly fistula formation, septicemia, acute renal failure, and acute lung injury may also occur. Retching and straining are some of the risk factors after surgery that increases the risk of pelvic hematomas.

Ultrasonography is the imaging modality of choice in detection and also demarcation of size and location of hematomas.

For a simple hematoma drainage with sinus forceps shall suffice undercover of prophylactic antibiotics. In difficult cases, surgical exploration under anesthesia may be required. If the hematoma is small sized and is not infected it can be allowed to gradually resolve with careful monitoring.

Nerve Injury

Neuropraxia: One of the complications of nerve compression during prolonged surgery. Lower limb is usually affected due to lithotomy position compressing either femoral or peroneal nerves. Most cases resolve spontaneously. Physiotherapy may be needed to prevent contractures.[11]

Post-traumatic neuropathy: It can occur due to nerve damage during surgery or at the injection site because of fault in injection technique.

Symptoms:
- Neuralgic pain
- Alterations in sensitivity
- Numbness, tingling, and weakness in the areas supplied by the nerves
- Effect on the sympathetic nervous system
- Allodynia (experiencing normal stimuli as painful).

Investigations include nerve conduction studies and cross-sectional imaging.

Treatment:
- Antidepressants and antiepileptics can be given for neuralgic pain, e.g. gabapentin and amitriptyline.
- Nerve block with local anesthetic injections and steroid injections can help in reducing scar hypersensitivity.
- Permanent blocks may cause relief initially but differentiation of pain occurs later.

- Whenever feasible, decompression of nerve by surgery, removal of suture material causing compression, and excision of neuroma has to be done.

WOUND SEPSIS AND WOUND DEHISCENCE

These are the most dreaded complications of abdominal surgery. The incidence of wound dehiscence varies from place to place and is up to 0.4%–3.5%.[12,13] The incidence of mortality is up to 45%.[14,15]

Wound sepsis and dehiscence will increase the duration of hospital stay and increase the morbidity and health expenditure of the patient.

Wound healing can occur by:
- *Primary intention:* When the wound edges are opposed
- *Secondary intention:* When wound edges are wide apart.

Wound dehiscence or disruption can be partial (rectus sheath or peritoneum not disrupted) or complete (all the layers are disrupted).

Risk Factors for Wound Sepsis and Dehiscence

- Poor nutritional status
- Old age
- Obesity
- Anemia
- Comorbidities like diabetes and hypertension
- Peritonitis
- Emergency procedures
- Vertical incisions
- Poor wound closing techniques
- Postoperative cough and vomiting
- Poor wound care postoperatively.

Measures to Prevent Wound Sepsis and Dehiscence

- Improvement of the nutritional status
- Aseptic precautions during surgery
- Antibiotic cover
- Nasogastric tube usage as and when needed during surgery
- Taking the appropriate incisions—preferably avoiding midline incisions
- Timely management of postoperative cough and vomiting
- Electrolyte balance maintenance.

Presenting Complaints

Wound sepsis is evident usually in the form of discharge from the wound that is often purulent in nature. When severely infected the wound edges tend to get necrosed which results in gaping of the wound.

A serous discharge from the wound often during the third or fourth postoperative day should be a warning sign of wound dehiscence. The more dramatic presentation of complete dehiscence by disruption of all the layers and protrusion of viscera outside is less common.

Treatment

Improvement of the nutritional status of the women plays a key role on treatment of both sepsis and dehiscence. Addressing the underlying risk factor for that particular patient like proper glycemic control will help in wound healing.

Management of Wound Sepsis

Wound sepsis requires isolation of organism causing sepsis by culture and sensitivity of the wound discharge or a swab from the infected site. Mild wound infections can be resolved by appropriate antibiotics alone but severe wound sepsis with necrosis and sloughing needs to be resutured again after antibiotics and excision of the sloughed tissue.

Management of Dehiscence

Partial dehiscence is managed conservatively by prophylactic antibiotics and resuturing of the wound under antibiotic cover. In case of complete dehiscence the wound and the protruding organs should be immediately covered with sterile towels, a narcotic agent should be administered and the patient should be operated on an emergency basis. Deep tension suturing should be applied in order to avoid tension over the sutures on the wound edges.

SUMMARY

- Thorough knowledge about the anatomy of operating area and optimum surgical skill will help in reducing the complications of surgery.
- Injury to urinary tract, bowel, blood vessels, uterus and cervix can occur in cases with distorted anatomy like fibroids, endometriosis, chronic PID, previous surgery, malignancy and tuberculosis.
- Proper identification of high risk cases and measures like preoperative ureteric stenting, bowel emptying will avoid injury to ureters and bowel respectively. In case of vascular injuries, resulting in primary or reactionary hemorrhage, resuscitation with fluids and/or blood transfusions will be necessary. Antibiotics will be needed in secondary hemorrhage.
- Pelvic hematoma can be diagnosed with the help of ultrasound. Simple hematomas can be managed by drainage undercover of antibiotics. Small hematomas can be allowed to resolve spontaneously.
- Addressing nutrition and comorbidities will avoid wound sepsis and dehiscence. Wound sepsis has to be managed by antibiotics and resuturing. Wound dehiscence is managed by simple resuturing or emergency tension suture application depending on the severity of the complication.

CONCLUSION

Gynecological surgeries like any other surgeries are not exempted from complications. Proper anticipation of the complications and timely identification and rectification of intra-operative injuries will help to avoid severe morbidity to the patient. Improvement of nutritional status and standard protocol for preoperative preparation, operative procedure and postoperative care will avoid wound sepsis and related complications.

REFERENCES

1. Wu HH, Yang PY, Yeh GP, et al. The detection of ureteral injuries after hysterectomy. J Minim Invasive Gynecol. 2006;13(5):403-8.
2. Hurt GH. Gynecologic injury to the ureters, bladder and urethra. In: Walters MD, Karram MM (Eds). Urogynecology and Reconstructive Pelvic Surgery, 2nd edition. St Louis, MO: Mosby; 1999. pp. 377-86.
3. Soong Y, Lim PH. Urological injuries in gynecological practice. When is the optimal time for repair? Singapore Med J. 1997;38(11):475-8.
4. Underwood P. Operative injuries to the ureter. In: Rock JA, Jones HW (Eds). TeLinde's Operative Gynecology, 10th edition. New Delhi: JB Lippincott; 1997. pp. 197-232.
5. Daly JW, Higgins KA. Injury to the ureter during gynecologic surgical procedures. Surg Gynecol Obstet. 1988;167(1):19-22.
6. Seibel BE. Postoperative complications and postoperative emergencies. In: Benrubi GI (Ed). Handbook of Obstetrics and Gynecologic Emergencies, 4th edition. Philadelphia:

Wolters Kluwer Lippincott Williams & Wilkins; 2010. pp. 316-28.
7. Mäkinen J, Johansson J, Thomás C, et al. Morbidity of 10110 hysterectomies by type of approach. Hum Reprod. 2001;16(7):1473-8.
8. Krebs HB. Intestinal injury in gynecologic surgery: A ten year experience. Am J Obstet Gynecol. 1986;155(3):509-14.
9. Reich H, McGlynn F, Budin R. Laparoscopic repair of full thickness bowel injury. J Laparoendosc Surg. 1991;1(2):119-22.
10. Thompson JD, Rock WA Jr. Control of pelvic hemorrhage. In: TeLinde's Operative Gynecology, 8th edition. Pennsylvania: JB Lippincott;1997. pp. 197-232 .
11. Cosson M, Lambaudie E. Boukerrou M, et al. Vaginal, laparoscopic or abdominal hysterectomies for benign disorders: Immediate and early post-operative complications. Eur J Obstet Gynecol Reprod Biol. 2001;98(2):231-6.
12. Webster C, Neumayer L, Smout R, et al. National Veterans Affairs Surgical Quality Improvement Program. Prognostic models of abdominal wound dehiscence after laparotomy. J Surg Res. 2003;109:130-7.
13. Gislason H, Grønbech JE, Søreide O. Burst abdomen and incisional hernia after major gastrointestinal operations—comparison of three closure techniques. Eur J Surg. 1995;161:349-54.
14. Fleischer GM, Rennert A, Rühmer M. Die infizierte Bauchdecke und der Platzbauch. Chirurg. 2000;71:754-62.
15. Poole GV Jr. Mechanical factors in abdominal wound closure: the prevention of fascial dehiscence. Surgery. 1985;97:631-40.

CHAPTER 21

Complications in Laparoscopy

Kavita Manchanda, Varsha Rengaraj

INTRODUCTION

Laparoscopic surgery has become widely accepted by surgeons and patients as an effective technique to treat gynecologic pathologies. Shorter duration of hospital stay, early recovery, lesser blood loss, and postoperative pain makes laparoscopic surgery superior to open surgeries.

As the technology has improved and surgical skills have increased, the nature and characteristics of laparoscopic procedures have also become more complex. Although the incidence of complications decreases as surgeons gain experience with laparoscopy, the growing difficulty of some procedures in gynecologic surgery may increase the frequency of severe complications (visceral and great vessel injuries).

The delay in recognition of complications and timely intervention increases morbidity and mortality. Incidence of complications during laparoscopic procedures range from 0.2% to 10.3%.[1] The majority of complications arise while introducing instruments for creating pneumoperitoneum. Two methods of entry (open-entry and closed-entry) have been compared for rates of complications. The open-entry has been associated with lesser incidence of complications, and the mortality resulting from delayed diagnosis can be avoided by intraoperative diagnosis. Apart from injuries upon entry, other possible sources of injuries include thermal injuries by use of cautery, operative manipulations, and suturing, and the presence of CO_2 in extraperitoneal spaces.

The complications seen are described in **Table 1**.

INTESTINAL INJURY

The bowel injury is reported to occur in 0–0.5%[2] of cases. Approximately half of these occur during introduction of trocar or while

Chapter 21: Complications in Laparoscopy

TABLE 1: Summary of complications of laparoscopic gynecologic surgery.

Complications	Rate (%)	Cause of complication	Clinical presentation	Management
Abdominal wall vascular injury	0.5	Entry related	Intraoperative blood dropping to operation field Postoperative hemorrhage and hematoma	Coagulation Tamponade Suturing
Intestinal injury	0–0.5	Entry related (laceration) Operative (thermal)	Usually diagnosed postoperatively with peritonitis-like finding.	Most cases required conversion to laparotomy. Thermal injury: Bowel resection *Trocar injury:* Primary repair or resection related with localization, extension and bowel preparation. *Veress injury:* Can be managed expectantly
Ureteral injury	0.025–2	Electrocautery (leading cause) Other (i.e. trocar, laser, dissection, staples, suturing)	Intraoperative diagnosis is very rare. Presentation may be delayed by the several weeks especially in thermal injury. Symptoms are variable	*Intraoperative diagnosed patients:* Intraoperative laparoscopic repair, double J-shaped catheter for focal injury *Postoperative diagnosed patients:* Laparotomic end-to-end anastomosis, ureteral implantation, ureteral reconstruction or ureteroneocystostomy
Bladder injury	0.02–8.3	Entry related Thermal During dissection	Most of cases diagnosed intraoperatively. Abdominal discomfort and oliguria are major findings postoperatively	Based on localization, extension and type of injury; Conservative management Surgical repair
Major vascular injury	0.04–0.5	Entry related Energy source Operative	Bleeding from trocar or veress Observation via laparoscope Retroperitoneal hematoma	Laparotomic vessel repair without removing veress or trocar Laparoscopic repair also reported

Contd...

Contd...

Complications	Rate (%)	Cause of complication	Clinical presentation	Management
Hernia at trocar site	0.17–0.2	Entry related	Bowel obstruction findings Incarceration	Laparoscopic or laparotomic hernia repair Bowel resection in incarcerated cases
Subcutaneous emphysema	2.3	CO_2 presence in subcutaneous tissue	Subcutaneous emphysema	Resolve spontaneously
Hypercarbia	5.5	Longer operative times High end-tidal CO_2 Older patient age	Acidosis	Ventilation
Cardiac arrhythmia	27	-	Sinus tachycardia, bradycardia, ventricular, tachycardia, and asystole	Stopping gas in-flow Anticholinergic agent for bradycardia Reinsufflation after the arrhythmia settles down
Pneumothorax/ pneumomediastinum	0.2–1.9	Pneumoperitoneum Diaphragmatic defect	Respiratory related symptoms	Discharging CO_2 from peritoneal cavity Inhalation with 100% O_2 Thorax tube
Port-site metastasis	1.1–2.3	Pneumoperitoneum and CO_2 related	Postoperative port-site tumor	Resection, chemotherapy, radiotherapy

creating pneumoperitoneum. These are mostly lacerations which can be superficial or deep. Rest of the injuries are thermal in nature, due to inadvertent contact with cautery or due to manipulations of instruments during operative procedure. Most of the injuries go unrecognized intraoperatively, leading to delayed intervention which may be life-threatening. Therefore, these have been reported to be the most common cause of laparoscopy-related mortality. There is significant increase in mortality if the diagnosis is delayed by more than 72 hours.[3]

The bowel injuries can be superficial or deep. Deep injuries can lead to exposure of bowel lumen with escape of bowel contents or gas through the rent. These types of injuries can be recognized intraoperatively. Superficial burns or lacerations can go unrecognized intraoperatively. In such cases, patients present in postoperative period with nonspecific symptoms like fever, mild abdominal pain and abdominal distension, which further delays diagnosis. Late sequelae include generalized peritonitis with collection of fecal matter in peritoneal cavity leading to septic shock.

Bowel injuries can be managed either expectantly or by surgical repair depending upon the nature, size, and location of injury. Expectant management can be done in injuries by veress needle. If the injury is in small bowel, primary closure in two layers is adequate.

In cases with large bowel involvement, the treatment options include primary repair, segmental resection and repair or diversion colostomy. Resection is mandatory in thermal injuries.

URINARY TRACT INJURY

Ureteral Injury

The most common cause of iatrogenic ureteral injury is pelvic surgery. There has been increase in number of cases due to increasing number of pelvic and retroperitoneal surgeries being performed laparoscopically. Though, no identifiable predisposing risk factors can be found in majority of patients. But cases with distorted pelvic anatomy like severe endometriosis, adhesions due to previous surgeries, broad ligament, and cervical myoma can be associated with higher risk. Incidence of ureteral injury during laparoscopic hysterectomy varies from 0.2% to 6.0%.[4] Injuries to ureter can occur with electrocautery, loop suturing or during sharp dissection with electrocautery identified as the leading cause. Ureters are most commonly injured at the following three locations:
- At the level of infundibulopelvic ligaments
- Ovarian fossa
- The ureteral canal.[5]

Injuries may include transection (partial or complete), ligation with suture, avulsion, crush injury from clamp, devascularization, and fulguration with cautery. These injuries are frequently undetected, as high degree of suspicion is required for timely recognition. The methods for identifying ureteral injury are:
- Retrograde ureteral dye injection
- Intravenous indigo carmine injection
- Intraoperative ureteral catheterization[6]
- Intravenous excretory urography
- Dissection of the ureter.

Intraperitoneal leak cannot be demonstrated intraoperatively in cases with coagulated or ligated ureter. These cases can be detected by cystoscopic examination which shows lack of a ureteral jet.

Patients can present in postoperative period with malaise, fever, abdominal distension, flank pain, ileus, nausea, vomiting, and frank peritonitis. Sometimes, collection of urine can be confined in retroperitoneal space forming urinoma, which presents as flank mass with other associated features. There can be leakage of fluid from trocar insertion point, which on biochemical analysis shows high urea and creatinine levels as that in urine. There can be rise in serum markers of inflammation like increased leukocyte count and elevated CRP levels.

Diagnosis

Diagnosis should ideally be made intraoperatively, which ironically is missed in 50–70% of cases. Postoperative diagnosis can be aided by ultrasonography, which can show collection of fluid in abdomen. Cystoscopy or cystotomy with retrograde pyelogram allows identification of site of injury and also can serve as a therapeutic measure in case there is slight obstruction or minimal injury. Computed tomography with intravenous pyelogram is preferred modality in cases where retrograde pyelogram cannot be performed. Leakage of contrast can be seen around the site of injury after injection of dye, it also delineates integrity of upper tract and relevant anatomy. Intravenous urogram aids in confirming the diagnosis in cases presenting with features of obstructive uropathy resulting from ligation of ureter during suturing or by thermal injury.[7] Management of ureteric injuries depends upon type, site, and extent of injury. In cases diagnosed intraoperatively, immediate repair can be done. Stenting can be done in cases of partial obstruction and for small defects, which heal spontaneously. In cases presenting late in postoperative period, ureteral stenting may not be useful. In these cases open repair is recommended.[8] Most of the iatrogenic injuries involve distal ureter. As there is extensive damage to blood supply of ureter with distal injury, ureteroneocystostomy is required. The cases with involvement of long segment of ureter can be managed by Vesico psoas hitch. Ureteroureterostomy is done in cases with proximal and mid-ureteric injuries where the length of involved segment is small or Boari flap repair if distal end is not available for anastomosis.

Prevention

Ureteric injury can lead to catastrophic complications, hence preoperative and intraoperative measures should be taken to minimize this complication. Meticulous dissection and delineation of course of the ureter in such cases depends on sound knowledge of pelvic anatomy and surgical skills. Intravenous pyelogram can be done preoperatively to delineate the course of ureter in cases with cervical and broad ligament fibroids and cases with malignancy. Preoperative stenting can be done in cases with suspected high risk cases due to distorted anatomy. Use of electrocautery should be minimized in the vicinity of ureter; instead sutures can be used to achieve hemostasis.

Bladder Injury

The incidence of bladder injury during laparoscopic surgeries range from 0.02% to 8.3%.[8] It is one of the most common urinary tract injury during gynecologic laparoscopic surgery. Most injuries occur during hysterectomy operations. Common risk factors are:
- Endometriosis
- Previous surgery
- Overdistended bladder
- Pelvic adhesions
- An inexperienced surgeon.

Direct injury to bladder may occur during entry process, especially with suprapubic trocar insertion. Most of the injuries occur during dissection of bladder from the cervix during hysterectomy. Thermal injuries with electrocautery can occur with inadvertent contact with tissue or poor insulation of the instrument.

Diagnosis

Intraoperative diagnosis can be made by leakage of urine from site of injury, hematuria or distension of urinary bag with gas. Hence, urobag should be examined frequently in cases with high risk of bladder injury. In suspected cases, cystoscopy with instillation of methylene blue dye to observe dye leakage helps in making the diagnosis along with delineating site and extent of injury. Almost half of the cases present in postoperative period with nonspecific symptoms like abdominal distension, suprapubic pain, ileus, leakage of urine through vagina, and decreased urine output.[9]

Management

Management depends upon the site, size, and time of recognition of injury. It may be conservative or surgical via laparoscopy, laparotomy, or vaginal approach. Immediate repair can be done in injuries identified intraoperatively. In full thickness injuries, two-layered watertight closure with 3-0 absorbable sutures is recommended, with first layer involving mucosa and second layer involving muscularis and serosa burying the first layer. In partial thickness injuries, only the muscularis and serosa are taken in a single layer. Cystoscopy is done post repair to check for leakage from the site. Patient is catheterized for 10–14 days.[10]

To prevent bladder injures:
- Thorough knowledge of pelvic anatomy and strict adherence to the surgical principles are of utmost importance in minimizing the risk of injury.
- In high-risk cases, delineation of boundaries of bladder before dissection by distending bladder with saline or saline containing methylene blue dye.
- Dissection of bladder adequately from vagina to minimize chances of injury during vaginal cuff closure
- Avoid suprapubic insertion of veress needle and placement of lateral ports under direct visualization[11] and strict adherence to electrosurgical principles to avoid thermal injury.

ABDOMINAL WALL VASCULAR INJURY

Abdominal wall has rich vascular supply, which is susceptible to injury during laparoscopic surgeries. These mostly occur during lateral port placement. It may involve both superficial and deep epigastric vessels and less commonly muscular vessels. The incidence of abdominal wall bleeding is 0.3–0.5%.[12] These can be recognized intraoperatively by dripping of blood in to operative field. Patients may also present in postoperative period with hematoma, extensive bruising over the skin, abscess formation due to infection of the hematoma, and life-threatening hemorrhage requiring blood transfusion and surgery for hemostasis.

Management: If diagnosed intraoperatively, coagulation of site of bleeding should be done. The site should be re-evaluated for hemostasis after decompressing pneumoperioneum.[13] Temponade and suturing either by *laparoscopy* or after enlarging the incision of trocar entry may be required in cases if bleeding is not controlled by coagulation.

Prevention: Placement of lateral ports lateral to rectus muscle sheath and under direct visualization by transillumination of the anterior abdominal wall may help in avoiding these types of injuries. All port sites should be inspected for any evidence of bleeding before withdrawing the laparoscope.

HERNIA AT THE SITE OF THE ABDOMINAL WALL TROCAR

Trocar site hernia is a preventable complication associated with laparoscopic surgeries, with incidence ranging from 0.17% to 0.2%.[14] Many factors have been evaluated for their association with development of hernia. >10 mm trocar entry points, incomplete or nonclosure of fascial defect have been found to be associated with development of hernia.

It may be early or delayed onset. Early onset hernia may contain loops of intestines, omentum and present with abdominal pain, distension and other features of obstruction in early postoperative period. Delayed onset hernia usually present with asymptomatic swelling at the site of trocar insertion and hernial sac is usually peritoneum.

Although repairing the hernia is enough in most of these cases, in patients with incarceration, intestinal resection may be required.

Hernias are repaired laparotomically or less commonly, laparoscopically. Trocar sites >10 mm should be sutured for prevention. To minimize the risk of herniation, secondary trocars should be removed under supervision before the primary one, valves should be kept closed to prevent a sucking effect, and 5 mm trocars should be preferred.

MAJOR VASCULAR INJURY

Retroperitoneal major vascular injuries are complications associated with high mortality and may be caused during insertion of Veress needle or trocar and by energy source. The incidence is estimated to range from 0.04% to 0.5%.[15] Most injuries were entry related and independent of the complexity of the surgery. In this situation, either the aorta, vena cava, or, more commonly, the common iliac vessel has been traumatized.

Bleeding from the Veress and trocars at the entry site may be an alert. Also intra-abdominal or retroperitoneal visualization (generally as a hematoma) with a laparoscope is possible. Therefore, visualization of the peritoneal cavity immediately after entry prevents any delay in diagnosis. Shock may develop directly due to abundant blood loss. Patients with anatomic detorsions and retroperitoneal manipulations are more prone to energy source injuries. Major vascular injuries may rarely remain unrecognized intraoperatively. The removal of the Veress needle or trocars in case of a vascular injury may result in abundant bleeding and the inability to locate the site of bleeding because of a retroperitoneal hematoma. Through a midline incision, access to the bleeding site should be achieved before these instruments are removed, and injury should be repaired.

PNEUMOPERITONEUM RELATED COMPLICATIONS

- Hypercarbia and therefore acidosis develop due to absorption of CO_2 in prolonged operations.
- Erroneous insertion of Veress needle into preperitoneal space during creation of pneumoperitoneum may result in subcutaneous emphysema, pneumomediastinum, and pneumothorax. It may also result from leakage of gas around cannula. Prolonged duration of surgery, higher maximum measured end-tidal CO_2, multiple surgical ports, and advanced age increase the risk.

  Subcutaneous emphysema may be localized or may extend to extremities, the neck, the mediastinum, and even the pericardium, which may result in cardiovascular collapse.

  To avoid these complications, proper preoperative assessment of the patient should be done. In obese patients, needle or trocar entry can be attempted at 90° angle, taking due care to avoid other major injuries like retroperitoneal vascular injuries. Alternatively, open-entry has been advocated to prevent preperitoneal emphysema without increasing other complications.[16]
- Intraoperative diaphragmatic injury or presence of congenital diaphragmatic hernia may result in migration of CO_2 into the mediastinum resulting in pneumothorax, pneumomediastinum or pneumopericardium. Management options include watchful observation after deflation of pneumoperitoneum with or without O_2 supplementation, simple aspiration or thorax tube drainage.
- Carbon dioxide is absorbed more rapidly than air, therefore chances of intra-abdominal air persistence are less as compared to laparotomy patients, and even less in obese than in lean patients. Generally, it does not persist after the 7th day.[17]

GAS EMBOLISM

Gas embolism is a rare but life-threatening complication, resulting from introduction of CO_2 into major vessel through the veress needle. It causes reduction in blood flow to the lungs resulting in fall in end-tidal carbon dioxide concentration (earliest sign). Blood spurting from the Veress needle is an alarming sign. Other features include increase in jugular venous pressure, cyanosis due to decreased perfusion, and sudden circulatory collapse necessitating cardiopulmonary resuscitation. Transesophageal echography has been found to be most sensitive for diagnosis.

Preventive measures include assessment of correct placement of veress needle by measures such as aspiration with a syringe prior to creating pneumoperitoneum and entry into abdomen at correct angle. The air in the insufflation tube should be flushed out to prevent room-air embolism, which is even more dangerous owing to lesser solubility than CO_2.[17]

The veress needle is kept in place and the patient is made to lie on left side in steep Trendelenburg position. Aggressive supportive measures like 100% O_2 administration and volume expansion are taken for resuscitation with continuous vital monitoring.

POSTOPERATIVE SHOULDER PAIN

Shoulder pain results from irritation of diaphragm by fluid or retained gas and is mediated through phrenic nerve. Trendelenburg position resulting in stretching of falciform ligament can also add to it. Complete removal of intraperitoneal gases at the end of surgery prevents this complication.

VULVAR EDEMA

Vulvar edema is thought to result from leakage of adhesion solution barrier used during surgery. The leakage can occur either through a patent canal of Nuck, or development of a fistulous tract at lower trocar puncture wound, which dissects downward through subcutaneous tissues by gravity.[18]

COMPLICATIONS RELATED TO ANESTHESIA AND PATIENT POSITION

Nerve Injury

Nerve injuries usually occur due to incorrect positioning resulting in compression or overstretching of nerve plexus. These are usually transient in nature and recovery is usually spontaneous over a period of time. Brachial plexus, common peroneal nerve, and the saphenous nerve are the most commonly involved ones.

Cardiac Arrhythmia

Various types of cardiac arrhythmias medications including bradycardia, sinus tachycardia, and ventricular tachycardia related to administration of anesthetic medications have also been reported in laparoscopy.

OTHER COMPLICATIONS

Venous Thrombosis

Venous thrombosis may occur in postoperative period. The risk factors include prolonged duration of surgery, associated predisposing conditions like advanced age, hypertension, and diabetes mellitus. The restricting effect of raised intraperitoneal pressure resulting in venous stasis may also lead to thrombosis.

Port-site Metastasis

The incidence of port-site metastases in patients with gynecological malignancies has been reported as 1.1–2.3%,[19] which is similar to the rate of wound metastasis seen in open surgeries.

Risk factors proposed for port-site metastasis are:
1. Advanced and metabolically aggressive tumor.
2. Carbon dioxide has been found to be associated with significantly increased tumor growth as compared with other insufflating agents.
3. Gasless laparoscopy reduces the risk as compared to pneumoperitoneum.
4. High efflux of gas from the abdominal cavity through the space around the trocars.

Recurrence of ovarian or primary peritoneal malignancies with ascites is associated with highest risk.

Port site lavage with cytotoxic agents like taurolidine, 5-fluorouracil, doxorubicin, *povidone*-iodine solution, and methotrexate have been suggested as a preventive measure.[19]

SUMMARY

Laparoscopic surgeries are preferred over open surgeries nowadays because of shorter postoperative hospital stay, reduced time to recovery and esthetic benefits. Laparoscopic surgeries differ from open surgeries in lack of tactile sensation of tissues and can be associated with a variety of complications like ureteral, bladder, bowel or vascular injuries. Most of these complications occur at the time of introduction of trocar into the abdominal cavity. Hence, surgeon should be aware of risk factors associated with an individual case. Another potential source of injury can be thermal injury with the use of cautery. Judicious and meticulous use of cautery with knowledge of basic thermodynamic principles can reduce such complications. Intraoperative recognition and prompt management can reduce postoperative morbidity.

CONCLUSION

Laparoscopic surgeries require experience to provide best possible outcome to the patient. It has been found that rate of complications plateau after a certain learning curve. Surgeon should be well aware of the anatomy and the challenges an individual case can present with. Prompt diagnosis and management of complications are main requisites to improve outcome.

REFERENCES

1. Magrina JF. Complications of laparoscopic surgery. Clin Obstet Gynecol. 2002;45(2):469-80.
2. Jansen FW, Kapiteyn K, Trimbos-Kemper T, et al. Complications of laparoscopy: A prospective multicenter observational study. Br J Obstet Gynaecol. 1997;104(5):595-600.
3. Reich H, McGlynn F, Budin R. Laparoscopic repair of full-thickness bowel injury. J Laparoendosc Surg. 1991;1(2):119-22.
4. Donnez O, Jadoul P, Squifflet J, et al. A series of 3190 laparoscopic hysterectomies for benign disease from 1990 to 2006: evaluation of complications compared with vaginal and abdominal procedures. BJOG. 2009;116(4):492-500.
5. Karaman Y, Bingol B, Günenç Z. Prevention of complications in laparoscopic hysterectomy: experience with 1120 cases performed by a single surgeon. J Minim Invasive Gynecol. 2007;14(1):78-84.
6. Tanaka Y, Asada H, Kuji N, et al. Ureteral catheter placement for prevention of ureteral injury during laparoscopic hysterectomy. J Obstet Gynaecol Res. 2008;34(1):67-72.
7. Ostrzenski A, Radolinski B, Ostrzenska KM. A review of laparoscopic ureteral injury in pelvic surgery. Obstet Gynecol Surv. 2003;58(12):794-9.
8. Hasson HM, Parker WH. Prevention and management of urinary tract injury in laparoscopic surgery. J Am Assoc Gynecol Laparosc. 1998;5(2):99-114.

9. Chan JK, Morrow J, Manetta A. Prevention of ureteral injuries in gynecologic surgery. Am J Obstet Gynecol. 2003;188(5):1273-7.
10. Oh BR, Kwon DD, Park KS, et al. Late presentation of ureteral injury after laparoscopic surgery. Obstet Gynecol. 2000;95(3):337-9.
11. Pillet MCL, Leonard F, Chopin N. Incidence and risk factors of bladder injuries during laparoscopic hysterectomy indicated for benign uterine pathologies: a 14.5 years experience in a continuous series of 1501 procedures. Hum Reprod. 2009;24(4):842-9.
12. Nezhat C, Childers J, Nezhat F, et al. Major retroperitoneal vascular injury during laparoscopic surgery. Hum Reprod. 1997;12(3):480-3.
13. Munro MG. Laparoscopic access: complications, technologies, and techniques. Curr Opin Obstet Gynecol. 2002;14(4):365-74.
14. Vilos GA, Ternamian A, Dempster J, et al; Clinical Practice Gynaecology Committee. Laparoscopic entry: a review of techniques, technologies, and complications. J Obstet Gynaecol Can. 2007;29(5):433-447.
15. Leron E, Piura B, Ohana E, et al. Delayed recognition of major vascular injury during laparoscopy. Eur J Obstet Gynecol Reprod Biol. 1998;79(1):91-3.
16. Murdock CM, Wolff AJ, Van Geem T. Risk factors for hypercarbia, subcutaneous emphysema, pneumothorax, and pneumomediastinum during laparoscopy. Obstet Gynecol. 2000;95(5):704-9.
17. Kalhan SB, Reaney JA, Collins RL. Pneumomediastinum and subcutaneous emphysema during laparoscopy. Cleve Clin J Med. 1990;57(7):639-42.
18. Pados G, Vavilis D, Pantazis K, et al. Unilateral vulvar edema after operative laparoscopy: a case report and literature review. Fertil Steril. 2005;83(2):471-3.
19. Nagarsheth NP, Rahaman J, Cohen CJ, et al. The incidence of port-site metastases in gynecologic cancers. JSLS. 2004;8(2):133-9.

Gynecological Oncology Emergencies

Ipsita Batra

INTRODUCTION

An oncologic emergency in a cancer patient is a potentially acute life-threatening condition that has developed as a result of malignant disease or its treatment. These may arise from direct local effects of their tumors, metastasis on involved tissues or paraneoplastic syndromes.[1,2]

With advances in cancer treatment, survival has increased and hence, it is crucial to manage the complications correctly. As cancer patients are often admitted through emergency with advanced disease and the frequency of visits increase near end of life, these patients need special attention.

A gynecologic cancer patient may present with emergencies which can be categorized broadly into medical, surgical, and psychiatric.

SURGICAL EMERGENCIES

For appropriate treatment, it is important to understand the underlying cause. Patient's performance status, severity of emergency, cancer stage and prognosis, and patient's wishes are important for decision regarding invasive treatment. Frequently used scores to determine performance status include Eastern Cooperative Oncology Group (ECOG) Score and World Health Organization Performance Status.[3]

Obstruction of Gastrointestinal Tract

Prevalence in ovarian cancer patients was found to be 5.5–42% in various studies.[4]

Causes

Causes of bowel obstruction in gynecological cancer patients can be divided into benign and malignant as shown in **Table 1**.

Carcinoma ovary and its associated postoperative adhesions and ileus are the most common causes. Carcinoma cervix can present with radiation enteritis-induced bowel obstruction.[5]

Chapter 22: Gynecological Oncology Emergencies

TABLE 1: Causes of bowel obstruction in gynecological cancer patients.

Benign	Malignant
Postoperative adhesions	Intraluminal tumor presence or invasion
Postradiation strictures or radiation enteritis	External compression by tumor mass
Strangulation or hernia	
Ileus	
Pseudo-obstruction (Ogilvie's syndrome)	
Volvulus	
Diverticulitis	
Intussusception	

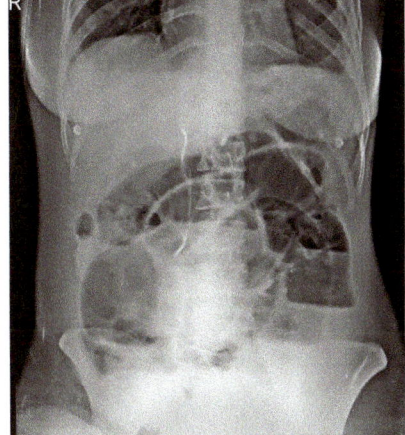

Fig. 1: X-ray abdomen showing bowel obstruction.

Postoperatively, occurrence of obstruction symptoms tends to be shorter for malignant causes (<3 months) and longer (around 5 years) for benign causes.

Presence of intestinal obstruction may be a sign of deteriorating health and failure of treatment.

Symptoms

Nausea, vomiting, abdominal pain, intolerance to food, constipation/obstipation or rarely loose stools.

Recurrent obstruction: Patients may present with recurrent intermittent obstruction typically due to adhesions.

Signs

Abdominal distention, high pitched bowel sounds, ascites, and abdominal tenderness may be present.

Hypovolemia, leukocytosis, anemia, and metabolic abnormalities are seen in laboratory findings.

Plain abdominal radiography and abdominopelvic computed tomography (CT) are the main imaging modalities helpful in diagnosis **(Fig. 1)**.

At times, a preoperative colonoscopy may be helpful in diagnosing primary colon cancer.

Treatment

Conservative
- Nil per oral
- Fluid and electrolyte correction
- Total parenteral nutrition/feeding tube postobstruction
- Nasogastric tube decompression
- Broad spectrum antibiotics
- Antiemetics (ondansetron, haloperidol, and octreotide).

Conservative management helps to gain time to identify origin and staging of disease.

Minimally invasive diagnostic modalities may be used.

Patients presenting with peritonitis, pneumoperitoneum, or signs of bowel ischemia should undergo urgent surgical exploration. The remainder can be managed nonoperatively for 48–72 hours.

Surgical management: Surgeries include laparotomy for adhesiolysis, bypass, bowel

Section 4: Emergencies in Gynecological Surgeries

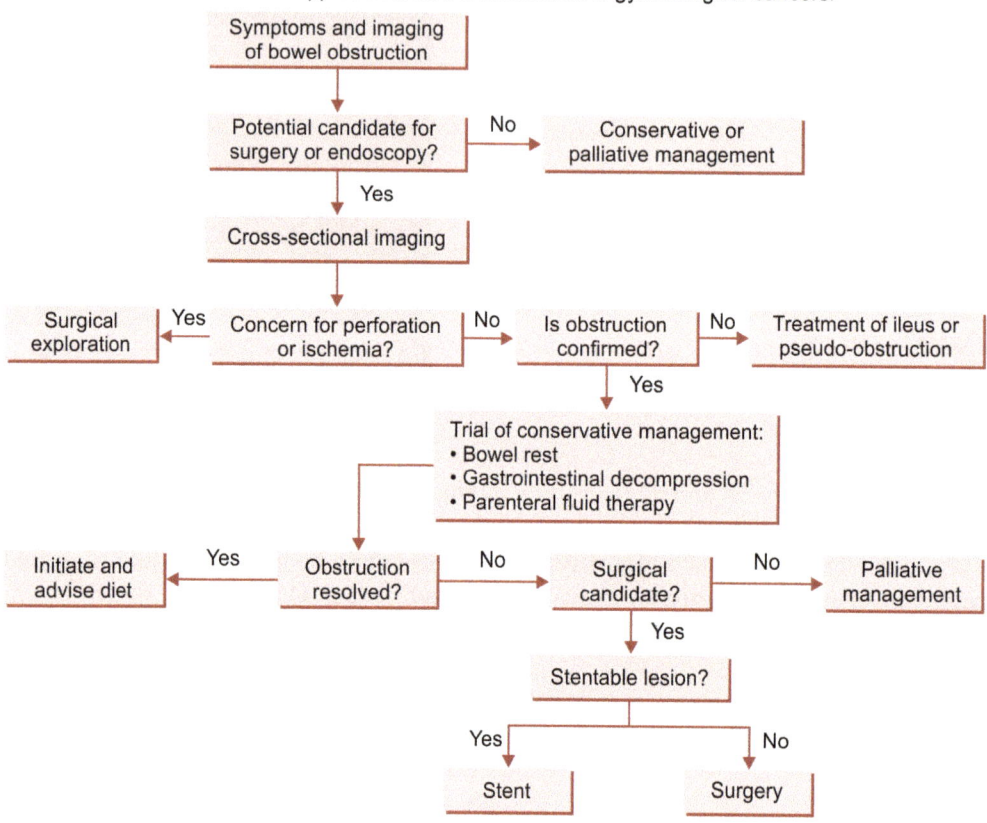

Flowchart 1: Approach to bowel obstruction in gynecological cancers.

resection, ileostomy or ileocolostomy and endoscopic detorsion, stent placement, decompression or ablation.

Complete surgical resection is desirable if the tumor can be resected with negative margins.

In ovarian cancer, initial cytoreductive surgery has shown a survival benefit when combined with chemotherapy.[6]

Radiation enteritis is amiable to surgery.[7]

Certain factors have been associated with poor surgical outcomes in various studies of cancer patients with bowel obstruction:
- Imaging evidence of residual primary or recurrent tumor
- Imaging evidence of peritoneal disease (carcinomatosis)
- Imaging evidence of multiple sites
- Patients with ascites
- Hypoalbuminemia (<3.5 g/dL)
- Old age (≥65 years old)
- Poor performance status.

Nomograms based upon some of these factors have been developed to predict 30-day mortality and select which patients may benefit from surgery. **Flowchart 1** can help to guide the plan of management.

Obstructive Uropathy

Causes
- Extramural compression
- Direct ureter invasion

- Fibrosis or pelvic inflammatory disease (PID) after surgery
- Catheter-induced edema
- Strictures after radiation therapy.

Stage III carcinoma cervix extends to the pelvic sidewall and/or involves the lower third of vagina causing hydronephrosis or a nonfunctioning kidney.

Symptoms

- Urinary retention
- Lumbar or back pain
- Hematuria, pyuria
- Chills/fever.

Signs

- Proteinuria, elevated blood urea nitrogen, raised creatinine, increased serum phosphorous, and serum potassium.
- Final pathogenesis includes hydronephrotic atrophy and renal insufficiency leading to renal failure.

Investigations

Ultrasonography (USG) of urinary tract, excretory urogram, radioisotope renogram, and CT of abdomen are helpful.

Treatment

Any urinary obstruction should be corrected before cancer treatment.

Immediate release of obstruction is essential. It is very important to decide about conservative or aggressive therapy.

Obstruction can be relieved by ureteral stenting.

Percutaneous nephrostomy (PCN) is a simple and cost effective procedure with minimal morbidity, used to relieve bilateral obstruction. The decision to do PCN should be individualized based on performance status.[8]

Hemorrhage

Causes

- Endometrial cancer, cervical cancer, vulval cancer, and gestational trophoblastic neoplasia may present with vaginal bleeding.
- Hemorrhage can also be a postsurgical acute complication requiring relaparotomy and further management.
- Radiation enteritis can lead to gastrointestinal bleeding.

Initial Management

Immediate resuscitation with intravenous (IV) fluids and blood products replacement.

Next step includes identifying the cause by careful history and examination.

History of intermenstrual and postcoital bleed may suggest Ca cervix. Per speculum and vaginal examination will help identify the cause. Pregnancy test should be considered in history suggestive of gestational trophoblastic neoplasia. Biopsy should be taken for confirmation of diagnosis.[9]

Definitive Management

Vaginal bleeding:
- *Minimal bleeding:* Evacuate clots and apply Monsel's solution
- *Moderate bleeding:* Vaginal tamponade
- *Profuse bleeding with failed conservative therapy:* Embolization or ligation of uterine or internal iliac arteries. High dose radiation therapy may be attempted in carcinoma vulva cases.

Gastrointestinal (GI) bleeding requires urgent endoscopy.

TABLE 2: Surgical emergencies with its associated cancer.

Surgical emergency	Causes
Bowel obstruction	• Carcinoma ovary tumor spread • Postoperative adhesions • Radiation enteritis
Obstructive uropathy	Locally advanced cancer cervix
GI fistulas/GI injury	• Cytoreductive surgery for ovarian cancer • Radiation enteritis
Urinary fistulas/Ureteral injury	• Radical hysterectomy for cancer cervix • Radiation therapy in cervical and vulval cancers
Operative hemorrhage	Intra- or postoperative
Vaginal bleeding	• Carcinoma cervix • Carcinoma vulva • Gestational trophoblastic neoplasia
GI bleeding	• Radiation enteritis • Ovarian metastasis
Vaginal cuff dehiscence	• Postradical hysterectomy for cancer cervix • Postcytoreductive surgery for ovarian cancer
Abdominal wall dehiscence	Postexploratory laparotomy for carcinoma ovary

Perforation and Fistulas

Causes

- Surgical injury
- Radiation enteritis.

Ureteral injury can occur during radical hysterectomy. Prophylactic stenting should be considered during preoperative planning. Stenting is useful as a secondary prevention measure.

Radiation enteritis can also lead to intestinal perforation or fistula formation.

Management

It can be conservative or surgical, depending on performance status.

Wound Dehiscence

- Healing of tissues is compromised in cancer patients. It usually presents within 5–7 days postoperatively.
- Evisceration or vaginal cuff dehiscence can be an emergent postoperative condition after surgery for gynecologic carcinomas.
- Abdominal laparotomy wound dehiscence can also be encountered. Laparoscopy and robotic surgery can avoid this complication.
- Radical vulvectomy for carcinoma vulva is associated with high chances of wound dehiscence. Prevention strategies include meticulous dry dressing.[10]

Surgical emergencies with its associated cancer have been summarized in **Table 2**.

MEDICAL EMERGENCIES

Infections and Febrile Neutropenia

- Oncology patients are more prone for opportunistic infections due to disruption of anatomy, poor blood supply, and radiations.
- Certain infections like necrotizing fasciitis and septicemia can present as emergencies.

Wound cellulitis and wound hematoma are common at vaginal vault site.
- Febrile neutropenia is defined when absolute neutrophil count is less than 0.5×10^9/L, with an accompanying fever. Fever is termed as an axillary or oral temperature more than 38.5° on one occasion or 38° on two occasions 12 hours apart.[11]
- Management includes blood counts with cultures, and proper antibiotic coverage.[11]

Deep Vein Thrombosis and Thromboembolism

Deep vein thrombosis (DVT) and thromboembolism are important preventable causes of morbidity and mortality in oncology patients. Various risk assessment scoring systems like Khorana Score and Padua Score are being used nowadays for selecting patients who require pharmacological therapy for prevention of DVT.[12]

Risk Factors

- Age
- Cancer-induced acquired coagulopathy
- Venous stasis due to pelvic mass
- Postoperative immobility
- Infection.

For hospitalized medical patients and in perioperative period, pharmacological thromboprophylaxis is recommended. LMWX is the preferred drug of choice.

Investigations

- Venous Doppler for DVT confirmation.
- CT angiogram of chest or VQ scan for confirmation of pulmonary embolism.

Treatment

Anticoagulant therapy is warranted in cancer patients with new or recurrent venous thromboembolism (VTE). Low molecular weight heparin therapy is recommended for 3–6 months.[13]

For patients at risk for bleeding, mechanical measures like inferior vena cava filters are recommended.[14]

Metabolic Abnormalities and Tumor Lysis Syndrome

- Hypercalcemia may be seen with ovarian cancer. Causes of hypercalcemia include direct lysis of bone by metastasis or ectopic parathormone production. Treatment involves intravenous fluids, alkalinization of urine, and bisphosphonate therapy in patients with adequate renal function.[15]
- Hyponatremia and syndrome of inappropriate antidiuretic hormone (ADH) secretion may be seen in cancer patients.
- Tumor lysis syndrome (TLS) is caused by massive tumor cell lysis and the release of large amounts of potassium, phosphate, and uric acid into the systemic circulation. It finally results in acute kidney injury with oliguria or anuria. It is most frequently seen in highly aggressive lymphomas and acute leukemias following chemotherapy, although it may also occur in other tumor types with a high proliferative rate, large tumor burden, or high sensitivity to cytotoxic therapy. For all patients with high risk, adequate hydration therapy and hypouricemic agents are recommended.[16]
- Acute kidney injury may need urgent dialysis.

■ PSYCHIATRIC EMERGENCIES

Cancer patients can present with acute psychiatric emergencies also. Being diagnosed with cancer along with the debilitating course of chemotherapy, radiotherapy, and prolonged stays in hospital can act as acute psychological stressors. Major depression with feelings of despair can lead to suicidal tendencies.

It is important as a clinician to identify these psychiatric illnesses and approach the patient with a multidisciplinary team for a holistic healing process.[17]

SUMMARY

- Gynecological oncology patients often have surgical and medical emergencies which may be life-threatening if they are not managed appropriately.
- Surgical emergencies include bowel obstruction, obstructive uropathy, hemorrhage, perforation and fistulas, and wound dehiscence. Medical emergencies include infections and febrile neutropenia, deep vein thrombosis and thromboembolism, metabolic abnormalities and tumor lysis syndrome and psychiatric emergencies among others.
- Each one is approached differently and if managed appropriately can be dealt with to improve the survival and/or the quality of life of the patient.

CONCLUSION

It is important to recognize emergent situations associated with gynecological cancers, early and accurately, so that correct investigations and treatment can be instituted to prevent morbidity and mortality. A clinician should also be adept at providing counseling, emotional support, and end of life care while maintaining the dignity of the patient.

REFERENCES

1. Bosscher MRF, van Leeuwen BL, Hoekstra HJ. Current management of surgical oncologic emergencies. PLoS One. 2015;10(5):e0124641.
2. Bosscher MR, Bastiaannet E, van Leeuwen BL, et al. Factors associated with short-term mortality after surgical oncologic emergencies. Ann Surg Oncol. 2015;23(6):1803-14.
3. Young J, Badgery-Parker T, Dobbins T, et al. Comparison of ECOG/WHO Performance Status and ASA Score as a Measure of Functional Status. J Pain Symptom Manage. 2015;49(2):258-64.
4. Ripamonti C, Mercadante S. Pathophysiology and management of malignant bowel obstruction. In: Doyle D, Hanks G, Cherny NI, Calman K (Eds). Oxford Textbook of Palliative Medicine, 3rd edition. New York: New York Oxford University Press; 2004. pp. 496-507.
5. Prost À la Denise J, Douard R, Malamut G, et al. Small bowel obstruction in patients with a prior history of cancer: predictive findings of malignant origins. World J Surg. 2013;38(2):363-9.
6. Ripamonti C, Easson A, Gerdes H. Management of malignant bowel obstruction. Eur J Cancer. 2008;44(8):1105-15.
7. Sher ME, Bauer J. Radiation-induced enteropathy. Am J Gastroenterol. 1990;85(2):121-8.
8. Carter J, Ramirez C, Waugh R, et al. Percutaneous urinary diversion in gynecologic oncology. Gynecol Oncol. 1991;40(3):248-52.
9. Munro M; Southern California Permanente Medical Group's Abnormal Uterine Bleeding Working Group. Investigation of women with postmenopausal uterine bleeding: clinical practice recommendations. Perm J. 2014;18(1):55-70.
10. Baggish MS, Lee WK. Abdominal wound disruption. Obstet Gynecol. 1975;46(5):530-4.
11. Richardson S, Pallot D, Hughes T, et al. Improving management of neutropenic sepsis in the emergency department. Br J Haematol. 2009;144(4):617-8.
12. Łukaszuk R, Dolna-Michno J, Plens K, et al. The comparison between Caprini and Padua VTE risk assessment models for hospitalised cancer patients undergoing chemotherapy at the tertiary oncology department in Poland: is pharmacological thromboprophylaxis overused? Contemp Oncol (Pozn). 2018;22(1):31-6.

13. Lee AY. Management of thrombosis in cancer: primary prevention and secondary prophylaxis. Br J Haematol. 2005;128(3):291-302.
14. Lyman G, Khorana A, Kuderer N, et al; American Society of Clinical Oncology Clinical Practice. Venous Thromboembolism Prophylaxis and Treatment in Patients With Cancer: American Society of Clinical Oncology Clinical Practice Guideline Update. J Clin Oncol. 2013;31(17):2189-204.
15. Stewart A. Hypercalcemia associated with cancer. N Engl J Med. 2005;352(4):373-9.
16. Cairo M, Coiffier B, Reiter A, et al; TLS Expert Panel. Recommendations for the evaluation of risk and prophylaxis of tumour lysis syndrome (TLS) in adults and children with malignant diseases: an expert TLS panel consensus. Br J Haematol. 2010;149(4):578-86.
17. Hodgkinson K, Butow P, Fuchs A, et al. Long-term survival from gynecologic cancer: psychosocial outcomes, supportive care needs and positive outcomes. 2007;104(2):381-9.

CHAPTER 23

Imaging in Gynecological Emergencies

Aradhana Kalra Dawar, Jahnavi Esanakula

INTRODUCTION

Acute pelvic pain, vaginal bleeding, vomiting, syncope, fever, and acute abdominal pain are some of the symptoms with which a patient can present to emergency owing to a gynecological cause. There may be an antecedent history of recent contact, trauma or surgery. Also, it is mandatory to know the date of last menstrual period and ascertain if there is any period of amenorrhea. Proper clinical history and examination are of utmost importance for diagnosis. Laboratory investigations and sonography adds to the diagnosis.

These gynecological emergencies include several diseases that result from adnexal and uterine disorders. *Adnexal disorders* may be classified into mainly three categories:
- Infection/pelvic inflammatory disease (PID), such as tubo-ovarian abscesses, pelvic peritonitis, and hydrosalpinx/pyosalpinx
- Hemorrhage from ruptured hemorrhagic ovarian cysts and ectopic pregnancies
- Tumors causing adnexal torsion and rupture of ovarian tumors.

Unusual adnexal torsion causing massive ovarian edema, isolated fallopian tube torsion, and paraovarian cyst torsion, has also been described.

Uterine disorders in gynecological emergencies may be classified into two categories:
1. Acute fibroid complications, including red degeneration of a uterine leiomyoma, torsion of subserosal myomas, and torsion of the uterus
2. Causes of acute uterine bleeding, including retained products of conception and uterine arteriovenous malformations.

Diagnosing gynecological emergencies may sometimes be challenging because of an overlap of symptoms with nongynecological conditions. Ultrasonography especially transvaginal sonography is the imaging modality of choice; however, when a definitive diagnosis cannot be established, computed tomography (CT) and/or magnetic resonance (MR) imaging may narrow the differential diagnosis. MR has high sensitivity and specificity and is well suited for pregnant patients due to no radiation exposure. But due to its high cost, increased time for examination and less availability it is utilized only when other modalities cannot yield a proper diagnosis.

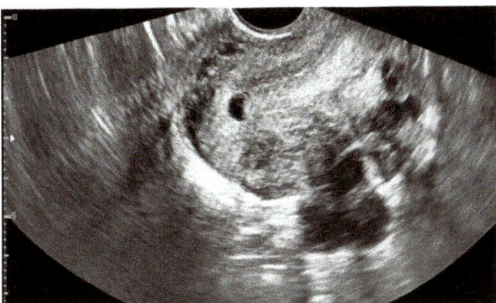

Fig. 1: Left tubo-ovarian mass in a patient presenting with infertility with fluid in the endometrial cavity.

IMAGING MODALITIES IN VARIOUS ACUTE EMERGENCIES

Pelvic Inflammatory Disease

Acute pelvic pain is one of the most common presentations of this acute PID. Patient may present with an acute emergency. Affected age group is usually 18–44 years (sexually active population). Patient may present with pain abdomen, fever, and vomiting. Disseminated peritonitis can be complicated by inflammation and obstruction of the bowel, ureteric obstruction, and perihepatitis (Fitz-Hugh-Curtis syndrome).

- Ultrasound may be normal initially. There may be hydrosalpinx with fluid in the endometrial cavity.
- Sonographic features diagnostic for hydrosalpinx include a tubular cystic mass separate from the ovary, with: "beads on a string" or "cogwheel" appearance (small round nodules less than 3 mm in size that represent endosalpingeal folds when viewed in cross section) **(Figs. 1 and 2)**.
- In advanced conditions, ultrasound may show thick endometrium with or without fluid in endometrial cavity, ovarian enlargement, and/or uterine enlargement with indistinct contours and free intraperitoneal fluid.[1] Ultrasound may diagnose tubo-ovarian abscesses and pyosalpinx.
- These tubo-ovarian abscesses appear as thick-walled, cystic areas containing septae and/or fluid-debris levels.
- On CT scan, tubo-ovarian abscess appears as complex fluid collections, with thickened, irregular wall which is contrast enhanced band like infiltrates.
- CT involvement is usually bilateral except in cases of postsurgical abscess or direct extension of infection from adjacent organ like appendix. Abscess has also been seen after an intrauterine insemination (IUI) or after puncturing an endometrioma after ovum pick up in in vitro fertilization (IVF).

Torsion

Adnexal torsion is the rotation of adnexal structures like ovary or fallopian tube on the vascular pedicle. Benign ovarian tumors like dermoid or mature cystic teratoma are often complicated by torsion. Rarely, it may occur in structurally normal ovaries too. Torsion of endometriotic cysts is uncommon due to associated adhesions. Ultrasound with Doppler is the first-line imaging modality.

- Sonographic features include enlarged ovary, whirlpool sign of twisted vascular

Section 4: Emergencies in Gynecological Surgeries

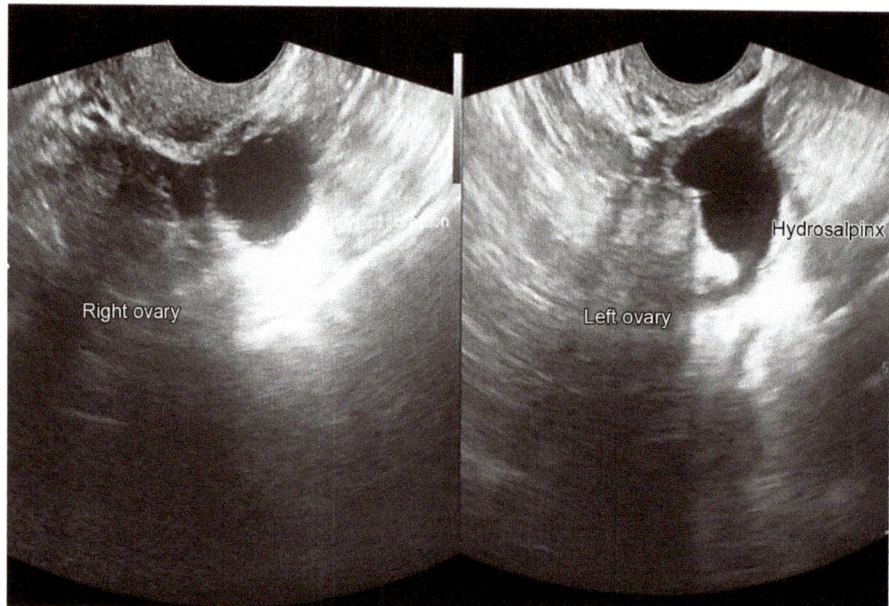

Fig. 2: Bilateral hydrosalpinx in a patient presenting with infertility.

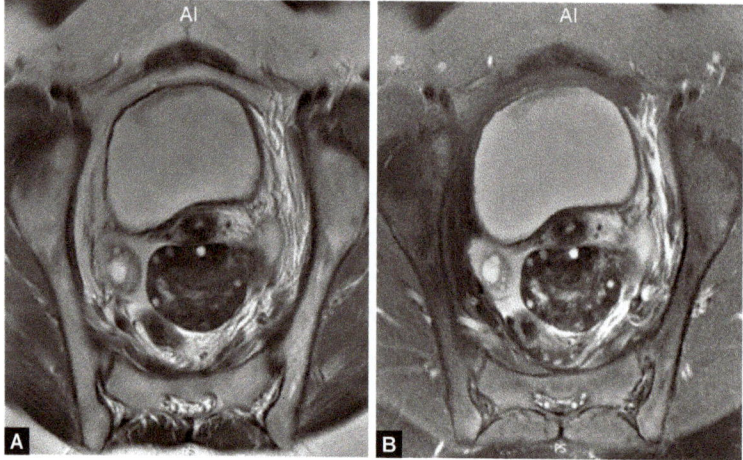

Figs. 3A and B: Axial T2W MRI and Axial T2-fat saturated images showing left ovarian torsion hemorrhagic ovary with peripherally displaced follicles. This is a surgically proven case. Patient presented to the ER with acute pain abdomen. Laparoscopy revealed ovarian torsion.
Courtesy: Mahajan Imaging and Diagnostic Center, Delhi.

pedicle, occlusion of venous and lymph drainage, and usually free pelvic fluid.
- Multiple cortical follicles with enlarged ovary are infrequent but specific sign of ovarian torsion[2] **(Figs. 3A and B)**.
- Ipsilateral uterine deviation may be observed due to shortened adnexal ligament.
- As ovaries have double vascularization (ovarian artery from aorta and ovarian

branch of uterine artery), complete absence of Doppler signal is not mandatory.
- However, absence of arterial flow or elevated RI, with absent venous flow and enlargement of ovaries is highly indicative of ovarian torsion.
- Cross-sectional examination shows smooth walls and wall thickening of the cystic lesion, thickened fallopian tube, ascites, and deviation of uterus to affected side. Thickened tube can be identified by sagittal MR.

Ovarian Hyperstimulation Syndrome

Ovarian hyperstimulation syndrome is a complication of ovarian stimulation, an iatrogenic disorder with increasing incidence which follows the increasing number of IVF procedures. Ultrasonography shows both ovaries enlarged with multiple cysts of different sizes. Presence of ascites and pleural effusion and/or pericardial effusion can be noticed **(Fig. 4)**.

Hemorrhage

Ectopic Pregnancy

Ectopic pregnancy is implantation of embryo outside endometrial cavity. Fallopian tube is the most common site of ectopic pregnancy followed by ovary (3%), cervix, scar of previous cesarean section, and broad ligament or abdominal cavity (<1%).

Risk factors include:
- Previous ectopic pregnancy
- Pelvic inflammatory disease
- Previous tubal surgery
- Ruptured appendix/appendicitis
- Artificial reproductive techniques
- IUCD in situ.

USG findings:
- The presence of a gestational sac in adnexa with or without fetal pole and cardiac activity is a specific but less sensitive sign of ectopic gestation present in 10–17%.[3]
- Adnexal rings (fluid sac with thick echogenic ring with yolk sac/fetal pole)

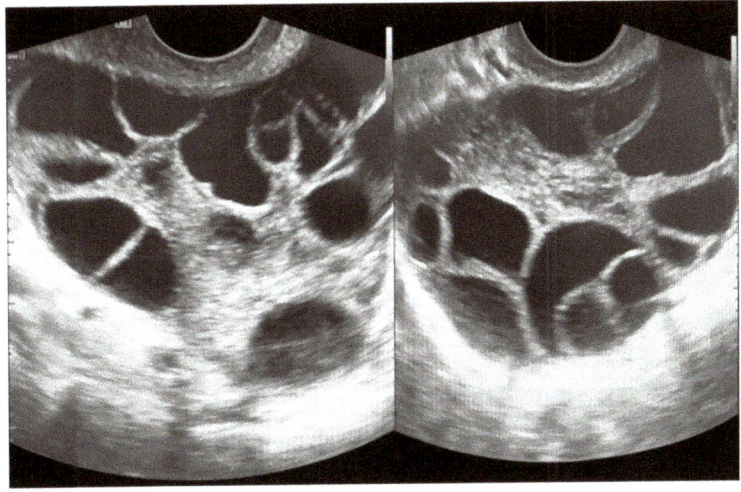

Fig. 4: Ultrasound picture of ovarian hyperstimulation showing enlarged ovaries with multiple follicles of varying sizes.

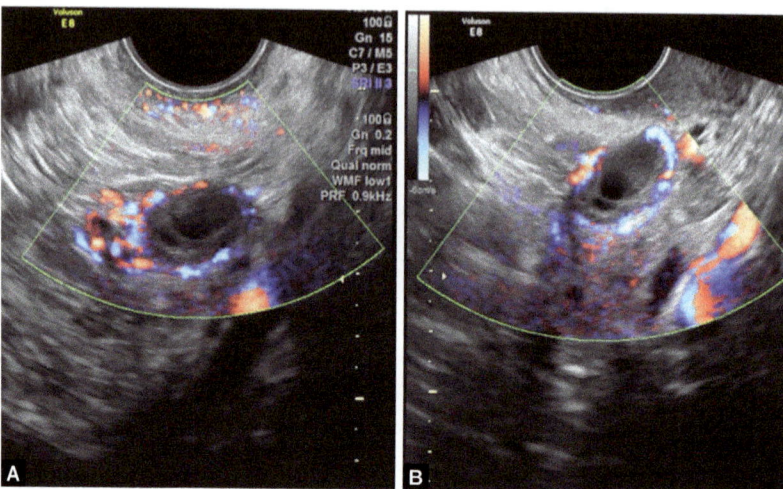

Figs. 5A and B: Profusely increased peripheral vascularity on TVS Doppler described as ring of fire appearance demonstrated in a case of ectopic pregnancy.

are present in 38% using transvaginal sonography (TVS) and 22% using transabdominal sonography (TAS).[4]
- Complex adnexal mass could also be a sign of ectopic gestation.
- *Decidualization* endometrium with tiny cystic spaces in the absence of an intrauterine pregnancy
- Doppler shows increased peripheral vascularity around the trophoblastic tissue termed "Ring of fire" **(Figs. 5A and B)**.
- The presence of fluid in pouch of Douglas is usually associated with ectopic gestation. It does not always indicate rupture of ectopic gestation.
- Hemorrhage from a ruptured ectopic may be seen as an avascular mass (hypo or hyperechoic). The presence of intra-abdominal free fluid should raise concerns about ruptured ectopic gestation.
- One of the most important differential diagnoses is a corpus luteal hemorrhage. A clearly demarcated extra ovarian mass in adnexa and a positive pregnancy test differentiates an ectopic from the latter.
- Ectopic gestation may be seen in other areas like cervix, cornu, ovary, rudimentary horn or interstitial or scar ectopic. Cesarean scar ectopic **(Figs. 6 and 7)**
- Heterotypic pregnancy is the presence of an intrauterine and extrauterine gestation. Incidence is 1 in 100,000 but its rising with the rise of infertility and ART **(Figs. 8 and 9)**.

Corpus Luteal Hemorrhage

A hemorrhagic ovarian cyst is usually corpus luteal hemorrhage. The reason for hemorrhage may be its increased vascularity.[5] It is physiological and usually self-limiting. Patient may present in the ER with features of hemorrhagic shock due to rupture of the corpus luteal cyst. Rupture is seen more commonly on the right because of the sigmoid colon presence on the left side which gives a cushioning effect **(Figs. 10A and B)**.

Endometriosis

Endometriosis is the presence of ectopic, hormone-sensitive endometrium, which proliferates and bleeds synchronously with

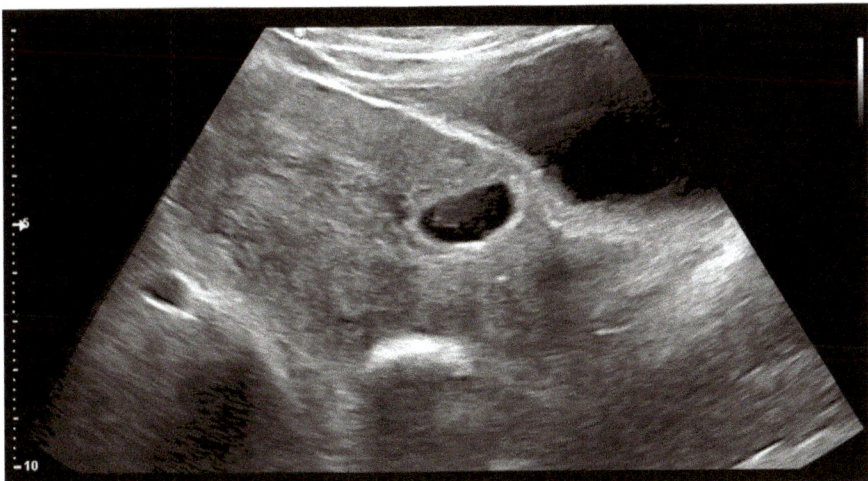

Fig. 6: A 32-year-old lady with spontaneous conception with previous cesarean 4 years back at 6 weeks with cesarean scar ectopic. Gestational sac with yolk sac fetal pole and cardiac activity seen in the enlarged previous cesarean scar. Note the bulge of the anterior uterine wall with thinned out myometrium between the ectopic and overlying serosa.
Courtesy: Sattva—The Fetal Medicine Center, New Delhi.

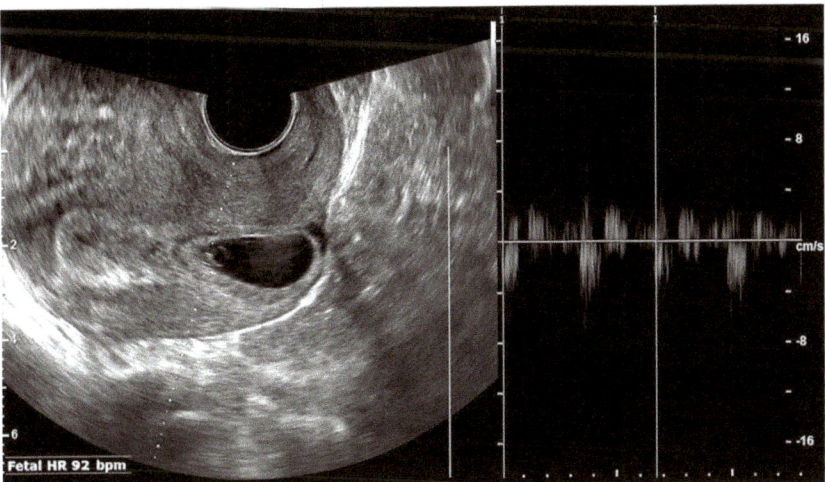

Fig. 7: Cardiac activity in the scar ectopic.

endometrium. The most prominent symptom is cyclic pelvic pain, while acute abdomen occurs in cases of massive bleeding, rupture or infection. Ultrasound reveals anechoic cyst with acoustic enhancement **(Fig. 11)**.

Endometriomas can be seen as cystic masses in MRI and show very high signal intensity and very low signal intensity on T1-weighted images and T2-weighted images, respectively.

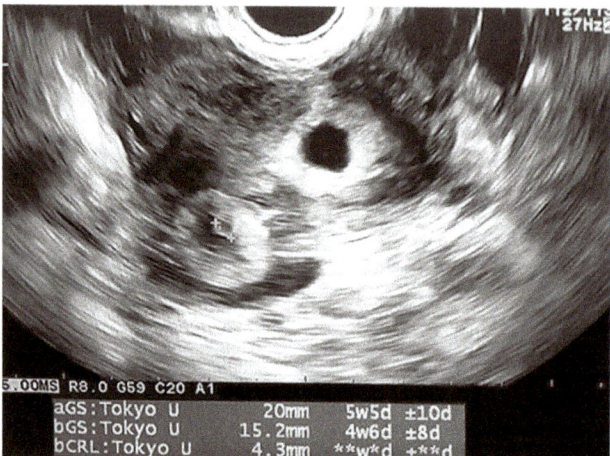

Fig. 8: A 36-year-old with IVF conception diagnosed at 6 weeks with heterotopic pregnancy. Ultrasound revealed an intrauterine gestation and gestational sac and fetal pole with cardiac activity in the posterior myometrium. Myomectomy was done 3 months prior. Patient presented within 24 hours with ruptured posterior wall and 1.5 L of hemoperitoneum. Posterior wall sutured and intrauterine pregnancy was salvaged.

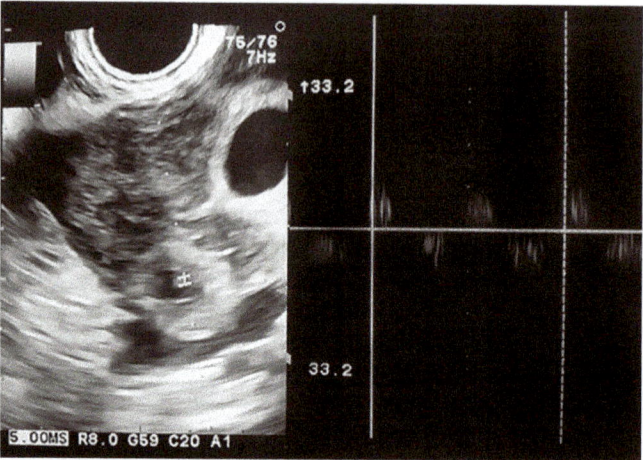

Fig. 9: Myometrial scar pregnancy with cardiac activity.

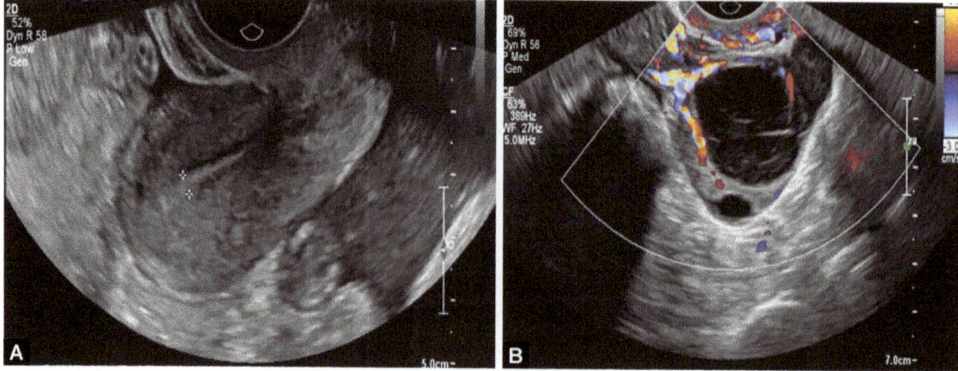

Figs. 10A and B: Ruptured adnexal cyst as seen by disruption of cyst wall and hemorrhagic free fluid on transvaginal ultrasound.

Chapter 23: Imaging in Gynecological Emergencies

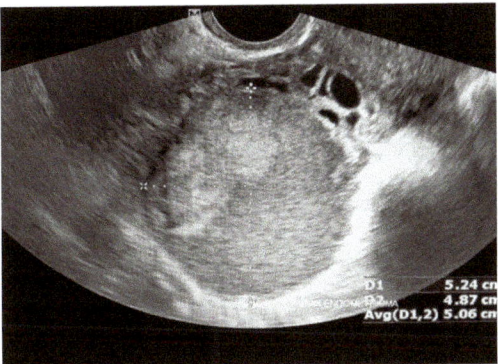

Fig. 11: A 25-year-old presenting with infertility and severe dysmenorrhea. Ultrasound picture reveals right ovarian endometrioma. Note the classical unilocular cyst with acoustic enhancement and homogeneous ground-glass appearance owing to hemorrhagic debris.

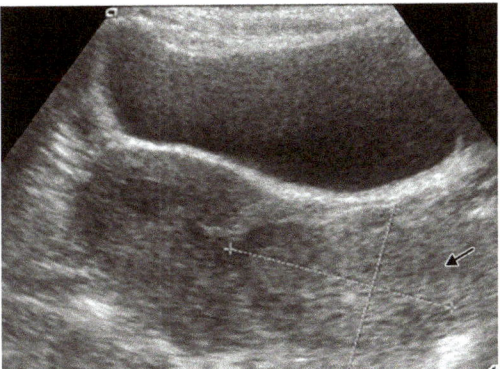

Fig. 12: Prolapsed fibroid in the vagina. Patient presented to the ER with ulcerated growth in the vagina with pain and urinary retention.

Acute abdomen occurs in cases of massive bleeding, rupture or infection. If an endometriotic cyst ruptures, the shape of the cyst may change, and the cyst fluid leakage may appear as loculated hyperintense fluid around the cyst on fat-saturated T1-weighted images.

Fibroids: Acute Presentations

Fibroids are one of the most common benign tumors in females. They are smooth muscle tumors seen in young women. They are estrogen sensitive and may remain asymptomatic for years. On ultrasound, they are seen as well-defined hypoechoic lesions. Acute pain may be caused by the following complications or secondary changes of fibroid.

- *Degeneration*: Degeneration may be hyaline (most common), fatty or red degeneration. It shows cystic areas surrounded by vascularity on Doppler. Degeneration in some cases may be quite extensive and the entire leiomyoma may mimic an ovarian mass being completely cystic and may become quite large. Patients present with acute pain and fever. MRI can be used in differentiating these lesions. Degenerated fibroids have variable MRI appearances composed of nonenhancing areas and/or cystic changes.
- *Prolapse of pedunculated fibroid*: Prolapse of pedunculated submucosal fibroid from the endocervical canal into the vagina can lead to acute pain **(Fig. 12)**. Sagittal T2-weighted images can identify the stalk.
- *Torsion of fibroid*: Torsion of a subserosal pedunculated fibroid is rare. The torted fibroid appears heterogeneous and lacks contrast enhancement. The adjacent ovaries will be normal.
- *Torsion of uterus*: Torsion of uterus is a very rare condition. Rotation of the uterus greater than 45° along the long axis is called uterine torsion. It occurs at the level of the uterine isthmus. Predisposing factors include a gravid uterus, myomatous uterus, congenital uterine anomalies, and adnexal masses. Presentation may be vague discomfort to shock. Preoperative diagnosis may be difficult due to the rarity.
  - An abnormal position of ovarian vessels across the uterus using color Doppler US may help diagnose uterine torsion.

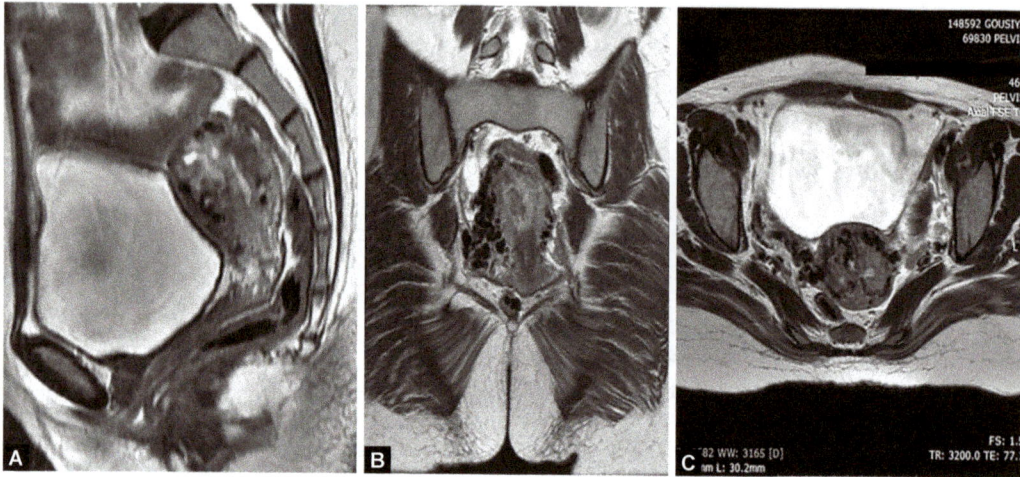

Figs. 13A to C: (A) Sagittal; (B) Coronal; (C) Axial view of uterine AV malformation
Courtesy: Mahajan Imaging and Diagnostic Center, Delhi.

- Axial T2-weighted MR image may show a whirlpool sign (of a twisted pedicle) at the level of the uterine corpus.

Arteriovenous Malformations

Uterine *arteriovenous* (AV) malformations may be congenital or more commonly acquired. They may rupture and cause sudden hemorrhagic shock in a young patient.
- Grayscale sonography may reveal subtle loss of myometrial homogeneity, tubular spaces can be seen in the myometrium, sometimes, a mass like region can be seen in the sonography.
- On Doppler tubular anechoic structures within the myometrium are noticed with a typical low resistance (RI ~0.2-0.5) and high velocity flow.
- MR imaging is a noninvasive method of confirmation of diagnosis.
- Multiple serpentine flow-related signal voids are typically seen in the uterine wall, endometrial cavity, and parametrium on T1- and T2- weighted images. Contrast-enhanced dynamic MR angiography can

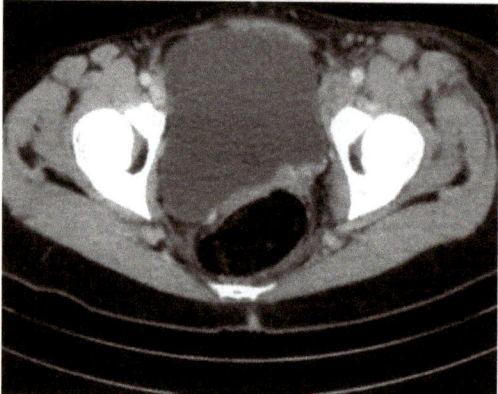

Fig. 14: Thrombosis of ovarian vein.
Courtesy: Mahajan Imaging and Diagnostic Center, New Delhi.

depict complex serpentine abnormal vessels that enhance as intensely as normal vessels and show early venous return **(Figs. 13A to C)**.

Puerperal Septic Thrombosis

Acute abdomen can be caused by postoperative or puerperal septic:
- Ultrasound may show tortuous noncompressible tubular structure, the thrombosed

vein with hypoechoic material. The structure may be seen from the adnexa, lateral to the IVC, till to renal hilus.
- Absent flow may be present on Doppler.
- CT demonstrates hyperdense wall and hypodense defect inside the contrast filled vein. It can cause septic pulmonary embolism, so CT examination of thorax is also recommended in such cases **(Fig. 14)**.

CONCLUSION

Pain in the pelvis and abdomen can be caused by a vast number of causes, both physiological and pathological. It is often a challenging task to differentiate gynecological causes from gastrointestinal and urological causes. Correlating the patient's history, pregnancy status, and radiological findings, a prompt diagnosis can be made which allows potential life-saving intervention. Being equipped with knowledge of variegated clinical presentation of individual pathological conditions and their US, CT, and MRI features, is necessary for making prompt and accurate diagnosis.

REFERENCES

1. Roache O, Chavan N, Aquilina J, et al. Radiological appearances of gynaecological emergencies. Insights Imaging. 2012;3(3):265-75.
2. Graif M, Itzchak Y. Sonographic evaluation of ovarian torsion in childhood and adolescence. Am J Roentgenol. 1988;150(3):647-9.
3. Nyberg DA, Hughes MP, Mack LA, et al. Extrauterine findings of ectopic pregnancy at transvaginal US: importance of echogenic fluid. Radiology. 1991;178(3):823-6.
4. Thoren MK, Lawson TL, Aiman EJ, et al. Diagnosis of ectopic pregnancy: endovaginal vs transabdominal sonography. Am J Roentgenol. 1990;155(2):307-10.
5. Bennett GL, Slywotzky CM, Giovanniello G. Gynecologic causes of acute pelvic pain: spectrum of CT findings. Radiographics. 2002;22(4):785-801.

SECTION 5

Miscellaneous Gynecological Emergencies

- Acute Retention of Urine
  Arveen Vohra
- Sexual Assault
  Priyanka Yadav
- Miscellaneous Gynecological Emergencies
  Sowmya Davuluri
- Medicolegal and Ethical Issues in Gynecological Emergencies
  Taswin Kaur Reddy

CHAPTER 24

Acute Retention of Urine

Arveen Vohra

INTRODUCTION

Urinary retention is the inability to empty the bladder. It may be acute or chronic. Acute urinary retention is a medical emergency requiring prompt action.

DEFINITION

Sudden inability to void, resulting in painful bladder, over distention and the need for catheterization to obtain relief is termed acute retention of urine.[1,2]

The causes of acute retention of urinary retention are outlined in **Table 1**.

A case report of a woman with acute urinary retention caused by a 17 × 9 mm urethral calculi, without any urinary anatomic abnormality, diagnosed by computed tomography (CT) and treated endoscopically has been recently cited.[11]

SYMPTOMS

- Incomplete voiding not enough to relieve symptoms
- Pain in the lower abdomen (pelvis) along with inability to urinate
- Inability to empty the bladder despite an urge to urinate
- Back pain, fever, and painful urination may indicate a urinary tract infection.[12]

EVALUATION (TABLE 2)

A detailed history and physical examination is necessary to know the cause of urinary retention.[12-14]

INVESTIGATIONS

- A urine routine and microscopic examination is necessary to check for signs of infection, stones or medical problems.[12,14,15]

TABLE 1: Causes of urinary retention.

Blockage of the urethra[1,3]	Scar tissue, organ prolapse (cystocele, rectocele, uterine prolapse), pelvic mass (gynecological malignancy, uterine fibroid, ovarian cyst), retroverted impacted gravid uterus, vaginal childbirth, injury, blood clots, infection, and stones
Disruption of the nervous system[3]	Spinal cord injury, spinal cord tumor, strokes, diabetes mellitus, herniated or ruptured disk in the vertebral column of the back, infection, multiple sclerosis, heavy metal poisoning or blood clot in the spinal cord
Infection and inflammation[4,5]	Cystitis, urethritis, vulvovaginitis, herpes
Surgery [3,6-8]	Direct result of the anesthetic or the surgery like hysterectomy and previous bladder surgeries, postpartum complications-postinterventions (vaginal instrumental delivery, cesarean section), relative immobility postsurgery
Medication[9,10]	Drugs like anticholinergics/antispasmodics like oxybutynin, alpha-adrenergic agonists, antihistamines such as diphenhydramine, chlorpheniramine and tricyclic antidepressants

TABLE 2: Evaluation of urinary retention.

History	Physical examination	Causes
Pelvic pressure, protrusion of pelvic organ from vagina	Prolapse of bladder, rectum or uterus on pelvic examination	Cystocele, rectocele, uterine prolapse
Pelvic pain, dysmenorrhea, lower abdominal discomfort, bloating	Enlarged uterus, ovaries, or adnexa on pelvic examination	Pelvic mass, uterine fibroid, gynecologic malignancy
Dysuria, vaginal itching, and discharge	Inflamed vulva and vagina, vaginal discharge	Vulvovaginitis
Dysuria, hematuria, fever, back pain, urethral discharge, genital rash, recent sexual activity	Suprapubic tenderness, costovertebral angle tenderness, urethral discharge, genital vesicles	Cystitis, urethritis, herpes, urinary tract infection, sexually transmitted infection
Painless hematuria	Gross hematuria with clots	Bladder tumor
Constipation	Abdominal distention	Fecal impaction
Constitutional symptoms, abdominal pain or distention, rectal bleeding	Palpable abdominal mass, positive fecal occult blood test, rectal mass	Advanced gastrointestinal tumor or malignancy
Existing or newly diagnosed neurologic disease, multiple sclerosis, Parkinson's disease, diabetic neuropathy, stroke, overflow incontinence	Generalized or focal neurologic deficits	Neurogenic bladder

- Complete blood count
- Renal function tests including electrolytes, serum blood glucose
- Abdominopelvic ultrasonography to rule out infection, tumors, calculi, and hydronephrosis and evaluate the urinary

tract (the kidneys, bladder and ureters). Postvoid residual urine is also measured.[16]
- CT scan or MRI of the spine can be done for further evaluation if history indicates neurological damage. Abdominopelvic CT scan or MRI is done to evaluate for suspected pelvic, abdominal, or retroperitoneal mass or malignancy causing extrinsic bladder neck compression
- Cystoscopy to examine the bladder, urethra for abnormalities that can cause urinary retention
- Urodynamic tests include uroflowmetry, cystometry, electromyography, urethral pressure profile, video urodynamics, and pressure flow studies of micturition. The pressure flow study helps to identify bladder outlet obstruction from cystocele. These also evaluate bladder function (detrusor muscle and sphincter) in patients with neurogenic bladder to help guide management.[3,12-15,17]

CO_2 cystometry gives as valid information as H_2O cystometry in estimating detrusor contractile function in patients with acute urinary retention.[18]

MANAGEMENT (FLOWCHART 1)

Definitive management of urinary retention will depend on the etiology and may include surgical and medical treatments.[19]

Interest in female urinary retention has increased recently because of improved understanding in the pathophysiology as well as the availability of specialized treatments such as sacral neuromodulation.

Catheterization

- Foley's catheter is inserted through the urethra into the bladder for immediate relief of the symptoms[3]
- Hematuria, hypotension, and postobstructive diuresis are potential complications of rapid decompression; however, there is no evidence that gradual bladder decompression will decrease these complications[20]
- Rapid and complete emptying of the bladder is therefore recommended
- Suprapubic catheters improve comfort and decrease bacteriuria and recatheterization in patients requiring catheterization for up to 14 days.[21]

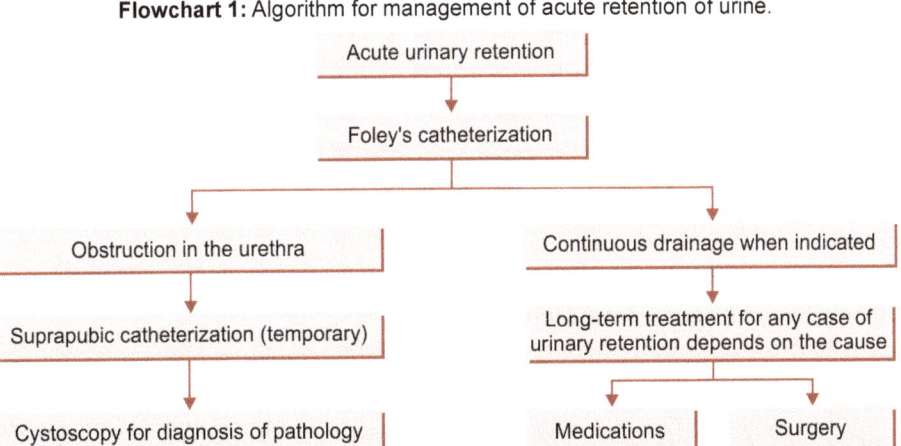

Flowchart 1: Algorithm for management of acute retention of urine.

Medications

- Alpha receptor blockers relax the muscles at the neck of the bladder, thus reducing the obstruction to the flow of urine
- Generally used for treating long-standing obstructive symptoms; may have a role in treating acute obstruction. [22-24]

Surgery

- The most common procedure for cystocele and rectocele repair is anterior colporrhaphy and pelvic floor repair
- Urethral stricture is treated by serial urethral dilation to widen the stricture
- An alternate method is to inflate a small balloon at the end of a catheter inside the urethra, placing a stent or by performing an internal urethrotomy, if indicated. [3,12,17,19,23,24]

COMPLICATIONS

- Permanent bladder damage and stones due to over distension.
- Urinary tract infection, sepsis, trauma, urethral strictures or erosions following catheterization.
- Chronic kidney disease and renal failure due to back pressure changes.
- Overzealous surgical correction causes incontinence.[12]

CONCLUSION

Acute retention of urine is an emergency that causes intense hypogastric pain as the urinary bladder over distends. If left untreated, the retrograde increase of pressure in the upper urinary tract can cause acute renal failure.

Identification of transient causes by detailed clinical evaluation can treat many women without unnecessary interventions.

REFERENCES

1. Rosenstein D, McAninch JW. Urologic emergencies. Med Clin North Am. 2004;88(2): 495-518.
2. Choong S, Emberton M. Acute urinary retention. BJU Int. 2000;85(2):186-201.
3. Curtis LA, Dolan TS, Cespedes RD. Acute urinary retention and urinary incontinence. Emerg Med Clin North Am. 2001;19(3):591-619.
4. Fuselier HA Jr. Etiology and management of acute urinary retention. Compr Ther. 1993;19(1):31-6.
5. Hemrika DJ, Schutte MF, Bleker OP. Elsberg syndrome: a neurologic basis for acute urinary retention in patients with genital herpes. Obstet Gynecol. 1986;68(3 Suppl):37S-39S.
6. Kim J, Lee DS, Jang SM, et al. The effect of pudendal block on voiding after hemorrhoidectomy. Dis Colon Rectum. 2005;48(3):518-23.
7. Glavind K and Bjørk J. Incidence and treatment of urinary retention post-partum. Int Urogynecol J Pelvic Floor Dysfunct. 2003;14(2):119-21.
8. Yip SK, Sahota D, Pang MW, et al. Postpartum urinary retention. Obstet Gynecol. 2005;106(3): 602-6.
9. Verhamme KM, Sturkenboom MC, Stricker BH, et al. Drug-induced urinary retention: incidence, management and prevention. Drug Saf. 2008;31(5):373-88.
10. Verhamme KM, Dieleman JP, Van Wijk MA, et al. Nonsteroidal anti-inflammatory drugs and increased risk of acute urinary retention. Arch Intern Med. 2005;165(13):1547-51.
11. Sungur M, Baykam M, Calışkan S, et al. Urethral calculi: A rare cause of acute urinary retention in women. Turk J Emerg Med. 2018;18(4):170-1.
12. Selius BA, Subedi R. Urinary retention in adults: Diagnosis and initial management. Am Fam Physician. 2008;77(5):643-65.
13. Dörflinger A, Monga A. Voiding dysfunction. Curr Opin Obstet Gynecol. 2001;13(5):507-12.
14. Stohrer M, Goepel M, Kondo A, et al. The standardization of terminology in

neurogenic lower urinary tract dysfunction: with suggestions for diagnostic procedures. International Continence Society Standardization Committee. Neurourol Urodyn. 1999;18(2): 139-58.
15. Bradway C, Rodgers J. Evaluation and management of genitourinary emergencies. Nurse Pract. 2009;34(5):36-43.
16. Stevens E. Bladder ultrasound: avoiding unnecessary catheterizations. Medsurg Nurs. 2005;14(4):249-53.
17. Ellerkmann RM, McBride A. Management of obstructive voiding dysfunction. Drugs Today (Barc). 2003;39(7):513-40.
18. Lin K-J, Fan Y-H, Lin AT, et al. Is CO_2 cystometry a reliable test in estimating detrusor contractile function in patients with acute urinary retention? Urological Science. 2017;28(1):27-31.
19. Ramsey S, Palmer M. The management of female urinary retention. Int Urol Nephrol. 2006;38(3-4):533-5.
20. Nyman MA, Schwenk NM, Silverstein MD. Management of urinary retention: rapid versus gradual decompression and risk of complications. Mayo Clin Proc. 1997;72(10): 951-6.
21. Niël-Weise BS, van den Broek PJ. Urinary catheter policies for short-term bladder drainage in adults. Cochrane Database Syst Rev. 2005;(3):CD004203.
22. Khastgit J, Khan A, Speakman M. Acute urinary retention: medical management and the identification of risk factors for prevention. Nat Clin Prac Urol. 2007;4(8):422-31.
23. Vilke GM, Ufberg JW, Harrigan RA, et al. Evaluation and treatment of acute urinary retention. J Emerg Med. 2008;35(2):193-8.
24. Newman DK. Managing Urinary Retention in the Acute Care Environment. [online] Available from https://www.verathon.com/wp-content/uploads/2019/05/BladderScan-Managing_Urinary_Retention.pdf. [Last accessed September, 2019].

CHAPTER 25

Sexual Assault

Priyanka Yadav

■ INTRODUCTION

There is a rising incidence of sexual assaults in developing countries. Approximately 13% of women and 3% of men worldwide, experience sexual assault.[1,2] There are severe effects on physical and mental health of female.[2,3] The survivors of sexual assault face the physical and psychological effects for a lifetime. Many survivors experience stigma from society and family.

■ FORMS OF SEXUAL ASSAULT

Sexual assaults are classified into various types:
- *Natural offences*: Rape, incest, and adultery
- *Unnatural offences*: Sodomy, tribadism, bestiality, and buccal coitus
- *Sexual perversions*: Sadism, masochism, necrophilia, fetichism, transvestism, exhibitionism, and masturbation
- *Sex-linked offences*: Stalking, voyeurism, sexual harassment, trafficking, and indecent assault

■ EFFECTS OF SEXUAL ASSAULT

Effects of rape can be categorized into the following:
- *Physical*: Injuries to genitalia and body parts, pregnancy, urinary tract infections, sexually transmitted diseases, and pelvic inflammatory disease.
- *Psychological*: Self-blame, depression, flashbacks, sleep and eating disorders, dissociative identity disorder, post-traumatic stress disorder, distrust of others, psychosexual disorders, substance abuse and rape trauma syndrome (RTS). RTS has two phases—acute disorganized phase with outward emotions or little emotions and a reorganization phase where lifestyle changes are done and there is manifestation of phobias.[4]

■ RISK FACTORS TO SEXUAL VIOLENCE

These are conditions or characteristics associated with an individual or surroundings

that increase the likelihood of the individual committing or being a victim of sexual assault.
- *Individual factors*: Being female, having special needs like chronic illness, handicap, mental disabilities, and young age
- *Family factors*: Broken families, lack of supervision by adults, mental disability in parents, families with drug and alcohol addiction in parents, and step father families
- *Community factors*: Social stigma which makes it difficult for the victim to be outspoken, leading to repeated assault
- *Social factors*: Hypersexualization of young, denial nature of society, social norms regarding gender roles, and social norms that support sexual abuse.

MANAGEMENT

Proper history regarding the nature of assault, any weapons or condoms used, time of assault, change of clothes, and documentation of the same is of utmost importance. Any drug taken voluntarily or involuntarily, specific events of assault, and post assault hygiene should be noted. Time of complaint and if there was any delay, the reason for delay should also be duly noted down. History regarding the relative positions of the victim and the person who committed the crime, whether there was any ejaculation and bleeding or any vaginal discharge has to be collected. Last menses date, previous intercourse, and information of current use of hormonal contraception should be noted.

Examination of Victim

Examination of victim should be done only after request from investigation police officer or magistrate. It should never be done against the victim's will. If the victim is intellectually disabled or a minor, consent of the parents must be taken. The goals of examination of victim are to search for injuries, to corroborate the injuries with the history, to collect and preserve the evidence for laboratory examination, and to treat the victim's physical and psychological effects.

Examination Proper

General examination for marks of violence, resistance, bruises, and bite marks should be done. The psychological state of the victim should also be observed and noted.

Genital examination: Only one-fifth of the victims have genital injuries. Genital injuries may be absent in females who were assaulted under submission owing to fear.

Steps: Rape is a legal definition. It is not a medical diagnosis.
- Victim should be positioned on a table with a good light, with her legs wide open and drawn up. Speculum can be used, if necessary.
- Injury to labia to be noted—finger nail scratches, inflammation, and edema of vaginal introitus and labia minora
- Nature of hymen and injuries to hymen—note down the position of tears. Glaister Keene rod can be used as and when necessary
- Tears and injuries of posterior vagina to be noted
- Presence of semen in the vagina and over the external genitalia should be noted
- Test for intoxication and sexually transmitted diseases
- Negative findings are as important as positive findings and have to be duly documented

- In a deflorate female, penetration may not cause injuries. Hence, lack of injuries does not indicate absence of penetration
- In young children no general injuries may be seen. Sometimes, there may be redness or edema of vulva.
- Colposcopic photo documentation should be done during vaginal examination.

Specimens to be collected:
- Avulsed head hairs
- Pubic hair combings and avulsed pubic hairs
- Swabs from bite marks for saliva and soiled areas of skin
- Blood—grouping and test for intoxication
- Nail scrapings
- Swabs from introitus, vagina, and cervical os

Test for seminal fluid: Florence test, Barberio's test, acid phosphatase test, sperm creatine phosphokinase test, prostate specific antigen detection, and fluorescence in situ hybridization (FISH) can be used for detection of seminal fluid. Microscopic examination is done for detection of spermatozoa.

Treatment:
- Manage these physical effects using antibiotics to prevent wound infection, TT boosts if required
- Medication for pain relief or anxiety
- Provide emergency contraceptive and present within 72 hours of assault
- Treat sexual transmit infections
    - Benzathine penicillins—1.2 lakh IU stat
    - Gentamycin 6 mg/kg single dose
    - Erythromycin 12.5 mg/kg every 6 hours for 7 days
    - Metronidazole 5 mg/kg every 8 hours for 7 days

Examination of Accused

Consent must be taken for examination. General history of medical illness must be taken. Details of the specific incident must not be taken from the accused. The physical and psychological state of the accused should be observed and duly noted.

General examination: General physical power of the accused should be assessed. Marks of struggle and injuries must be documented.

Genital examination:
- Development of genital organs should be observed
- Injuries to genitalia and pubic hair avulsion must be noted
- Accused penis is cleaned with saline and washings should be examined for vaginal cells, cervical cells, and Barr bodies
- Absence or presence of smegma has to be documented

Specimens to be collected from accused:
- Pubic hair—combings and avulsed pubic hair
- Head hair
- Loose hair elsewhere in body
- Nail scrapings
- Swabs from prepuce, urethral orifice, and penile shaft
- Test—sexual transmitted disease and blood grouping

COUNSELING

Support services for victims and family with psychosocial therapy is essential.[1,5,6]
- Define and acknowledge the assault
- Psychoeducation
- Emphasis on confidence and coping with problem
- Building trust in others
- Psychosexual counseling
- Cognitive behavioral therapy

Rape crisis centers, community centers, support groups, and volunteer medical and other professional groups can work in harmony to counsel the sexual assault victim.[7]

SUMMARY

Thorough history examination, screening, referral, Follow-up is required for support of victim along with psychosocial therapy for victims and families.

CONCLUSION

- The rising incidence of sexual assault in developing countries affects the physical and more importantly the mental health of the survivor.
- Management of these cases require detailed examination and specific specimen from the survivor as well as accused.
- Victims should be supported medically and socially with behavioral therapy.

REFERENCES

1. Spitzberg BH. An analysis of empirical estimates of sexual aggression victimisation and perpetration. Violence Vict. 1999;114(3):241-60.
2. Hurst C, MacDonald J, Say J, et al. Routine questioning about non-consenting sex: a survey of practice in Australasian sexual health clinics. Int J STD AIDS. 2003;14(5):329-33.
3. Krug EG, Dahlberg LL, Mercy JA, et al. Sexual violence. In: Krug EG, Dahlberg LL, Mercy JA, Zwi AB, Lozano R, (Eds). World report on violence and health. Geneva, Switzerland: World Health Organization; 2002. pp. 141-81.
4. Burgess AW, Holmstrom LL. Rape trauma syndrome. Am J Psychiatry. 1974;131(9):981-6.
5. Poirier M. Care of the female adolescent rape victim. Pediatr Emerg Care. 2002;18(1):53-9.
6. Tomlinson DR, Harrison J. The management of adult male victims of sexual assault in GUM clinic: a practical guide. Int J STD AIDS. 1998;9(12):720-5.
7. Walker LEA (Ed). Rape and Sexual assault. In: Abused women and survivor therapy: A practical guide for the psychotherapist. Washington, DC: American Psychological Association; 1994. pp. 23-53.

CHAPTER 26

Miscellaneous Gynecological Emergencies

Sowmya Davuluri

INTRODUCTION

Early recognition and timely management of gynecological emergencies such as ectopic pregnancy, urinary retention, ovarian torsion, etc. helps reducing the gynecological morbidities. Other gynecological conditions which may present as emergencies are menstrual disorders, bleeding gynecological malignancies, coital laceration and sexual assault. Acute abdominal pain, bleeding per vagina are the most common presenting complaints. Advances in the ultrasound, minimal access surgeries have helped in the early diagnosis of these conditions. This chapter gives an overview of the conditions and their management.

URINARY RETENTION

Definition

Sudden inability to void, resulting in painful bladder, over distention, and the need for catheterization to obtain relief is termed acute retention of urine.[1,2] The causes of acute retention are enumerated in **Flowchart 1**.

Difference between Acute and Chronic Retention

	Acute retention	Chronic retention
Urination	No urine	Overflow and incontinence
Pain	Severe	No pain
Obstruction	Complete	Partial
Suprapubic tenderness	Present	No tenderness

Evaluation and Management of Acute Urinary Retention

Evaluation and management of acute urinary retention is given in **Flowchart 2**.

Complications of Unsafe Abortions

Unsafe abortions are the leading cause of maternal morbidity and accounts for 13% of

Chapter 26: Miscellaneous Gynecological Emergencies

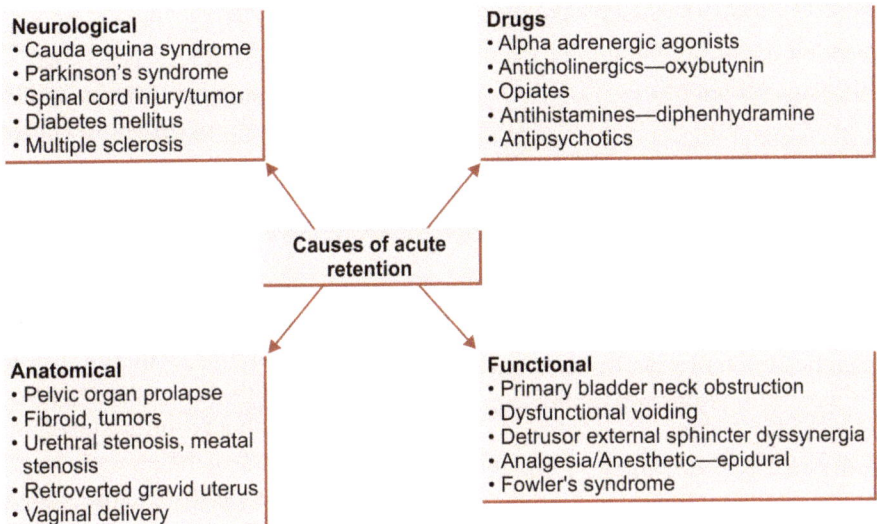

Flowchart 1: Causes of acute retention.

Neurological
- Cauda equina syndrome
- Parkinson's syndrome
- Spinal cord injury/tumor
- Diabetes mellitus
- Multiple sclerosis

Drugs
- Alpha adrenergic agonists
- Anticholinergics—oxybutynin
- Opiates
- Antihistamines—diphenhydramine
- Antipsychotics

Anatomical
- Pelvic organ prolapse
- Fibroid, tumors
- Urethral stenosis, meatal stenosis
- Retroverted gravid uterus
- Vaginal delivery

Functional
- Primary bladder neck obstruction
- Dysfunctional voiding
- Detrusor external sphincter dyssynergia
- Analgesia/Anesthetic—epidural
- Fowler's syndrome

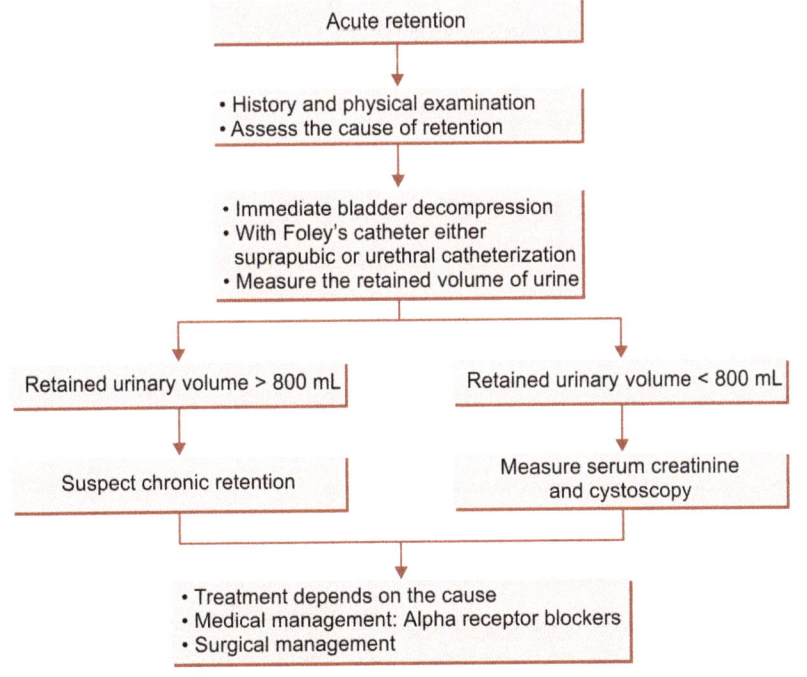

Flowchart 2: Evaluation and management of acute urinary retention.

Acute retention
- History and physical examination
- Assess the cause of retention

- Immediate bladder decompression
- With Foley's catheter either suprapubic or urethral catheterization
- Measure the retained volume of urine

Retained urinary volume > 800 mL → Suspect chronic retention

Retained urinary volume < 800 mL → Measure serum creatinine and cystoscopy

- Treatment depends on the cause
- Medical management: Alpha receptor blockers
- Surgical management

the maternal deaths and are mostly seen in the developing countries.[3-5] Severe hemorrhage and infections constitute the main causes of morbidity in unsafe abortion.

To avoid complications due to abortions, a proper postabortion care has to be implemented:
- Availability of emergency services for treating the complications of abortion
- Counseling and delivery of contraceptives or sterilization
- Comprehensive reproductive healthcare
- Use of safer techniques and improving the provider skills
- Prompt and appropriate treatment of complications.

Manual vacuum evacuation is the best treatment option for a safer abortion.[6]

RAPE AND SEXUAL ASSAULT

Any form of nonconsensual act even without penetration of any orifices is defined as sexual assault and nonconsensual penetration of either vagina or anus is defined as rape. Victims usually present with genital injury and the incidence ranges between 10% and 80% and nongenital injuries range between 31% and 82%.[7] Pregnancies following rape have been accounted to 5%.[8] Adolescents, children, and physically challenged women are the most vulnerable group.

Management of these cases includes a detailed history and a detailed examination starting with physical appearance of the victim, genital injuries, and collection of swabs from the vulva, vagina, cervix, perineal, and the rectal areas.

Prophylactic antibiotics should be started to cover the common sexually transmitted diseases (STDs) and postexposure prophylaxis for human immunodeficiency virus (HIV) should be started. Emergency contraception should be prescribed to the victim. Psychological support is the most important as most of the victims suffer from post-trauma stress disorders.[7]

TORSION OVARIAN CYST

Ovarian torsion refers to the rotation of the ovary to the extent of occluding an artery or vein resulting in ischemia of the ovary. Torsion is the fifth main cause of gynecological emergencies and accounts for 2.7% of the cases. About 50% of the torsions demonstrate an ovarian mass and 2% of these are ovarian malignancies.[9] Ovarian torsion in pregnancy is common around 10–17 weeks gestation and usually the size of the mass is >4 cm and accounts for 10–22%.[10,11]

Patients with torsion present typically with acute abdominal pain, vomiting, abdominal tenderness, guarding, and tachycardia.

Evaluation

Ultrasound with Doppler study is the gold standard though not confirmatory. A torsed ovary is enlarged due to edema or vascular engorgement. On Doppler, either absent or decreased blood flows are noted. Whirlpool sign—where there is twisted vascular pedicle, and circular vessels within the mass is highly sensitive for ovarian torsion.[12] Magnetic resonance imaging (MRI) demonstrates the components of the mass. Only direct visualization gives a definite diagnosis.

Management

Management of torsion ovarian cyst is given in **Flowchart 3**.

Chapter 26: Miscellaneous Gynecological Emergencies

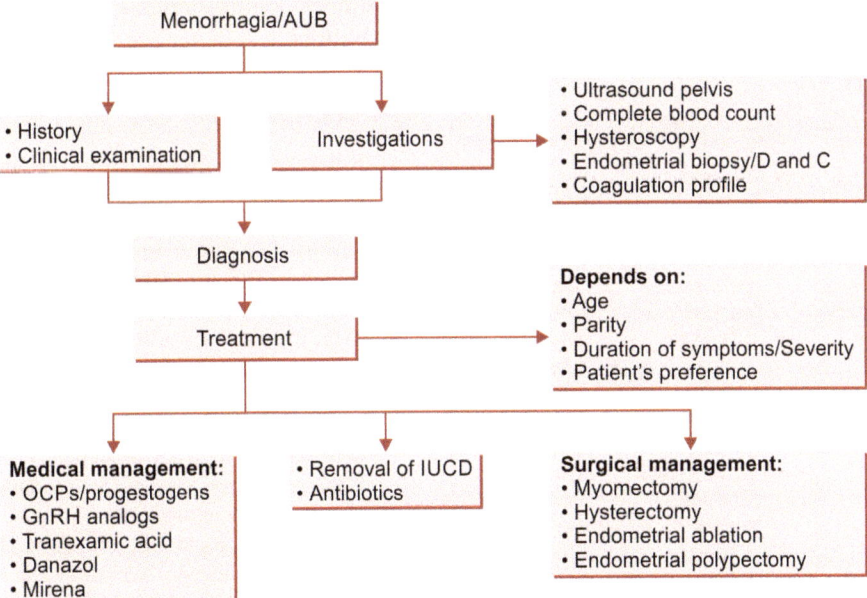

Flowchart 3: Management of torsion ovarian cyst.

Flowchart 4: Management of abnormal uterine bleeding.

(AUB: abnormal uterine bleeding; IUCD: intrauterine contraceptive device; OCPs: oral contraceptives)

■ MITTELSCHMERZ PAIN

It is most commonly seen in reproductive age group and is unique to the ovulatory cycles. The co-relation of pain to the menstrual cycle is important for the diagnosis. This pain is usually unilateral and lasts less than 24 hours. The severity ranges from mild to moderate. This pain can be due to irritation of the periovarian peritoneal tissue by the follicular fluid. This condition can be treated with analgesics/nonsteroidal anti-inflammatory drugs (NSAIDs) and reassurance.

ABNORMAL UTERINE BLEEDING

Definition

Bleeding from the uterine corpus that is abnormal in volume, regularity, timing that has been for the last 6 months or more.[13]

Abnormal uterine bleeding accounts for 20–30% of all cases and is the most common cause of emergency admissions.[14,15] The goal is to decrease the bleeding and to prevent the woman to either develop anemia or prevent the worsening of existing anemia. Severe bleeding is commonly accompanied by tachycardia and hypotension.

Etiology

Systemic	*Anatomical*	*Endocrinological*
• Stress • Chronic liver and kidney disease • Medications	• Fibroid uterus • Endometrial hyperplasia/cancer • Cervical cancer • Polyps • Perimenopausal • IUCD in situ • Endometriosis • Endometritis	• Hypo/Hyperthyroidism • Obesity • Polycystic ovaries • Anovulatory cycles • Pituitary tumors • Puberty • Cushing's syndrome • Diabetes mellitus

Management

Management of abnormal uterine bleeding is given in **Flowchart 4**.

SUMMARY

Acute urinary retention, ectopic pregnancy, and PID are common conditions seen in the emergency room. There is now more robust evidence, based on randomized controlled trials (RCTs) and meta-analysis, that allows clinicians and their patients to decide on expectant, medical and conservative surgical management to minimize morbidity while preserving physical, reproductive and emotional wellbeing.

CONCLUSION

Acute gynecological emergencies are common causes of morbidity and mortality. Early recognition and timely management of gynecological emergencies such as ectopic pregnancy, urinary retention, ovarian torsion, etc. helps reducing the gynecological morbidities.

REFERENCES

1. Rosenstein D, McAninch J. Urologic emergencies. Med Clin North Am. 2004;88(2):495-518.
2. Choong S, Emberton M. Acute urinary retention. BJU Int. 2000;85(2):186-201.
3. Okonofua F. Abortion and maternal mortality in the developing world. J Obstet Gynecol Can. 2006;28(11):974-9.
4. World Health Organization. Unsafe abortion: global and regional estimates of the incidence of unsafe abortion and associated mortality in 2000, 4th edition. Geneva, Switzerland: World Health Organization; 2004.
5. Singh S. The incidence of unsafe abortion: A global review. In: Warriner IK, Shah IH (Eds). Preventing Unsafe Abortion and its Consequences: Priorities for Research and Action. New York: Guttmacher Institute; 2006.
6. Rogo K. Improving technologies to reduce abortion-related morbidity and mortality. Int J Gynecol Obstet. 2004;85 (Suppl 1):S73-82.
7. Gribbin C. Sexual assault and rape. Curr Obstet Gynecol; 2004.
8. Holmes MM, Resnick HS, Kilpatrick DG, et al. Rape related pregnancy: estimates and descriptive characteristics from a national

sample of women. Am J Obstet Gynecol. 1996;175(2):320-4; discussion 324-5.
9. White M, Stella J. Ovarian torsion: 10-year perspective. Emerg Med Australas. 2005;17(3):231-7.
10. Johnson TR Jr, Woodruff JD. Surgical emergencies of the uterine adnexae during pregnancy. Int J Gynaecol Obstet. 1986;24(5):331-5.
11. Yen CF, Lin SL, Murk W, et al. Risk analysis of torsion and malignancy for adnexal masses during pregnancy. Fertil Steril. 2009;91(5):1895-902.
12. Valsky DV, Esh-Broder E, Cohen SM, et al. Added value of the gray-scale whirlpool sign in the diagnosis of adnexal torsion. Ultrasound Obstet Gynecol. 2010;36(5):630-4.
13. Whitaker L, Critchley HO. Abnormal uterine bleeding. Best Pract Res Clin Obstet Gynaecol. 2016;34:54-65.
14. Matteson KA, Weitzen SH, LaFontaine D, et al. Accessing care: Use of a specialized women's emergency care facility for non-emergent problems. J Womens Health (Larchmt). 2008;17(2):269-77.
15. Curtis KM, Hillis SD, Burney AK, et al. Visits to emergency departments for gynecologic disorders in the United States, 1992–1994. Obstet Gynecol. 1998;91(6):1007-12.

CHAPTER 27

Medicolegal and Ethical Issues in Gynecological Emergencies

Taswin Kaur Reddy

INTRODUCTION

The health services in the country has transformed leaps and hurdles over the past decades at the present ranking 112 out of 190 countries; according to the World Health Organization (WHO).[1] Although the allocated amount for health services is minute,[2] the facilities provided are at par of those at developing countries. In this process, there is a tectonic shift in the way the general population perceives health and ethics.

Long gone are those days where doctors were looked upon as saints or as a step lower, if not equivalent than the creator himself. The recent explosion and propagation by the media have made doctors stand in the limelight for any blame game in a hospital setting. With the increasing accessibility, publicity, and advancement of health services, there are numerous gray areas especially in the legal aspects that a medical practitioner can be held responsible for in the court of law and this is no exception for the gynecologist. It is alarming to note that there is 110% rise in number of medical negligence cases in India yearly and 60–66% of these cases are based on improper consent from patients and relatives prior to a procedure or improper documentation![3]

It is impossible to describe in this chapter all the laws of ethical and the medicolegal issues that can arise in all the countries of the world especially since the rules, regulations, and legislations regarding these issues are different in between countries. Hence, this chapter aims at providing an overview of the medicolegal and ethical aspects based on the current laws of the land, especially in India.

Although obstetrics steals the limelight from its twin sister when it comes to medicolegal litigation claims, gynecology has its own share of litigant claims.

GRAY AREAS FOR MEDICOLEGAL AND ETHICAL PROBLEMS IN GYNECOLOGY[4]

Consent and documentation	Failure to recognize complications
Confidentiality	HIV transmission
Intraoperative problems	Research
Failure to diagnose/ delay in diagnosis	

Gynecology patients with an exception of those with cancer are mostly younger women seeking a better quality of life by regulation of their menstrual cycle, treatment of nonlife threatening infection or pelvic floor dysfunction, fertility preservation/control or treatment. Hence, their expectations of a good outcome are relatively high.

Medical practitioners via the Hippocratic Oath[5] vow to perform an ethical practice and abide by the five principles of ethics,[6] i.e. beneficence, autonomy, nonmaleficence, justice, and confidentiality.

- *Beneficence*—is to act in the best of interests of the patient and to balance the risks against the benefits. The benefits that medicine is competent to seek for patients are the management and prevention of disease, handicap, injury and unwanted pain and agony; and the prevention of preventable death.
- *Autonomy*—to respect the right of the individual. The informed consent in clinical practice is an example of respect of autonomy.
- *Nonmaleficence*—commonly known as "primum non nocere" or first do no harm. The gynecologist should prevent harm and this is best understood as expressing the limits of beneficence.
- *Justice*—to treat all patients equally without unfair discrimination. There should be fairness in distribution of risks and benefits. Medical needs and benefits should be weighed properly.
- *Confidentiality*—is a basis of trust between the health personnel, i.e. gynecologist and the patient.

PREVENTION OF MEDICOLEGAL PROBLEMS[7,8]

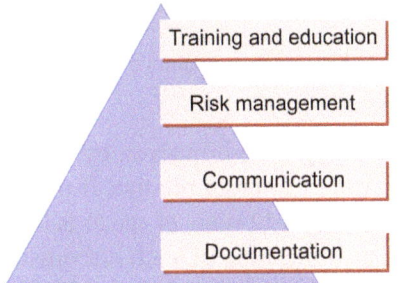

CONSENT AND DOCUMENTATION

Consent is defined as a process during which the professional provides adequate and accurate information concerning a procedure to a patient that allows them to reach a considered decision. The process of obtaining consent is understood to have three elements—disclosure by the physician to the patient of her condition and its management options, understanding of that information by the patient, and followed by a voluntary decision by the patient to authorize or refute treatment **(Fig. 1)**.

The concept of consent comes from the ethical issue of respect of individual integrity, autonomy, and self-determination. Every individual has a right to determine what should be done to his body. In the court of law, a legally valid consent for a procedure or treatment is one that is:

- *Given by the person himself*, if above 12 years of age (Sec. 88 IPC), conscious and

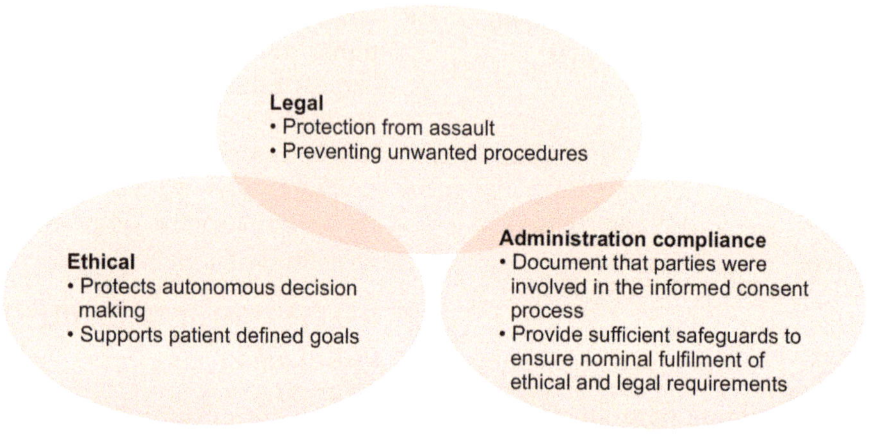

Fig. 1: Venn diagram showing the multiple overlapping purposes of informed consent.[9]

Legal
- Protection from assault
- Preventing unwanted procedures

Ethical
- Protects autonomous decision making
- Supports patient defined goals

Administration compliance
- Document that parties were involved in the informed consent process
- Provide sufficient safeguards to ensure nominal fulfilment of ethical and legal requirements

mentally sound or given by the parent, guardian or close relative, if the patient is less than 12 years of age or is insane or is unconscious. In such circumstances, consent given by parent, guardian or close relative is known as "substitute or proxy consent".

- *Informed expressed written consent*
- *Given before* actually doing the *procedure*
- Given in the present of *two witnesses*
- Given freely, voluntarily, and directly
- Given without fear, fraud or force
- *Signed by the doctor, patient (or guardian), and witnesses*
- Should be written in patient's own handwriting

It is important to ensure that the consent includes the nature of the diagnosis, the nature of the planned treatment, foreseeable risks of the treatment, prognosis if the treatment is not carried out and if any alternative therapies are available.

Blanket consent is one that is taken on a printed form that covers almost everything the doctor or hospital might do to a patient without mentioning anything specifically. Blanket consents are usually legally inadequate for any procedure that has risks or multiple alternatives.

In any clinic, consent taking is very essential and consent from preferably both the partners—husband and wife, is mandatory prior to treatment. It is very crucial to counsel, document, and to take necessary consents involved in part of the treatment to avoid unforeseen legal complications.[10]

The patient and their attendees should be made to understand that there is no guarantee on the success of the treatment and all the possible complications of the procedure and the alternatives of the procedure should be documented and discussed beforehand. This is important as many patients especially in developing countries for example India, assume that they will walk home disease free once they step into a doctors chamber.

A consent should not be overlooked or taken as a substitute for a detailed discussion regarding the intended intervention and its alternatives, allowing the patient and her family to take part in the decision making process of her own care.

With the exception of an unanticipated emergency, the practitioner should never exceed the scope of the authority given by the patient. An example commonly quoted is when an abdominal hysterectomy is planned but however on table the surgeon decides to perform an unindicated bilateral salpingo-oophorectomy without a prior informed consent. This shall be an unethical practice and the surgeon shall be liable in the court of law for performing a surgery without the patient's consent. An example of an unanticipated emergency is an abdominal hysterectomy for postpartum hemorrhage to save life. In such cases, the opinion of an experienced colleague or specialist must be sought before undertaking an additional intervention. In an emergency, if the patient is unable to give consent, her next of kin should be involved. Although not legally binding, this is a good practice that may help avoid future tussle and litigation.

Written informed consent is preferred. However, under most circumstances, during a gynecological examination or an ultrasound examination, written consent is not considered necessary but women should be provided sufficient information and a verbal consent is mandatory especially if she is being examined by the opposite sex. If required, the information of such a discussion may be documented in the patient records.

In the era of technology, numerous multimedia images are captured and stored for future use, if required. It is essential to note that these images of laparoscopic findings, ultrasound pictures and X-rays do not require additional consent for use as part of the care record as the consent for care purposes is an implicit in the consent given for the intervention. The consent form should propose that the image may be used for education or teaching. However, if the woman may and will be recognizable from the images, this must be made clear to her before she gives consent and the same is to be documented in the patient's records.

The failure to obtain consent in cases where it should be and the patient has come to harm could lead to legal claims for assault and negligence which may proceed to criminal charges with a heavy impact on rare instances.

Documentation

Apart from necessary consent taking, documentation at each and every step is essential. Clinicians should be made aware that "if it is not documented, it was not done". From a medicolegal standpoint view, "good documentation is good defense, poor documentation is poor defense, and no documentation is no defense."

Thus, it is important to document the patient's visits, complaints, medication given, options offered to the woman, and the intervention performed. It is essential to document the discussion with the patient and the management plan that has been jointly agreed upon. As described above, the consenting process should be robust, detailed, and the risks should be clearly explained and documented.

To maintain confidentiality, codes can be used while alerting the healthcare professional of the need of special care and precaution. These codes can be used when handling cases complicated by HIV infection or Hepatitis B. During an operative intervention, it is mandatory to document the swab and instrument count in the operation notes.

It is mandatory that all clinics maintain detailed records legibly written or computerized, including all operative cases. Records should be stored in the medical records department.

Communication

Effective and good communication skills are the cornerstone in today's health care practice. With doctors being frequent victims of litigations and assaults, it is of utmost importance to build an exceptional patient-doctor relationship from the outset. This process will definitely have a positive impact on history taking, informed choices, and the consenting process. The patient/women should be involved in every stage of the management and treatment process. Information leaflets may be provided to help patient to make an informed choice and decision. When counseling by the doctor themselves seems to be difficult, the help of an independent counselor can be taken and is vital. Witnesses are also counseled and made aware of the ongoing process.

Another vital element of counseling is the debriefing process after the procedure especially if an unexpected or an untoward outcome and it is essential to explain honestly what went wrong. It is evident that apart from financial compensation, patients resort to legal action because they want to find out what exactly went wrong and why it occurred. Hence, to spare the rod; honesty, timely explanation, and empathy shown during an unexpected outcome irrespective of liability and efforts to identify what went wrong may go a long way to prevent litigations.

In respect to communication skills, the healthcare providers should be a supporting and an active team member and every effort should be taken to improve "team building". Difficult and unexpected outcomes should be discussed and an internal enquiry should be held. The findings as well as the actions taken are brain stormed to prevent similar incidents in the future. Multidisciplinary meetings and ward rounds can not only help improve knowledge, understanding but also improves communication and creates respect of each other's roles. Staff involved should be aware of the protocols implemented in the hospital setup. Communication irrespective of an emergency or otherwise must be unambiguous and effective.

RISK MANAGEMENT

Components of Risk Management

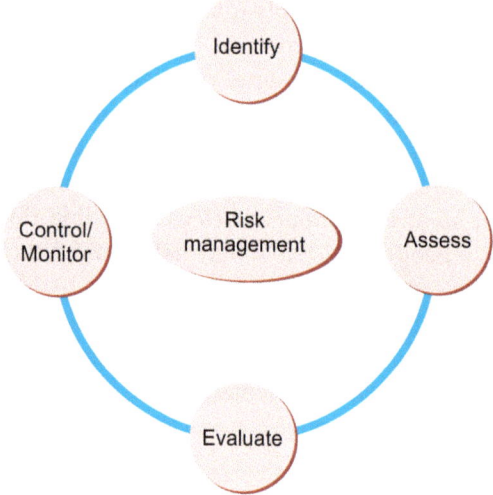

Healthcare setting is equivalent to other services where risk management is an important integral part of a gynecology clinic. The process of risk management cycle involves identifying the involved risks, assessing the situation and the risks involved, evaluating the options in hand as well as the changes that can be implemented and lastly monitoring the diversity of tweaks executed. Clinical incident reporting is essential and includes near-misses and actual adverse outcome. These cases should be discussed in an open, detailed, and no blame atmosphere with a feedback to the team members so that the lessons learnt and the message delivered can be put into practice with preference to the patient's safety.

TRAINING AND EDUCATION

Clinical skills and effectiveness should be improved by the use of evidence-based guidelines and protocols. Hence, training, support, and mentoring should be readily available for those who require them. The use of simulators and role plays aid in improvement and practice of these vital skills. It is also essential to update the guidelines according to the recent evidence and national guidelines which shall definitely assist the healthcare provider if a litigant situation arises.

The significance and distinction of clinical audit should be used to assess the quality of care and at the same time deficiencies to be identified and recommendations made to improve practice.

It is the duty of the gynecologist themselves to acquaint themselves with the laws of the land. In the process, some have specialized in the field of medicolegal research on litigation and risk management, and their help can definitely be sought in the days of need.

FORENSIC GYNECOLOGY[11]

Many gynecologists have limited contact with forensic scenarios. Although, when a situation arises they will work with the forensic medicine experts; it is essential that they have some knowledge of this discipline in case they are caught unaware. Rape and sexual assault cases must be handled in a fragile and sensitive manner while respecting the laws and acts of the nation. In the recent days with the increasing crime rate, diligent consent taking and evidence preservation is indispensable to avoid future unexpected negative implications.

SPECIFIC PROBLEM AREAS

- *Female sterilization*: Historically, failed sterilization and a consequent pregnancy was the single most frequent surgery likely to give rise to litigations. As per experts, there are two aspects of sterilization failure that provide scope for litigants to find limelight—the inadequate consent and a defective surgery.

  Rarely, spontaneous recanalization may occur. However, more commonly an incomplete or traumatic occlusion of the fallopian tube may give rise to failure. Another common base for a stand in the court of law is when sterilization was done without diagnosing an existing pregnancy or when it is done in the secretory phase where implantation may have just taken place. Often, especially when performed by amateurs, ligation of the wrong structures (e.g. Round ligament) can be a high legal threat. Throughout the years, it has been confirmed that the risk of legal episodes are more common when sterilization is done in an emergency setting without an adequate counseling.

- *Contraception:* Many gynecology patients walk into the clinic for temporary fertility control and birth spacing. A plethora of options are available today and women are given a bag of potpourri to pick and choose from after explaining the pros and cons about the options available.

  The possible cornerstones of squabbling after an IUCD insertion are unintentional perforation of uterus, expulsion of the device, complication post insertion like bleeding and pain or even an IUCD failure. These instances can be a possible ground for a medicolegal claim if the patient was not counseled prior.

  While using an oral contraceptive pill, it is essential to explain to the woman the requirement of consuming the pill daily. A pill failure or a missed pill is not an unusual reason behind a contraception failure. A common example of possible prosecution is if oral contraceptive pills are given to women with history of a thromboembolic disorder.

Injectable contraception may lead to irregular menstruation and amenorrhea should be informed prior to acceptance of this method by the women.

Women should also be made aware of the possible long- and short-term side effects of the contraceptive methods chosen by them and a free choice is adopted for selection of the preferred method provided the women has no contraindications.

- *Injuries*: Gynecological procedures may be complicated by injuries to the surrounding structures like the bowel, bladder, large blood vessel or the rectum; though not very common. To safeguard, preprocedure consent should mention the minute risks of complications in order to decrease the risk of a legal problem. The patient and her party should be made aware with utmost honesty and empathy of the occurred complication and the measures taken to revert the incident.
- *Endoscopic surgery*: The era of day care surgeries, minimally invasive surgeries have taken an upper hand. Laparoscopic and hysteroscopic procedures are performed frequently.

    Hysteroscopy is considered a relatively safe procedure. Nevertheless, rarely, perforations, false passages, and hemorrhage can occur. These scenarios are more commonly encountered during an operative laparoscopy compared to a simple diagnostic procedure.

    Laparoscopy is the main modality today for almost all gynecological procedures. Unexpected organ damage may occur which shall require a laparotomy for inspection and further repair. Operative laparoscopy requires a long learning and training curve for a competent, correct, safe technique with the prompt and diligent recognition of complications. Like any other procedure, any unexpected outcome should be communicated to the patient and her kin.
- *Hysterectomy*: A commonly performed procedure with a high litigation radius. Today's medicolegal claims are usually for unwarranted unnecessary hysterectomy or the removal of ovaries without prior consent. Infrequently, allegations are lodged for unanticipated ureter injury or premature ovarian insufficiency post hysterectomy.
- *Urogynecology*: Day by day numerous new mechanics are cropping up, revolving around urinary incontinence and cosmetic gynecology. It is becoming more complicated for the general gynecologist to treat patients of this subspecialty. There is leeway where miss diagnosis or mismanagement may occur, leading to obstacles in one's clinical practice.
- *Assisted reproduction*: In an infertility clinic, consent taking is very essential and consent from both the partners—husband and wife, is mandatory prior to treatment. It is very crucial to counsel, document, and to take necessary consents especially when donor gametes or when a surrogate mother is involved in part of the treatment to avoid unforeseen legal complications. The use of gametes of the partner without their consent amounts to forgery.

    The couple should be made to understand that there is no guarantee on the success of the ART procedure. This is important as many patients especially in developing countries for example India, assume that they will walk home with a baby in their arms once they step into an infertility clinic.

In India, the Assisted Reproductive Technology (ART) Bill 2010[12] by the Ministry of Health and Family Welfare, Government of India and the Indian Council of Medical Research has laid down guidelines to be followed by the ART clinics and banks.

- *HIV transmission*: Women should be made aware that during their course of treatment especially with donor gametes, HIV transmission cannot be completely prevented. However, all precautions are implemented to prevent the transmission of infective diseases. All patients are screened for transmissible diseases especially HIV, Hepatitis B, and Hepatitis C. It is of utmost importance to inform the partner if one of them on routine testing is found to be seropositive. Universal precautions should be maintained at all times in the laboratory.

SUMMARY

- Ethical practices abiding by the hippocratic oath should be each practitioners goal.
- Principles of ethics—beneficence, autonomy, nonmaleficence, justice, confidentiality to be maintained at all times.
- A perfect consent and documentation is the cornerstone for prevention of medicolegal issues.
- A clear, concise and complete information should be provided to the patient.

CONCLUSION

The volcanic explosion of technology in healthcare has not only given hopes and smiles to millions of women suffering from gynecological problems but this double-edged sword has also opened its doors to a myriad of legal, ethical, and social challenges or controversies. Healthcare especially with respect to the mother and child is a Pandora's Box which has doors that are yet to be opened. It is an atom bomb that can be used as a germ warfare if not used with care. In the 21st century where doctors are the main targets of litigations, it is wise to look at both the sides of the coin before making a decision or treatment. The best way to handle a medicolegal problem is by preventing them. Above all practices, a good consent and neat documentation shall always be the cornerstone that speaks up in the court of law.

As said by Plato a long time ago, "Good people do not need laws to tell them to act responsibly and bad people will find ways around them".

REFERENCES

1. World Health Report 2000-Country Profile India.
2. Mathew J. 2018. Budget 2018: Insufficient allocation for the health sector. [online] Available from https://www.businesstoday.in/union-budget-2018-19/news/budget-2018-insufficient-allocation-health-sector-heathcare-scheme/story/269449.html. [Last accessed September, 2019]
3. Singh S. 2016. Alarming rise in medical negligence: Study. The Times of India. [online] Available from https://timesofindia.indiatimes.com/city/nagpur/alarming-rise-in-medical-negligence-litigation-study/articleshow/55484635.cms. [Last accessed September, 2019].
4. 2012. Ethical issues in obstetrics and gynecology by the FIGO Committee for the Study of Ethical Aspects of Human Reproduction and Women's Health. [online] Available from https://www.figo.org/sites/

default/files/uploads/wg-publications/ethics/English%20Ethical%20Issues%20in%20Obstetrics%20and%20Gynecology.pdf. [Last accessed September, 2019].
5. Encyclopedia Britannica. 2018. Hippocratic Oath Ethical Code... [online] Available from https://www.britannica.com/topic/hippocratic-oath. [Last accessed September, 2019]
6. Schröder-Bäck P, Duncan P, Sherlaw W, et al. Teaching seven principles for public health ethics: towards a curriculum for a short course on ethics in public health programmes. BMC Med Ethics. 2014;15:73.
7. Edozien L. Medico-legal issues in gynaecology. Obstet, Gynaecol Repro Med. 2012;22(10):273-8.
8. Edozien L. Medico-legal issues in gynaecology. Obstet, Gynaecol Repro Med. 2015;25(11):327-32.
9. Hall DE, Prochazka AV, Fink AS. Informed consent for clinical treatment. CMAJ. 2012;184(5):533-40
10. Raveesh BN, Nayak RB, Kumbar SF. Preventing medico-legal issues in clinical practice. Ann Indian Acad Neurol. 2016;19(Suppl 1):S15-S20.
11. Argent V. Medico-legal problems in gynaecology. Curr Obstet Gynaecol. 2006;16(5):289-94.
12. Ministry of Health & Family Welfare Government of India, New Delhi, Indian Council Of Medical Research New Delhi; 2010. The Assisted Reproductive Technologies (Regulation) Bill-2010. New Delhi: [online] Available from https://www.icmr.nic.in/sites/default/files/guidelines/art%20regulation%20draft%20bill1.pdf. [Last accessed September, 2019].

Index

Page numbers followed by *b* refer to box, *f* refer to figure, *fc* refer to flowchart, and *t* refer to table.

A

Abacavir 99
Abdominal aortic aneurism 110
Abdominal bloating 120, 169
Abdominal distention 207
Abdominal examination 3, 18
Abdominal pain 93, 110, 134, 149, 181
  acute 236
  causes of 54
Abdominal tuberculosis 146
Abdominal wall 192
  trocar 201
  vascular injury 197, 201
Abnormal uterine bleeding 26, 69, 72, 109, 240
  acceptable terminology 70*t*
  bleeding diagnosis 70
  classification 69
  classification acute 69
  classification chronic 70
  classification intermenstrual 70
  etiology 240
  management 72, 72*fc*, 239, 240
  terminology 69
Abortions 23, 31
  lead to 23
  management of 25
  repeated 25
  unsafe, complications of 236
Abruptio placentae 54
Abscess large 82
Abscess smaller 82
Acid-fast bacillus staining 94
Acid phosphatase test 234
Acquired immunodeficiency syndrome 32, 97
Actinomycin-D 43, 44
Acyclovir 101
Adenocarcinoma 114, 117, 168

Adenofibroma 133, 134
Adenomyomectomy 113
Adenomyosis 71, 63, 65, 110*t*, 111
  management of 111*fc*
  suspicion of 72
Adnexal disorders 214
Adnexal mass 25
Adnexal rings 217
Adnexal torsion 126, 215
Adolescent females 3
  gynecologic problem 3
  history taking 11*b*
  urinary problems 3
Adolescent population, problems in 11*b*
Adrenal hyperplasia, congenital 7, 11
Albumin 121
Alkaline 8
Alkalinization of urine 211
Alpha-fetoprotein 136
Alpha receptor blockers 230
Ambiguous genitalia 3
Amenorrhea 47, 70, 93
American College of Obstetricians and Gynecologists 10, 66, 160
Ampicillin 28
Amsel's criteria 84
Anaerobic bacteria 9
Androblastoma 168
Anemia 39
  correction of 72
Anesthesia, complications related 203*t*
Anorectal swab culture 18
Antecedent pregnancy 39
Antiemetics 122
Antiprogesterone (RU486) 30
Antiretroviral drugs 99

Antituberculosis drugs 95*t*
Antiviral chemotherapy 100
Appendicitis 90, 128, 217
Appendicular abscess 13, 110
Arachidonic acid 61*fc*
Arteriovenous 77
  malformations 222
Ascites, presence of 135
Assault in pediatric patient 17
Assisted reproductive technology 249
Atherogenic lipoprotein profile 147
Atopic dermatitis 3
Atrophic endometritis 160
Atypical proliferating tumor 133
Autonomy 243
Azithromycin 97, 101, 102

B

Bacterial vaginosis 83, 96
Bacterial vaginosis, treatment regimen for 84
Bacteroides 89
Bacteroides species 157
Barberio's test 234
Bartholin's
  abscess 83
  cyst 114
  gland 104
    infections of 82
Bartholinitis, recurrent 83
Beneficence 243
Benign cystic
  lesions 114
  teratoma 127
Benign disorders 34
  management of 164
Benign endometrial patterns 164
Benign fibroid polyp 183
Benign ovarian mass 138

Benign solid lesions 115
Benign tumor 110, 134
Benzathine penicillins 234
Beta-human chorionic
    gonadotropin 35, 38,
    40, 50, 51
Biopsy 78, 90, 114, 115
Birth control devices 147
Bisphosphonate therapy 211
Bladder injury 187, 197, 200
    incidence of 200
    types of 188
Blanket consent 244
Bleeding 147, 148
    abnormal uterine 70
    heavy menstrual 70
    high-dose progesterone 72
    intermenstrual 70
    per vagina 3, 79, 236
    postmenopausal 70
    prolonged menstrual 70
    shortened menstrual 70
Bleomycin 176
Blood grouping 25, 234
Boari flap repair 200
Body mass index 65
Bone density 146
Bowel injury 187, 189
    postoperative ileus 190
Bowel obstruction 207f
    in gynecological cancer 207t
Breast cancer 31, 73, 113, 137, 146
Breast examination 3
Breast tenderness 147
Brenner tumor 168
Burst abdomen 146

C

Calcium 65
Calymmatobacterium
    granulomatis 100
Canal of Nuck 203
Cancer antigen-125 136, 140
    level 173
    profile 137
Cancer treatment 206
Candida albicans 84
Carbohydrate antigen 19-9 137

Carbon dioxide 204
Carcinoembryonic antigen 137, 170
Carcinoma ovary 206
Cardiac
    activity 219f, 220f
    arrhythmia 198, 203
Cardiovascular effect 147
Carpopedal spasm 146
Catheter-induced edema 209
Causative organism 82
Cecum cephalad 171
Cefixime 19
Ceftriaxone 29, 87
Centers for Disease Control and
        Prevention 19, 20, 48
Central nervous system 61, 62
Cervical cancer 155
    prevalence of 76
    risk of 77t
Cervical culture 18
Cervical injury 190, 191
Cervical intraepithelial
        neoplasia 76, 77
Cervical polyps 76
Cervical stenosis 63
Cervicitis 76
Cervix, infections of 86
Cesarean scar ectopic 219f
Cesarean section 228
Chancroid 102
    clinical features 102
    diagnosis 102
    treatment 102
Chemotherapy 174
    neoadjuvant 173
    postoperative 173
    radiotherapy after first-line 173
Child sexual assault 17
Chlamydia 19, 82
Chlamydia trachomatis 9, 12, 82, 87
Chlamydial infections 87, 96
    clinical features 87
    complications 87
    diagnosis 87
    treatment regimen for 88t
Chlorpromazine hydrochloride 3

Choriocarcinoma 36, 136
Chromosomal analysis 13
Ciprofloxacin 101-103
Cisplatin 176
Clindamycin 84
Clindamycin cream 84
Clinical skills 247
Clomiphene citrate 73, 74
Colicky pain 26
Colorectal carcinoma 110
Colposcopy
    diagnosis and management 78
    indications for 79f
    role of 78
Combined oral contraceptives 73, 113
Communication skills 246
Complete hydatidiform mole 35
    biparental 36f
Complex ovarian cyst,
        management of 140f
Conception, retained products
        of 26
Condyloma acuminata 96, 102
Confidentiality 243
Conjugated equine estrogen 73
Consent 243
Constipation 181
Contraception 247
    advice: postabortion 32
    complications 144
    concept of 144
    effectiveness and safety of 145
    emergencies 144, 149
    evolution 144
    major complications 145
    practice implications 145
Corpus luteal hemorrhage 218
Cul-de-sac, posterior 170
Culdocentesis 90
Culture methods 94
Cycle cancellation 121
Cyclic endoperoxides,
        biosynthesis of 61fc
Cyclical oral progesterones 73
Cyclooxygenase-2 64
Cyclophosphamide 43, 44, 176

Index

Cyst wall, removal of 139
Cystadenocarcinoma 168
Cystadenoma 127, 133
Cystic and solid lesions 114t
Cystitis acute 103
Cystitis recurrent 103
Cystocele 116
Cystocele repair 230
Cystoscopy 199
    to examine bladder 229
Cystotomy 199
Cytomegalovirus 89
Cytoreductive surgery,
    secondary 172

D

Danazol 73, 74, 66, 113, 139
Debulking surgery 172
Decidualization endometrium 218
Decubitus ulcer 181
Deep tension suturing 194
Deep vein thrombosis 211
Dehiscence, management of 194
Delavirdine 99
Deoxyribonucleic acid 35, 94
    amplification technique 18
Depo-Provera, injectable 66
Depot medroxyprogesterone acetate 147
Dermoid cyst, spillage of 139
Diffuse macular erythroderma 86
Diphtheroids 9
Diseases, transmissible 249
Disseminated intravascular coagulation 27
Diverticular abscess 110
Diverticulitis 90, 128, 207
Documentation 245
Donovanosis 100
Dopamine agonists 121
Doxorubicin 19, 44, 176, 204
Doxycycline 87, 97, 101
Duphaston 73
Dysfunctional uterine bleeding 11, 14, 69
Dysmenorrhea 11-13, 53, 59
    assessment 63
    classification of 59
        membranous 62
        ovarian 63
        primary 59
        secondary 62
        secondary, causes of 62
    differential diagnosis of 63
    effects of recurrent 61, 62fc
    epidemiology 63
    for practice 67
    management of 64fc, 65
    pathogenesis 59
    risk factors for 63, 63t
    severe 221f
    sudden onset of 63
Dyspareunia 53, 65, 89
Dyspareunia, cases 76

E

Eastern Cooperative Oncology Group score 206
Ectopic pregnancy 47, 95, 146, 147, 217
    case of 218f
    clinical presentation 47
    diagnosis 48
    management of 50, 50fc
    site of 47
Ectropion 76
Efavirenz 99
Embryonal carcinoma 168
Embryos 121
Encephalitis 146
Endodermal sinus tumor 168
Endogenous human chorionic gonadotropin 119
Endometrial
    ablation 74
    biopsy 71, 77, 90, 163
    cancer 146, 155, 160, 209
    cavity 215
    fluid collection 156f
    hyperplasia 160, 164
    polyps 63
    sampling 161, 163
    thickness 77
        measurement of 162f
Endometrioid borderline tumor 134
Endometrioid stromal sarcoma 168
Endometrioid tumor 134
Endometrioma 110
Endometriosis 63, 65, 115, 127, 218
Endometriotic cyst 135, 139
Endoscopic surgery 248
End-tidal carbon dioxide 203
Enfuvirtide 99
Enterococcus species 81, 104
Enzyme-linked immunosorbent assay technique 88
Enzymes 61fc
Epithelial ovarian cancer 167
    classification 167
    diagnosis 170
    early-stage 172t
    epidemiology 167
    histologic types of 169
    management of 170
        advanced-stage disease 172
        early stage disease 172
        recurrent disease 174
    pathogenesis 169
    risk factors 168
    routes of metastasis 169
    signs 169
    spread pattern 169
    staging 170
    symptoms 169
Epithelioid trophoblastic tumor 40
Erythromycin 101, 234
Escherichia coli 9, 28, 81
Estrogen-progestin oral contraceptive pills 66
Ethambutol 95
Ethamsylate 73
Etoposide 43, 44, 176
Exogenous estrogens 160
External genitalia, examination of 3

F

Fallopian tube 47, 92, 215
    torsion of 126
Famciclovir 101

Female sterilization 247
Fertility preservation 243
Fetal loss 23
Fibroepithelial polyp 115
Fibroid
    acute presentations 221
    in pregnancy leads 53
    polyp 116
    red degeneration of 53
    torsion of 54, 221
    uterus 111
        management algorithm of 112fc
        with retroperitoneal abscess 54fc
FIGO
    scoring system 42t
    staging for primary carcinoma of ovary 171
    staging of ovarian tumors 142
Fish oil supplements 65
Fitz-Hugh-Curtis syndrome 215
Florence test 234
Fluid
    in abdomen 199
    replacement 122
    sac 217
Fluorescence in situ hybridization 234
Foley's catheter 229
Folinic acid 43, 44
Foreign body 115
    placement of 8
Forensic gynecology 247
Foul-smelling discharge 182
Fractional curettage 163, 164
Freezing 121
Freund's complete adjuvant 50
Functional cyst 135
Furunculosis 81

G

Gangrenous ovary 129f
Gardnerella vaginalis 83, 89
Gartner duct cyst 114
Gas embolism 202
Gastrointestinal tract,
    obstruction of 206

signs 207
symptoms 207
treatment 207
Genetic mutations 169
GeneXpert 94
Genital examination 233
Genital trauma 77
Genital tuberculosis 92, 155
    bacteriological evaluation 94
    causative organism 92
    clinical presentation 93
    diagnosis 93
    genital organs 92
    incidence 92
    investigations 93
    mode of spread 92
    pathogenesis 92
Genital warts 102
    diagnosis 102
    prevention 102
    treatment 103
Genitourinary infections 81
Gentamicin 28, 234
Germ cell tumor 168
Germline mutation 175, 176
Gestation 30
Gestational age, pregnancies of 31
Gestational sac 219f, 220f
Gestational trophoblastic disease 34, 45
    classification of 34fc
    clinical features 35
    genetics of 35
    pathogenesis of 34
    pathology 35
    risk factors associated with 35t
Gestational trophoblastic neoplasia 39
    chemotherapy for low-risk 43b
    investigations to determine treatment 42t
    management of
        high-risk 43
        low risk 43, 44fc
    regimens for treatment of high-risk 44t
    stages of 41f
    treatment of 41

Gestational trophoblastic tumor 34, 35, 40t
Gestational tumors, origins of 36t
Gestrinone 73
Ginger 65
Gonadoblastoma 168
Gonadotropin dose 120
Gonadotropin-releasing hormone agonists 7, 72-74, 111, 112, 113, 120, 121
Gonorrhea 19, 96
Granuloma inguinale 96, 100
    clinical features 100
    diagnosis 100
    treatment 100, 101
Granulosa cell tumor 175, 176
Granulosa-stromal cell tumor 168
Group B *Streptococcus* 81
Gynecological problems 10
    in adolescent population 8
Gynandroblastoma 168
Gynecological
    causes 109
    complaints 3b, 8fc
    conditions, treatment for 13t
    disorders 59
    emergency 126, 180, 236, 242
        imaging in 214
        medicolegal and ethical issues 242
    malignancy 158
    oncology 206
        bowel obstruction 208fc
        emergencies 206
        medical emergencies 210
        psychiatric emergencies 211
        surgical emergencies 206, 210t
    procedures 248

H

Haemophilus ducreyi 102
Haemophilus influenzae 9, 89

Index

Headache 149
Health and welfare draft
    medical termination
    of pregnancy bill, 2014
    32
Healthcare setting 246
Hematocolpos 13, 116
Hematogenous 92, 170
Hematomas 187
Hematometra 109
Hemodynamic shock 53
Hemorrhage 145, 209, 217
  causes 209
  definitive management 209
  initial management 209
Hemorrhagic cyst 127
Hemorrhagic infarction 55
Hemorrhoids 161
Hemostatics, roles of 26
Hepatitis B
  immunization 19
  surface antigen 18, 25
Hereditary ovarian carcinoma 174
Hernia 146, 201
Herpes genitalis 100
  clinical features 100
  diagnosis 100
  treatment 100, 101
Herpes simplex virus 12, 86
Herpesvirus 1 and 2 9
Hilus cell tumor 168
Hodgkin's lymphoma 110
Homogeneous 84
Hormonal contraceptives 147
Hormonal therapy 161, 174
Hormone replacement therapy 78, 96
Human chorionic gonadotropin 23, 49, 136
Human endometrial stromal cells 26
Human immunodeficiency virus 19, 25, 85, 97, 98, 238
  diagnosis of 99
  infection 12
  test 20
  transmission 249

Human papilloma virus 19, 102
Human placental lactogen 40
Hydatidiform mole 36
  complications of 39
  early complete 36*f*
  genetic origins of 36*f*
  immunohistochemistry in 37
Hydrosalpinx 109
  bilateral 216*f*
Hydrothermal ablation 74
Hydroureteronephrosis 182
Hydroxyethyl starch 121
Hydroxyprogesterone caproate 26
Hydroxyurea 44
Hypercalcemia, causes of 211
Hypercarbia 198
Hyperthyroidism 39
Hypoglycemia 146
Hypomenorrhea 69
Hyponatremia 211
Hypotension 86
Hypothalamic-pituitary-ovarian 11, 14
Hysterectomy 67, 74, 113, 158, 248
Hysterosalpingogram 93
Hysteroscopic procedure 74
Hysteroscopy 163, 248

I

Iatrogenic complication 122
Ibuprofen 66
Illness, severe 91
Impetigo 81
Implantation bleeding 24
In utero diethylstilboestrol 114
In vitro fertilization 47, 119, 215
Inappropriate antidiuretic hormone 211
Indinavir 19, 99
Infections 81-104
  and febrile neutropenia 210
Inferior vena cava 145
Infertility 95, 126, 216*f*
Inflammatory bowel disease 63
Informed consent 244*f*
Infundibulopelvic 126

Inhibin 136
Initiate antiretroviral therapy 99
Injury 248
  to urinary tract 187
Inotropes 29
Inpatient care, treatment regimen 91*t*
Integrase inhibitor 99
Intermenstrual bleeding 76
International Ovarian Tumor Analysis Rules 138
Interstitial cystitis 63
Intestinal injury 196, 197
Intraluminal tumor 207
Intraperitoneal
  chemotherapy 172
  instillation 173
  therapy 173
Intrauterine contraceptive device 30, 77, 147, 239
  failure 148
  forgotten 156*f*
Intrauterine insemination 215
Intrauterine pregnancy 49
Intrauterine walls, perforation of 148
Intravenous urography 189
Ionization-time of flight 137
Irritable bowel syndrome 63
Ischiorectal fossa 192
Isoniazid 95

J

Japanese herbal remedy 65
Jaundice, symptoms of 39
Justice 243

K

Khorana score 211
Kidney disease
  acute 211
  chronic 230
Klebsiella granulomatis 100
Krukenberg tumor 176

L

Labia minora 233
Labial agglutination 3
Lactate dehydrogenase 136

Lactobacilli 9, 83
Lamivudine 19, 99, 100
Laparoscopy 48, 90, 248
   and hysteroscopy 93
   complications in 196
   gasless 204
   gynecologic surgery,
       complications of 197*t*
   hysterectomy 199
   oophorectomy 129*f*, 130
   revealed ovarian torsion 216*f*
   surgery 196
   uterine nerve ablation 67
Laparotomy 191
Leiomyoma 25, 115, 155
   complicating pregnancy 56
   pedunculated 55*f*
   subclassification system 71*f*
   subserosal 55
   uterus 53, 56
      carneous degeneration 53
      impacted fibroid 56
      red 53
      torsion of fibroid 54
Leukorrhea 13
Leuprolide acetate 66
Levonorgestrel intrauterine device 73, 99
Levonorgestrel-releasing intrauterine system 66
Leydig cell tumor 168
Lichen planus 3
Lichen sclerosus 3
Lichen simplex lichenification 3
Lifestyle changes 65
Lipid cell tumors 168
Liver disorders 147
Liver function, impaired 113
Lymph nodes, enlarged 135
Lymphatic 92
   dissemination 170
Lymphogranuloma venereum 96, 100
   clinical features 101
   diagnosis 102
   treatment of 102, 102*t*

M

Magnesium 65
Malignancy 77, 180, 183
   index, risk of 137, 140, 170
Malignant cells 139
Malignant cyst features 135
Malignant disorders 34
Malignant endometrioid tumor 168
Malignant lesions 117
Malignant mucinous tumor 168
Malignant ovarian cancer
   classification of 168*t*
   management of 141
Malignant serous tumor 168
Malignant tumor 110, 141
Mantoux test 94
Mass per abdomen 13
   causes of 11*b*
Mass per vaginum 180
Massive tumor cell lysis 211
Maternal chromosome, loss of 36*f*
Matrix-assisted laser desorption 137
Matrix metalloproteinases 26
Medical termination of pregnancy 25, 30
   above 12 weeks of gestation 31
   Act, 1971 31
      eugenic grounds 31
      humanitarian grounds 31
      medical grounds 31
      social grounds 31
   authorized place for conducting 32
   between 9 weeks and 12 weeks 30
   methods for medical abortion in situations 31
   protocol 30
   up to 9 weeks gestation 30
Medicolegal problems, prevention of 243
Medroxyprogesterone 113
Mefenamic acid 66, 111
Meigs' syndrome 134

Melphalan 44
Menometrorrhagia 148
Menorrhagia 53, 69, 93
Menstrual abnormalities 13
   cases of 12
Menstrual
   changes 146
   cycle 243
   disorders 11
   disturbances 93
   dysfunction in adolescents 11*b*
   fluid 59, 61
   history 76
   pain, mechanism of 65
Menstruation duration of 76
Meperidine 3
Metabolic abnormalities 211
Metabolic effects 147
Metastasis, port-site 203
Metastatic deposits 135
Metastatic tumors 176
Metformin 120
Methicillin-resistant *S. aureus* 82
Methotrexate 43, 44, 50, 204
   contraindications 51
   single-dose protocol for 51*t*
Metronidazole 19, 28, 29, 84, 86, 234
Metrorrhagia 69
Micronized progesterone 26
Mifepristone 30, 31, 149
Migraine 147
Minimally invasive methods 74
Ministry of Health and Family Welfare 249
Mirena 66
Miscarriage 23
   case of 24
   early pregnancy 23
   types of 24, 24*t*
      complete 24, 25
      incomplete 24, 27
      induced 30
      inevitable 26
      missed 24, 27
      septic 24, 27
      spontaneous 24
      threatened 24, 25

Index

Misoprostol 27, 30, 31
Mittelschmerz pain 239
Mixed epithelial tumor 134, 168
Mobiluncus species 83
Mobius syndrome 30
Molar pregnancy
   metastases of 39
   pre-evacuation
      investigations 38*t*
   treatment of 38
      chemotherapy 38
      hysterectomy 38
      suction and evacuation 38
Molecular methods 94
Molluscum contagiosum 9, 96, 103
   treatment 103
Mucinous ascites 134
Mucinous carcinoma 134
Mucinous tumors 133
Multidrug-resistant disease 96
Mycobacterium genitalium 89
Mycoplasma hominis 9, 83, 89
Myoma 110*t*
   nonsurgical management 57*f*
   uterine fundus 56*f*
Myomectomy 74, 113, 220*f*
Myometrial scar pregnancy 220*f*
Myometrium, derived from 53

N

Nail scrapings 234
Naproxen sodium 66
Neisseria gonorrheae 9, 12, 82, 87
Nephrolithiasis 128
Nerve injury 192, 203
Nervous system, disruption of 228
Neuralgic pain 192
Neuroblastoma 110
Neuropathy, post-traumatic 192
Neuropraxia 192
Nevirapine 99
Nifedipine 66
non-Hodgkin's lymphoma 110
Nonhysteroscopic procedure 74
Nonmaleficence 243
Non-nucleoside reverse transcriptase inhibitors 99
Nonsteroidal anti-inflammatory drugs 14, 54, 64, 66, 72-73, 111-112, 121-122, 139
Norethisterone enanthate 147
Nucleic acid amplification test 88, 87
Nucleoside reverse transcriptase inhibitors 99
Nugent criteria 84
Nulliparity 63, 190
Nulliparous 168
Numbness 192

O

Obstetrical puerperal sepsis 155
Obstructed hernia 110
Obstructive uropathy 208
   causes 208
   investigations 209
   signs 209
   symptoms 209
   treatment 209
Obstructive vaginal disorders 3
Ogilvie's syndrome 207
Oligomenorrhea 69, 93
Omental prolapse 146
Oncologic emergency 206
Oocytes 121
Oophorectomy
   bilateral 129
   unilateral 142
Open gynecological surgery, complications in 187
Oral contraceptive pill 14, 64, 66, 78, 112, 137, 169
Oral sex 83
Ormeloxifene 73, 74
Ovarian borderline tumors 175
   management of 175
Ovarian cancer 109
   genetic counseling 137
   genetic risk assessment 137
   indications for 137
   lifetime risk of dying of 109
Ovarian cyst 111
Ovarian cyst management of 112*fc*
Ovarian hyperstimulation syndrome 119, 122, 217
   classification of 120
      critical 120
      mild 120
      moderate 120
      severe 120
   management 121
   pathophysiology 119
   prevention 120
Ovarian ligament 126
Ovarian malignancies 167
Ovarian mass 11
   guidelines on management of 177
   management of 133, 138, 167
Ovarian origin 110
Ovarian peritoneal malignancies 204
Ovarian reserve markers 120
Ovarian sex cord-stromal tumors 175
Ovarian stimulation parameters 120
Ovarian torsion 110, 126, 127
   clinical features 127
   diagnosis 128
   differential diagnosis 128
   etiology 127
   hemorrhagic, left 216*f*
   imaging features 128
   management 128
Ovarian tumors
   borderline 141
   classification 133
Ovary
   detorsed 129*f*
   endometriotic cyst of 136*f*
   malignant lesion of 136*f*
   normal anatomy of 126, 127*f*
   simple cyst of 135*f*

Ovulation induction 119
Ovulatory cycles 61
Ovulatory pain 59, 63

P

P57KIP2 gene 37
P57KIP2 immunostaining 37
Padua score 211
Pain, mechanism of 53
PALM COEIN system 71*t*
Pap smear 78
Papillary cystadenocarcinoma 168
Para-aortic lymph nodes 170
Paramesonephric duct cyst 114
Paraovarian cyst torsion 214
Paravesical space 192
Partial hydatidiform mole 36, 37
Partial thickness defect 188
Pediatric patient
   examination of 3
   management of 10*t*
Pediatric population
   management in 9*t*
   problems in 4-7*t*
Pedunculated fibroid, prolapse of 221
Pelvic adhesions 63
Pelvic adhesive disease 90
Pelvic examination 8, 25
Pelvic floor dysfunction 243
Pelvic hematoma 192
Pelvic inflammatory disease 47, 63, 87, 88, 89, 127, 146, 148, 209, 214, 215
   chronic 63
   diagnostic criteria for 90
Pelvic mass 109
   classification 114
   etiology 109
   investigations 110
   management 111
   symptoms 110
Pelvic organ injury 146
Pelvic organ prolapse 180
   emergencies 181*t*
Pelvic pain
   acute 214
   chronic 61, 62, 90

Pelvic side wall 192
Pelvic spleen 110
Pelvic structure in primary dysmenorrhea 60*f*
Pelvic tumors 53
Pelvic ultrasound 25
Penicillin allergy 97
Penile shaft 234
Peptic ulcer disease 51
Peptococcus species 89
Percutaneous nephrostomy 209
Perforation and fistulas 210
   causes 210
   management 210
Peritoneal fluid aspiration 90
Peritoneal masses 135
Peritoneal serous carcinoma, primary 176
Persistent nonhealing fistula 96
Physical abuse 18
Placental site trophoblastic tumor 40
Ploidy, determination of 37
Pneumoperitoneum related complications 202
Polycystic ovary syndrome 14, 71, 168,
Polymenorrhea 69
Polymerase chain reaction 88
Postcoital bleeding 65, 76
   etiology 76, 77*f*
   examination 77, 78*fc*
   management 76
Postexposure prophylaxis 19, 99
Postmenopausal bleeding 159
   causes of 160
   complications 164
   diagnostic pathways for 162*fc*
   etiology of 160*t*
   evaluation of 160
   significance of 159
Postmenopausal women 167, 177
   gynecological emergencies in 180
Postmolar surveillance 39
Postradiation strictures 207
Pouch of Douglas 28

Povidone-iodine solution 204
Pregnancy 13, 23, 53, 149
   adolescent 12
   biochemical 23
   loss early 24
   loss late 24
   teenage 11
   unknown location 24, 49*fc*
Premenopausal ovarian cysts, management of 139
Premenopausal women 133
Premenstrual tension syndrome 63
Preterm births 26
Progesterone 111
Progesterone only contraceptives 47
Progesterone, use of 121
Progestin-only 26
   long-acting reversible contraception 26
Progestogens 26, 72, 73
Promethazine hydrochloride 3
Prostaglandins 30, 59, 64
Prostate specific antigen detection 234
Protease inhibitor 99
Proteomics 137
Pseudo-Meigs' syndrome 135
Pseudomyxoma peritonei 134
Pseudosac 48
Psoriasis 3
Pubic hair 234
Puerperal septic thrombosis 222
Pulmonary embolism 146
Pyelonephritis, acute 104
Pyogenic infection 81
Pyometra 77, 93, 109, 155
   common causes of 155
   diagnosis 156
   differential diagnosis 156
   etiology 155
   investigations 157
   management of 157, 157*fc*
   pathogenesis 156
   signs and symptoms 156
Pyosalpinx 109, 146
Pyrazinamide 95

Index

Q
QuantiFERON-TB gold 94

R
Radiation
  enteritis 207, 208
  exposure 215
  therapy 174
    postoperative 172
Raltegravir 99
Rape 233
Rape and sexual assault 238
Rape crisis centers 235
Rectal bleeding 169
Rectal examination 8
Rectocele repair 230
Rectosigmoid colon 171
Renal tumor 110
Reproductive age group 69
Reproductive tract
    abnormalities 12
Retroperitoneal major vascular 202
Rh typing 25
Rifampicin 94, 95
Ring of fire 218
Ring worm 82
Risk management, components of 246
Ritonavir 99
Round ligament 247
Ruptured adnexal cyst 220*f*

S
Saline infusion sonography 161
Salpingo-oophorectomy, bilateral 171
Salpingotomy, case of 51
Saquinavir 99
Scabies 96, 103
Scar ectopic 219*f*
Seborrheic dermatitis 3
Self-help techniques 65
Seminal fluid, test for 234
Senile
  cervicitis 155
  endometritis 155
Septate vagina 3
Septic abortion 27
  case of 28
  investigations 29*fc*
  management of 29*fc*
  types of 28
Septic shock 198
Septicemia 90
Serologic tests 99
Seromucinous tumors 134
Serous tumors 133
Serum progesterone 48
Sex cord-stromal tumors 168, 175
Sex during menses 83
Sex partners, multiple 83
Sexual abuse 17, 20
  clinical manifestation 18
  examination 18
  incidence 17
  investigation 18
  management 18
Sexual active population 215
Sexual assault 11, 12, 232
  counseling 234
  effects of rape 232
  forms of 232
  incidence of 232
  management 233
  types 232
  with evidence of penetration 19*fc*
Sexual behavior 14
Sexual contact date 17
Sexual intercourse, early age 83
Sexual practices, safe 14
Sexual transmitted diseases 9, 11, 12, 14, 77, 234, 238
  organisms causing 12*t*
Sexual transmitted infection 19, 32, 87, 96
Sexual violence, risk factors to 232
Shigella 9
Shoulder pain, postoperative 203
Simple ovarian cyst
  management of 140*fc*
  unilateral 177
Small extraperitoneal defect 188
Smooth muscle cells 53

Speculum examination 27
Sperm creatine phosphokinase test 234
Spermatozoa, detection of 234
Spinal cord injury 228
Spontaneous abortion, cause of 23
Staphylococcus 81, 82, 104, 157
Staphylococcus aureus 9
Staphylococcus epidermidis 9
Staphylococcus saprophyticus 103
Sterilization 145
  immediate complications 145
  long-term complications 146
Steroids 29
Streptobacillus 102
Streptococcus 82
Streptococcus pyogenes 9
Streptococcus species 157
Streptomycin 95
Stromal hypercellularity 37
Stromal karyotypic debris 37
Submucosal fibroids 74, 113
Submucous fibroid polyp 155
Submucous myoma 180
Submucous polyp 182
Suprapubic tenderness 236
Surface-enhanced laser desorption 137
Surface papilloma 133
Swabs from prepuce 234
Syndrome of inappropriate antidiuretic hormone 211
Syphilis 96
  diagnosis 97
  serology test 89
  test 20
  treatment 97
  treatment regimen for 98

T
Tamoxifen 163, 164
Taurolidine 66, 204
Tetanus toxoid 28
Thiamine 65

Thiozine 3
Thread worm 82
Thromboembolism 119, 211
Thrombosis of ovarian vein 222f
Thyroid-stimulating hormone 25
Tingling 192
Tinidazole 84
Tissue culture 88
Tissue necrosis 53
Tissue retrieval in endobag 129f
Torsion ovarian cyst 90, 238
  evaluation 238
  management 238, 239fc
Torsion ovarian
  pathophysiology of 127
  pathophysiology of 127f
  pedicle 127
Toxic shock syndrome 86
Training and education 247
Tranexamic acid 72, 73
Transcutaneous electrical nerve stimulation 64, 65
Transitional cell tumor 134
Transvaginal sonography 37, 161, 170
Transverse septum 3
Transverse sinus thrombosis 146
Treitz ligament 171
Trendelenburg position 203
Treponema pallidum 96
Trichomonas vaginalis 9, 85, 104
Trichomoniasis 12
Trimethoprim-sulfamethoxazole 101, 103
Trophoblastic tissue 218
Tubal ectopic 47
Tubal origin 109
Tubal scarring leading 88
Tubal stump bleeding 146
Tubectomy 145
Tuberculosis of
  endometrium 92
  fallopian tube 92
  ovary 93
  pelvis 92

Tubo-ovarian
  abscess 13, 109
  mass, left 215f
Tumor lysis syndrome 211
Tumor markers 136

U

Upper genital tract, infections of 88
Ureaplasma urealyticum 9, 83, 89
Ureter, dissection of 199
Ureteral injury 188, 197, 199, 200
  diagnosis of 189, 199
  incidence of 199
  prevention 200
Urethra, blockage of 228
Urethral
  caruncle 116
  culture 18
  orifice 234
  prolapse 6
  stricture 230
Urethritis 103
Urinary frequency 169
Urinary infection 181
Urinary output 188
Urinary problems 47
Urinary retention 146, 181, 227, 236
  acute 227, 236
    causes of 237
    evaluation and management 237fc
  causes of 228
  chronic 236
  complications 230
  evaluation 227, 228t
  investigations 227
  management of 229, 229fc, 236
  symptoms 227
Urinary tract infection 102, 128
Urinary tract injury 199
Urodynamic tests 229
Urogenital malformations 11, 14
Urogynecology 248

Uterine and cervical injuries 187, 190
Uterine arteriovenous malformations 222
Uterine artery embolization 57, 74, 112, 113
Uterine cavity 47, 48, 110
  pus in 155
Uterine cervix 55f
Uterine disorders 214
Uterine fibroids 109
Uterine inversion 116, 180, 182
  causes 182
  diagnosis of 182
  main clinical symptoms 182
Uterine leiomyoma 128
Uterine myomas 63
Uterine origin 109, 110
Uterine perforation, management of 191
Uterine prolapse 180
Uterine torsion 56
Uterine vessels 59
Utero-ovarian ligament plication 130
Uterovaginal prolapse 117, 155

V

Vagina
  infections of 83
  normal 83
  prolapsed fibroid in 221f
Vaginal
  bleeding 25, 183, 214
    irregular 47, 182
  culture 18
  discharge 11, 65, 77, 84
  douching 85
  epithelial cells 83
  examination 65
  instrumental delivery 228
  introitus 233
  leiomyoma 115
  masses 113
  mucosa 8
  pH 8
  pressure 182
  swabs 13, 25, 157
  vault 192

Index

Valacyclovir 101
Vascular endothelial growth
    factor 119
Vascular injuries 187, 191
  major 197, 202
  primary hemorrhage 191
  reactionary hemorrhage 191
  secondary hemorrhage 192
Vascular permeability 119
Vascular thrombosis 113
Vasopressin 61
Vasopressors 29
Vasovagal reaction 148
Venereal disease research
    laboratory 18, 25
Venous thromboembolism 147
Venous thrombosis 203
Verapamil 66
Veress needle, insertion of 202
Vincristine 43, 44
Violin string 90

Volvulus 207
Vulva 192
  infections 81
    causes of 82*t*
Vulval
  region 78
  skin 8
  ulcers 78
Vulvar
  abscess 81
  edema 203
Vulvovaginal candidiasis 84
  classification of 85*t*
Vulvovaginitis 3, 8, 9
  organisms causing 9*t*

W

Wet mount 85, 86
Whiff test 84
Wound cellulitis 211

Wound dehiscence 187, 193, 210
Wound healing 193
  primary intention 193
  secondary intention 193
Wound hematoma 211
Wound infection 145
Wound sepsis 187, 193
  management of 193
  measures to prevent 193
  risk factors for 193
  treatment 193

Y

Yolk sac fetal pole 219*f*

Z

Zalcitabine 99
Zidovudine 19, 99, 100
Ziehl-Neelsen 94

EU GSPR Authorised Reprsentative
Logos Europe, 9 rue Nicolas Poussin
1700, La Rochelle, France
Phone: +33 (0) 6 67 93 73 78
E-mail: contact@logoseurope.eu

www.ingramcontent.com/pod-product-compliance
Ingram Content Group UK Ltd.
Pitfield, Milton Keynes, MK11 3LW, UK
UKHW050429150426
5217IPUK00019B/1304